CANCER, RESEARCH, AND EDUCATIONAL FILM AT
MIDCENTURY

ROCHESTER STUDIES IN MEDICAL HISTORY

Series Editor: Christopher Crenner
Robert Hudson and Ralph Major Professor and Chair Department of History
and Philosophy of Medicine
University of Kansas School of Medicine

Additional Titles of Interest

Sickness in the Workhouse:
Poor Law Medical Care in Provincial England, 1834–1914
Alistair Ritch

Of Life and Limb:
Surgical Repair of the Arteries in War and Peace, 1880–1960
Justin Barr

The Hidden Affliction:
Sexually Transmitted Infections and Infertility in History
Edited by Simon Szreter

China and the Globalization of Biomedicine
Edited by David Luesink, William H. Schneider, and Zhang Daqing

Explorations in Baltic Medical History, 1850–2015
Edited by Nils Hansson and Jonatan Wistrand

Health Education Films in the Twentieth Century
Edited by Christian Bonah, David Cantor, and Anja Laukötter

The History of the Brain and Mind Sciences: Technique, Technology, Therapy
Edited by Stephen T. Casper and Delia Gavrus

The Filth Disease: Typhoid Fever and the Practices of Epidemiology in
Victorian England
Jacob Steere-Williams

A complete list of titles in the Rochester Studies in Medical History series
may be found on our website, www.urpress.com.

Cancer, Research, and Educational Film at Midcentury

The Making of the Movie
Challenge: Science Against Cancer

David Cantor

UNIVERSITY OF ROCHESTER PRESS

First published 2022

University of Rochester Press
668 Mt. Hope Avenue, Rochester, NY 14620, USA
www.urpress.com
and Boydell & Brewer Limited
PO Box 9, Woodbridge, Suffolk IP12 3DF, UK
www.boydellandbrewer.com

ISBN-13: 978-1-64825-029-3 (paperback)
ISSN: 1526-2715; v. 50

Library of Congress Cataloging-in-Publication Data
Names: Cantor, David, 1957– author.
Title: Cancer, research, and educational film at midcentury: the making of the movie
    "Challenge: science against cancer" (1950) / David Cantor.
Other titles: Rochester studies in medical history. 1526-2715
Description: Rochester, NY: University of Rochester Press, 2021. | Series: Rochester
    studies in medical history, 1526-2715; 50| Includes bibliographical references
    and index.
Identifiers: LCCN 2021020102 (print) | LCCN 2021020103 (ebook) | ISBN
    9781648250293 (paperback; alk. paper) | ISBN 9781800103665 (ebook) | ISBN
    9781800103672
Subjects: MESH: Challenge (Motion picture: 1950) | Neoplasms—history | Motion
    Pictures—history | Research Personnel—history | Career Choice | History, 20th
    Century | United States | Canada
Classification: LCC RC267.5 (print) | LCC RC267.5 (ebook) | NLM QZ 11 AA1
    | DDC 362.196/9940072—dc23
LC record available at https://lccn.loc.gov/2021020102
LC ebook record available at https://lccn.loc.gov/2021020103

Cover image: Publicity photo, *Challenge: Science Against Cancer*: Shooting the radium therapy for
lip cancer sequence, Toronto General Hospital. *From left*: Grant McLean (looking into camera),
unknown film crew member, two unknown actors (doctor, patient), Morten Parker (below
patient), unknown actor (nurse), unknown member of film crew. Photo by Christian Lund,
October 1949. Source: NCI archives, AR-4900-010785.

S | H   **The Sustainable History Monograph Pilot**
M | P   Opening Up the Past, Publishing for the Future

CONTENTS

ACKNOWLEDGMENTS

This book has had a long gestation. It began by chance when I was working as a historian for the Division of Cancer Prevention at the US National Cancer Institute (NCI). One day in the early 2000s, Nancy Brun, then chief of the Information Resources Branch of the NCI's Office of Cancer Communications, came into my office to show me a scrapbook about a publicity campaign for a film that the NCI had released in 1950 called *Challenge: Science Against Cancer*. Neither of us knew much about this film, but the scrapbook documented a significant effort to promote it, with a wealth of primary sources between its covers: publicity pamphlets, press releases, clippings, photos, correspondence, invitation cards, plans for the campaign, and even the seating arrangements for one of the premieres of the film, along with other documentation such as the film script and narration. Nancy and I spent time leafing through the pages, and it seemed to me that it might one day be the basis for a journal article. It was not a priority, however, and I filed the scrapbook away.

A few years later, I disinterred the scrapbook when I was working for the History of Medicine Division (HMD) of the National Library of Medicine (NLM). Paul Theerman, Mike Sappol, and I had persuaded HMD to develop a series of DVDs on historical medical and health films in the NLM's collection. My DVD was to be a selection of the historical cancer films in the NLM's collection (along with an introductory essay and notes on the individual films) and was to include *Challenge*. The DVD series never came about, and eventually mutated into the NLM website *Medical Movies on the Web*, now *Medicine on Screen*, but it revived my interest in *Challenge*. Paul, then HMD's head of Images and Archives, agreed, with the blessing of Elizabeth Fee (then chief of HMD), to fund a visit to the National Film Board of Canada (NFB), which had produced the film, and the Library and Archives Canada to get some background material. It was then that my research life changed.

The NFB had kept almost everything on the film so that it was possible to know, sometimes on a day-to-day basis, how the film came about and how it was sponsored, made, and promoted. It was clear to me that this offered the opportunity for much more than a single academic paper or the liner notes for a DVD, and that a book on the making of cancer educational films was possible. The Library and Archives Canada in Ottawa confirmed this impression. It contained rich documentation on the history of cancer educational film in Canada and *Challenge* in particular, and on the perspectives of the Department of Health and Welfare, the Canadian Cancer Society, and National Cancer Institute of Canada on these developments. Paul also sanctioned a trip to interview Colin Low, one of the two animators of the film, and to visit York University, outside Toronto, where the composer Louis Applebaum's papers are held.

When I moved to the History Office of the National Institutes of Health (NIH) in 2007 my new boss, Robert Martensen, agreed to fund a further research trip to New York to visit the UN archives and to interview Morten Parker, the director of the film. Now, rather than being part of a proposed DVD series, the film was to be a gateway into the history of the NCI, part of the NIH, the focus of the office's mandate.

So this book is indebted to Nancy for starting the whole thing off; to Paul, Elizabeth, and Robert for financing key research trips; and to Michael Gottesman, Deputy Director for Intramural Research at the NIH, for giving me space to make a start on writing following Robert's untimely death. It is also indebted to the many archivists who helped me locate records. At the NFB, Bernard Lutz transformed my research direction by opening the door to the board's extensive collection and allowing me to photocopy virtually everything, and after his retirement André D'Ulisse continued my research transformation. Suzanne Dubeau, then Assistant Head, Clara Thomas Archives and Special Collections, York University, helped me review the Louis Applebaum papers, which include the score for *Challenge*. Judy Grosberg of the NCI's Office of Cancer Communications unlocked the NCI's archival collections during the period when these documents were being scanned into the LION database, where the scrapbook now resides. Paul Theerman, Nancy Dosch, Stephen Greenberg, and John Rees at the NLM helped me with access to its film and manuscript collections. Other archivists and librarians across the US and Canada answered my many email queries and are acknowledged in the endnotes.

I was lucky enough to meet some of those involved in the film. Colin Low (*Challenge's* co-animator) and Morten Parker (director) both generously invited me to their homes, talked about their careers and involvement with the movie and watched it with me, patiently explaining to this film tyro how it was put together. Low identified many of the animation techniques used in the film, how the work was divided between him and his co-animator, Evelyn Lambart, and how they imagined the audience they wanted to reach; and he sketched some of *Challenge's* animation images for me to show how they were made and the technical issues involved. Parker identified many of the actors in the film, helped me understand how he and Guy Glover (producer) divided their tasks, provided much other information on the making of the film, especially the live action, and loaned me his documentary records on its making. Parker identified the man in Figure 3.1 as Maurice Constant, a point confirmed by Constant's sons John and David. Dallas Johnson Read (formerly Helen Dallas and Dallas Johnson), the information officer who started the whole thing off at the NCI, graciously allowed me to interview her. At the time she was all but forgotten at the NCI, even though she had lived close by in Bethesda for many years. I would also like to thank Randy Bazilauskas, who shared memories of the life of his father, Vito, and his involvement in the film.

Many colleagues and friends have helped with this book. I had many conversations with my NLM colleague Mike Sappol, and he and Eva Åhrén watched the movie with me and helped me identify some of the iconographic references in the animation. Michael O'Brien, Bonnie Cohen, and Maurice Saylor helped me understand more about the role of music in film, and all three listened to and read the score, which Maurice also played for me on the piano. Anja Laukötter and Christian Bonah probably heard far more about this book than they wished to while we were ostensibly working on our jointly edited health education film book. Their invitations to several scholarly meetings in Strasbourg provided me with opportunities to buttonhole other historians interested in visual culture and film.

The book has benefited from the comments of participants at various seminars and conferences. I thank Thomas Söderqvist, who was the first to invite me to present on this film at a mini-symposium: "Perspectives on Cancer Research, 1950–2000," Forum for Tværvidenskabelig Medicinhistorie, Medicinsk Museion, Copenhagen University, Denmark, February 10, 2005; and Zoë Druick, who invited me to participate in a workshop on "Canada's National Film Board and the World: Proposals for a Research Agenda," Society for Cinema and Media Studies, Annual Meeting, Montreal, March 25–29, 2015. Papers based on this project were also given at the National Library of Medicine's History of Medicine Seminar, March 16, 2005; the Association of American Medical Colleges, Washington, DC, June 29, 2005; and the 2008 Biennial Film and History Conference, "Film and Science: Fictions, Documentaries, and Beyond," Chicago, October 30–November 2, 2008. Finally, I also discussed this film at a film presentation and lunchtime session I organized—"Canadian Persuasion: The National Film Board of Canada and the Post-Second World War Development of the Health Education Movie"—at the Annual Meeting of the American Association for the History of Medicine, Montreal, Quebec, May 3–6, 2007.

The series editors of Rochester Studies in Medical History, Ted Brown and later Chris Crenner, were unfailingly enthusiastic about the book through its long gestation. At the University of Rochester Press, Sonia Kane and Tracey Engel shepherded the manuscript through the review and production process. Sonia not only commissioned the book, but also arranged for the open access edition through the Sustainable History Monograph Pilot funded by the Mellon Foundation and administered by Longleaf Services. At Longleaf Services, I must thank Ihsan Taylor and Lisa Stallings. Finally, thanks are due to my copyeditor, Elsa Dixler, who ruthlessly cut my over-wordy prose, and significantly improved the text.

In regard to the website that accompanies this book, I must thank Sarah Eilers, who approved the idea very quickly, ensured that the NLM's copy of *Challenge* was re-digitized to a better quality than the existing one on the NLM's website, and that the other versions of the film and the filmstrip were incorporated into the new website. Sarah, Beth Mullen, and Oliver Gaycken at the University of Maryland, College Park, ensured that the website came together in time for publication of the book.

Several personal votes of thanks. My wife, Judith Freidenberg, has heard far too much about this seemingly never-ending project, and must have despaired of it ever reaching publication. It has been with us in one way or another since we met and has taken too much time away from our lives together. I cannot thank her enough for her love and support during its gestation and look forward to making up for lost time. Finally, I wish my parents, John and Elizabeth, could have seen the book into print. Unfortunately, both retired into dementia during its writing and died long before its completion. The book is dedicated to them.

As of April 2022, copies of *Challenge, Alerte,* and *Cancer* are available in the National Library of Medicine's NLM Digital Collections and on the NLM *Medicine on Screen* website, along with several of the publications associated with this film. *The Fight* and *The Outlaw Within* are currently available on the National Film Board of Canada website, and will eventually be added to NLM holdings, as will the filmstrip.

Medicine on Screen (NLM): https://medicineonscreen.nlm.nih.gov/

Digital Collections (NLM): https://collections.nlm.nih.gov/

Office national du film du Canada: https://www.onf.ca/explorer-tous-les-films/

National Film Board of Canada: https://www.nfb.ca/explore-all-films/

Some of the other films listed in the filmography are available at the above links and at the following websites:

MEDFILM database: https://medfilm.unistra.fr/

Moving Image Archive (Internet Archive): https://archive.org/details/movies

ABBREVIATIONS

AAMC	American Association of Medical Colleges
ABC	American Broadcasting Company
ACS	American Cancer Society
ASCC	American Society for the Control of Cancer
CBC	Canadian Broadcasting Corporation
CCPI	Consultative Committee on Public Information (United Nations)
CCS	Canadian Cancer Society
CDC	Communicable Disease Center (US)
CSCC	Canadian Society for the Control of Cancer
DNHW	Department of National Health and Welfare (Canada)
FSA	Federal Security Agency (US)
FY	fiscal year
GPO	Government Printing Office (US)
ISD	Information Services Division (of the Department of National Health and Welfare, Canada)
MFI	Medical Film Institute (of the American Association of Medical Colleges)
MPAA	Motion Picture Association of America
NACC	National Advisory Cancer Council (of the US National Cancer Institute)
NBC	National Broadcasting Company (US)
NCI	National Cancer Institute (US)
NCIC	National Cancer Institute of Canada
NFB	National Film Board of Canada
NIH	National Institutes of Health (US)
PHS	Public Health Service (US)
RCA	Radio Corporation of America (US)
RCMP	Royal Canadian Mounted Police
UN	United Nations
UNESCO	United Nations Educational, Scientific and Cultural Organization

UPA   United Productions of America
WHO   World Health Organization

CURRENCY

CAN$ Canadian dollar
US$ US dollar
$ Dollar: used where it is unclear whether the dollar is US or Canadian.

Introduction

I N 1949, THE US National Cancer Institute (NCI) and the Canadian Department of National Health and Welfare (DNHW) commissioned a film, eventually called *Challenge: Science Against Cancer*, as part of a major effort to recruit young scientists into cancer research. Both organizations were concerned that poor recruitment would stifle the development of the field at a time when funding for research had grown significantly and was expected to continue to grow in the foreseeable future. The fear was that there would not be enough new young scientists to meet the demand, and that the shortfall would undermine cancer research and the hopes invested in it. *Challenge* aimed to persuade young scientists to think of cancer research and biomedicine as careers. *Cancer, Research, and Educational Film at Midcentury* is the story of that film: why it was commissioned, how it was made, and how it was promoted and packaged.

Today *Challenge* is a largely forgotten film. It receives an occasional mention in histories of cancer control, and film historians and critics sometimes refer to its innovative animation sequences, and to the original score by Louis Applebaum.[1] And that is about it: *Challenge* is barely a footnote in the historiography of medicine and film. However, for much of 1949 the movie was a major focus of an international collaboration between the Americans and Canadians, and by the early 1950s it had come to be regarded as a triumph by the two government health agencies and had gained recognition in the film world. It won first prize in film competitions in Venice and New York, and a theatrical version was nominated for an Academy Award in 1951. The prospect of the award generated huge excitement among officials in both health agencies. Some hoped for a trip to the Oscar ceremony. Thus, by 1951, the NCI and the Department of National Health and Welfare proclaimed themselves satisfied that their money was well spent, despite a lack of evidence that it had done much to aid recruitment. Like many, if not most, educational films on medical subjects, however, *Challenge* had a short screen life. By the 1960s the film was rarely shown, displaced by newer films, newer people within the sponsoring agencies, and newer agendas.

The film might have been quietly forgotten by the sponsors, but memories of it remained alive in the organization that made it, the National Film Board of Canada (NFB), Canada's state-funded film producer and distributor. The board, founded in 1939, was a pioneer of documentary and animated film, as well as a propaganda arm of the Canadian government during the Second World War.[2] Despite internal doubts about the quality and effectiveness of the film, the NFB presented it as one of the best produced after the war, a harbinger of NFB Oscar nominations achieved by those involved in the film in the 1950s, and of future NFB technical innovations in documentary film and animation.

The influence of *Challenge* lingered on in other ways as well. The animation techniques in the film formed part of a genealogy that would eventually lead to the director Stanley Kubrick's film *2001: A Space Odyssey* (1968). In *Challenge*, the cell is portrayed as a universe in miniature in which the viewer is in the position of a traveler through outer space, the celestial bodies passing by comprising the inner parts of the cell. One of the two animators, Colin Low, later adapted ideas and techniques used in *Challenge* to make *Universe* (1960), an NFB educational film in which the viewer is again in the position of a traveler through outer space, the celestial bodies passing by representing stars, planets, and constellations. (Not the inner parts of the cell in this case.) It was *Universe* that caught the eye of Kubrick, who used it as inspiration for *2001*, tempted Low to work for him on the film, and used the narrator of *Universe* as the voice of the malfunctioning computer, HAL.[3]

Themes

In telling the story of *Challenge* this book has several aims. A first is to contribute to the story of post-Second World War cancer research. It is well known that funding for cancer research in both the United States and Canada expanded as never before after the war, the beginning of a vast research endeavor against this group of diseases, and the foundation for what became the US "War on Cancer" in the 1970s, and for smaller Canadian efforts.[4] What is less well known is the concern in those early years that the expansion might falter because young scientists were not entering the field. *Challenge* was a central part of government responses to such concerns in both Canada and the US and marked a major change in public cancer education programs in both countries. Until its release, such programs had focused more on recruiting patients into programs of cancer control than on recruiting scientists into cancer research. However, as funding for research increased after the war the balance began to shift. With the increase in funding, government and private initiatives against cancer came to focus on the recruitment of scientists and on generating public support for and understanding of research and its possibilities.

The book also highlights the role of government administrators in both Canada and the US who have not received much attention from historians: information or public affairs officers, struggling in different ways in each country to establish themselves within their agencies. Most historiographical attention has focused on the roles of leading philanthropists, politicians, scientists, physicians, and administrators in the growth of cancer research after the Second World War.[5] Yet information officers were crucial to the efforts of both national agencies. They labored to justify new federal commitments to research with their special focus on cancer and helped to recruit both patients and physicians and scientists. Individual information officers never achieved the kind of recognition accorded to those who ran the two major federal agencies. Nor would they ever achieve the prominence of a figure like the philanthropist Mary Lasker, who is often credited with helping to expand research. Instead, they worked behind the scenes, often anonymously, setting the stage for their more visible colleagues. This book is thus revealing of a relatively unknown side of the postwar expansion of cancer research.

A third aim of this book is to explore the history of post-Second World War cancer educational filmmaking.[6] As funding for cancer expanded dramatically after the war, so too did cancer filmmaking, especially in the US, which also came to target new audiences and new genres of film. Before the 1940s, filmmakers had used melodrama, primarily aimed at women, as a part of mass multimedia campaigns to promote programs of early detection and treatment of cancer. Through the 1940s, such campaigns came increasingly to address men as well, supplementing melodrama with genres such as cartoon comedies and detective stories. At the same time, films aimed at women now included how-to movies such as instructions for breast self-examination. In addition, children and young adults—alongside older adults—became the target of films that sought to explain the biology of cancer, the nature of research, and what needed to be done.

Challenge fell into this latter category of film, but unlike the others made at this time, it was produced in Canada for distribution in the two countries. As this book will show, until then Canada had made very few educational films about cancer and had largely relied on US films for its cancer education campaigns. *Challenge* turned this situation around and for the first time the Americans were to be reliant on Canadian filmmakers. Moreover, unlike in the US where cancer filmmaking was often farmed out to commercial filmmakers, *Challenge* was to be made by Canada's state-funded NFB. The NFB had developed a close relationship with the Canadian DNHW and was making a growing number of educational films to feed the department's new enthusiasm for film.[7] Among these were the highly acclaimed *Mental Mechanisms* series of films, the success of which was a factor in tempting the Americans to turn to the NFB to make *Challenge*.[8]

A final aim of this book is to examine the place of health education films within broader public education programs. Films had been incorporated into such programs from the early twentieth century, starting in the 1920s for cancer.[9] Enthusiasts for film argued that movies would be a transformative educational medium, a key to the success of future of health campaigns. But organizers came to recognize that films by themselves could not achieve their educational goals. Even the best could do as much harm as good. Critics argued that some produced in audiences an excessive optimism about therapeutic interventions that undermined faith in the film's message when the expected cure failed to come through. Others, they suggested, created an excessive fear of diseases or interventions against them that paralyzed audiences into inaction and so undermined programs of disease control. So if films were to transform health education campaigns, those campaigns had to compensate for such problems. Few, if any, saw films as so much of a problem that they should be abandoned. Instead, it was suggested that embedding them within broader multimedia campaigns might compensate for films' limitations. Books, magazines, newspapers, radio, pamphlets, posters, medical lectures, and face-to-face encounters between doctor and patient could direct people to watch the film, expand on points raised within it, answer concerns of patients, or counter misunderstandings or unwarranted fears or hopes generated by a film.

Challenge illustrates the persistence of such concerns in the postwar period. On the one hand, the book aims to show how the filmmakers sought to transform the concerns of their sponsors about science recruitment into something that would work as a film. Such efforts were shaped by a filmmaking culture within the NFB that established the themes of the film by mobilizing iconic figures such as the scientist and patient, alongside symbols such as the use of darkness to evoke ignorance. On the other hand, it also shows how sponsors did not feel that the film—however good it might be—could do all the work expected of it. They planned for several different versions of the film as part of a broader media campaign organized around film premieres in the US and Canada. They additionally produced books and pamphlets designed to help get the film into the classroom. Indeed, the film and the broader information and educational campaign were themselves part of even wider campaigns within the US and Canada to expand and reorganize research funding.

In the end, the NCI and the DNHW commissioned between them five different versions of the film: *Challenge: Science Against Cancer* (thirty minutes)and a French version, *Alerte: Science Contre Cancer* (thirty minutes), both targeted at students; *The Fight: Science Against Cancer*, a twenty-minute theatrical release aimed at a general cinema audience (only in English); and *The Outlaw Within* (English) and *Cancer* (French), ten-minute versions of the same film for the NFB's Canadian film circuits. For the NCI and the DNHW, these films were to be part of package that would eventually include Lester Grant's award-winning book, *The Challenge of Cancer* (1950), which explained to a general audience the state of scientific and medical knowledge about cancer and what could be done about it, a teacher's guide to facilitate the classroom use of the film and the book, and a filmstrip available in French and English versions—*What We Know About Cancer* and *Ce Que Nous Savons du Cancer*. The filmstrips were intended at first to be made from stills from the *Challenge* or its companion films, an intention abandoned in favor of using specially made images.[10] They also launched an intense media campaign to advertise the film package and influence audience perceptions by shaping reporting of it in television, radio, and print. Both Americans and Canadians—often the information specialists within the NCI and DNHW—saw the film as a powerful means of getting a message to the public, but both also saw limitations to its power. The media and educational campaigns in which it was embedded were intended to counter such limitations.

Sources

One of the frustrations of working on the history of sponsored films can be the dearth of artifacts and records. The films themselves have often crumbled to dust, and the paper trails that recorded why they were commissioned, how they were made, distributed, or shown have disappeared. *Challenge* is different. Not only do all five versions of the movie still exist, but so also do major collections of papers from the various organizations and individuals that sponsored, made, and evaluated the movie. At times it is possible to know what was happening day-to-day, and from multiple, sometimes opposing, viewpoints: why certain choices were made, how tensions between different stakeholders were addressed, how the filmmakers went about making the movie, and how it fit into the politics of the organizations that sponsored or made the film.

Nor do the records stop with the commissioning and making of the film. The broader multimedia package is also well documented. Lester Grant's book, the teaching guide, and the filmstrip have all survived, as have records of those who commissioned or made them. These records preserve the smallest details, from the seemingly mundane (debates over paper quality, typography, font, print runs, and costs, not to mention the problems of working during a Washington DC summer without air conditioning) to bigger questions about how best to ensure such publications would inspire an audience of high school science students. At the same time, the information specialists at the NCI and the DNHW compiled a large scrapbook for their agencies documenting the media campaigns around this film, which includes clippings of various media reports along with internal documents on the planning of the campaign. This scrapbook was likely assembled as part of institutional efforts to demonstrate the success of the film and perhaps to provide a model for future campaigns. In combination with other documentary and oral sources, the scrapbook allows us to explore not only the media plans devised by information specialists but also their views. It provides a rare glimpse into institutional process, documenting the steps in planning campaigns; the strategies adopted to approach different media and institutions; the response to these strategies; and the attempts to manage the responses.

Such rich evidence provides a unique opportunity to explore the roles of sponsors, filmmakers, and the media in such campaigns. In particular, it permits us not only to trace why the sponsors wanted a film to educate and recruit, but how and why the NFB transformed these ideas into something that they thought would work as a film. We can follow the institutional agendas of the Film Board and explore how information specialists, the media, and educators sought to transform these ideas through media and educational campaigns. *Cancer, Research, and Educational Film at Midcentury* is, in short, an exercise in reconstructing the contingencies of putting a health/science education film together in the 1940s and early 1950s, and how its form, uses, and reception were shaped by various stakeholders: the sponsors, the filmmakers, and those who promoted and viewed it. It shows how such contingencies ensured that control of the film and its argument remained elusive, and that it was a continual struggle to stimulate interest among sponsors, to define what they wanted of it, to produce the film itself, to shape its argument, and to influence its reception. Sometimes groups and individuals succeeded in their goals, sometimes they did not, but mainly they adjusted them as the film project developed.

Three projects

Challenge was one of thousands of films commissioned by medical, biomedical, and public health organizations after the Second World War. Unlike most Hollywood productions, such films did not aim primarily to entertain but to serve the agendas of their sponsoring agencies by educating, training, and informing various audiences and (crucially) transforming or reinforcing their beliefs and behaviors. Thus, like the industrial films studied by Vinzenz Hediger and Patrick Vondrau, these types of pictures must be understood in terms of their specific, usually organizational, purpose, in the context of power and organizational practice in which they were sponsored, created, and shown. They were a form of *utility film*, as Hediger and Vondrau put it, sponsored and produced in particular situations, for particular organizational reasons, and targeted at particular audiences.[11] Films such as *Challenge* thus required more than the technical work of scriptwriting, camerawork, animation, music, sound, editing, and direction. They also involved other forms of work: administrative and managerial, marketing and educational, political, and institutional. In writing a history of this film, I divide such work into three overlapping projects—sponsoring, making, and packaging—each a work in progress that involved intersecting, sometimes antagonistic, groups and individuals, with different interests, skills, and agendas, distributed across a variety of organizations. In this way we can trace the evolution of the film, its multiple aims, how the filmmakers sought to transform a biomedical project into film, and how the sponsors sought to cultivate audiences and shape their responses to it.

The chapters that document the first project—*sponsoring*—explore the two major sponsors, the NCI and the Canadian Department of National Health and Welfare, and their different interests and concerns. While both wanted to increase recruitment of young scientists to biomedical research and were fearful that competition for recruits from industry and from atomic physics would undermine plans, the Canadians were also wary of the Americans who seemed to be poaching some of their best scientists. *Challenge* was therefore a mixed blessing to the Canadians.

If the two sponsoring organizations had different agendas, it was also the case that groups and individuals *within* each sponsoring agency had different interests and agendas. Two key groups need to be highlighted. The first was composed of government scientists and physicians, some included formally as advisers to the film, overseeing its scientific content, and others who offered advice regardless, muttering at times in discontent at their exclusion. Not all scientists, physicians, and administrators were in favor of spending money on a film, but once the money was committed advocates and (former) malcontents were generally united in claiming that they wanted to ensure scientific and medical accuracy. All involved shared the concern that the film not cause untoward effects such as dissuading the public from seeking medical help or turning away would-be biologists from a career in cancer research. But they did not always agree on what constituted accuracy, and most were also keen to ensure adequate representation within the film of their own specialty or institution (and perhaps themselves), which led to complaints such as that one field of science was overrepresented (generally not the field of the complainant), while another suffered by neglect (generally the field of the complainant). Such disciplinary and professional struggles thus found expression in disputes over the cinematic representation of science and shaped efforts to recruit scientists into cancer research in the late 1940s and early 1950s.

Working alongside these government scientists and physicians was the second group, the information officers—sometimes called public affairs officers—whose role it was to promote the agendas of their sponsoring organizations, rather as their counterparts in public relations sought to promote and protect businesses and corporations. The book pays special attention to this group, for it was the directors of the information offices of the NCI (Dallas Johnson) and the DNHW (Lt. Col. C. W. Gilchrist) who were the film's principal advocates. Yet both Johnson and Gilchrist often found themselves in a similar, awkward situation, caught between the demands of scientists, physicians, and other administrators and those of the filmmakers, both uneasy with their dependence on the other. The issue was true for both Gilchrist and Johnson, but was particularly important for Johnson whose office, the NCI's Cancer Reports Section, had been created only recently in 1948, and who found herself at times struggling to keep both the NCI's scientists, physicians, and administrators and the filmmakers happy. Johnson might have been hired for her knowledge of the public and how best to reach it, but such knowledge was not sufficient to manage the relations between sponsors and filmmakers. That would involve considerable political footwork, in particular because of the importance of this film to the future of the Cancer Reports Section in the NCI. The film was the largest and most visible project undertaken by the section, and if the scientists, physicians, and other administrators were not happy with the outcome, it would complicate other public education efforts and undermine the place of the section within the agency.

The problem for Johnson was twofold. First, NCI scientists, physicians, and administrators were sometimes divided over the film and, second, the filmmakers sometimes seemed tempted to disregard NCI advice, since this film was a one-off without clear lasting consequences. In Johnson's view, the fallout from both problems would be borne by her Cancer Reports Section, and she therefore spent much of her time struggling to reconcile these differences, and to keep everyone on board. The Cancer Reports Section is the institutional origin of what would become cancer communications at the NCI, and this book is the first account of its beginnings, and the importance of *Challenge* to its history. It also provides the first account of the origin of what would become the Office of Communications and Public Liaison at the NIH and its sometimes difficult relations with its NCI counterpart. It is a paradox of this story that Johnson sometimes had better relations with her counterpart in Canada, Lt. Col. Gilchrist, than with her counterpart at the NIH, Judson Hardy. A focus on the work of Johnson and Hardy helps to answer the question of why the NIH and the NCI felt it necessary to bring in specialists in communications and to create communications offices after the Second World War, while a focus on Gilchrist helps to answer the question of why pre-existing health communications efforts within the DNHW were reorganized after the war.

The chapters that explore the second project—*making*—focus on the production of the film itself, both its political and technical aspects: how the filmmakers sought to turn the biomedical commission into something they thought would work as a film. This commission was something of a coup for the Canadians, since until then educational films about cancer had been produced largely in the United States, and "Canadianized" for home audiences. *Challenge* both allowed the Canadians to trumpet their own expertise in educational filmmaking and helped the NFB to address some of its postwar political problems. The story of *Challenge* thus allows us to examine the development of cancer educational films in Canada. It also allows us to explore the political meanings of this film for the NFB at a time when it was trying to find a role for itself, fend off criticism from Ottawa, and develop new means of financing movies. One example of the latter was the creation of international coproduction deals where the NFB partnered with other organizations abroad: *Challenge* was among the first of such deals.

Challenge provides insights into these political and institutional struggles, and into the cultures of filmmaking within NFB and how they shaped this film. The task of the NFB filmmakers was to turn the sponsors' goal of producing a recruitment film into something that worked cinematically for the intended audiences, but the sponsors changed, and the NFB adjusted its film to reflect this change. The film had started out as a commission from the Canadian DNHW, for which the NFB quickly produced a script. However, the NFB also saw the script as an opportunity to bring in international cosponsors, and when eventually they recruited the NCI, the script had to be revised. Despite Johnson's worries that the NFB might disregard the concerns of NCI scientists, the NFB's desire to develop coproduction deals meant that it saw the film as a very malleable project, one that had to address the interests and agendas of the sponsors. For this reason, the script was written and rewritten many times, in part to make the film work better, but also to adapt it to the addition of a new sponsor.

For those readers who wish to know how the final version of the film turned out see Chapter 4. Table 4.3 gives an outline of the film's final structure. You may also watch the film by following the NLM link provided above in "Viewing the Films." But it is worth holding off and reading through the first few chapters before seeing the film, for this version was a long time coming. The final version was quite different than that in the first iterations of the script, and there was no certainty in the beginning that table 4.3 would be the outcome (for comparison with earlier versions see tables 3.1, 4.1 and 4.2). Not only did the nature of the film change during the rewrites of the script but it was further modified as the filmmakers got down to making the movie itself, deploying skills and equipment available within the organization. The NFB used its own staff to make the film, and they employed techniques and practices that had been developed at the NFB since the 1940s (along with one key imported animation technique). It is here that the richness of the archival record is telling. The chapters on this project—*making*—explore how the NFB brought together the skills of in-house animators, cameramen, editors, scriptwriters, actors, and others to construct the film, along with technologies such as an optical printer or a motorized zoom used in the creation of visual effects.

The book not only traces how the script was shaped by the political and institutional goals of the NFB and the technical skills of staff, it also shows how the sponsors' desires to attract young recruits to cancer research were inflected through the approach to filmmaking of the founder of the NFB, John Grierson[12] For Grierson, the aim of documentary film was not to capture the phenomena that paraded before a camera, but to use the phenomena to reach a more abstract or generalizable reality, the essence of the age. For Grierson this meant that naturalistic representation had to be subordinated to symbolic expression. With an educational film such as *Challenge* this approach involved deploying a variety of symbols: the patient and scientist representative of these categories, the representation of the cell-as-universe, the use of light and darkness to symbolize knowledge and ignorance, the rain to symbolize environmental dangers to the cell, among others. Such symbols aimed to represent the patient as respectful, obedient, and subject to science; the scientist as a hero, explorer, and ordinary man; the cell as a universe or outer space to evoke the wonder of its biology and the huge scale of the cancer problem; and, in the case of the rain, the dangers of cancer in the environment. Such symbols would be evoked through the live action and the animation, and also in the musical score, the ambient sound, and the narration. The music, for example, included evocations of cell division, embryological growth, the work of science, the wonder of nature, the fear of cancer, and the harmony of the body; the ambient sound invoked the calm hope of a hospital waiting room and the constant work of science; and the writers of the narration tried to hold these visual and aural symbols together, often ditching scientific precision for poetic expression. The film thus emerged as a complex of symbols and ideas that aimed to argue for a subjugation of the body and cancer to science. *Challenge* aimed to educate its audience on the science of cancer, while portraying cancer research as an enterprise filled with wonder and excitement.

It would, however, be a mistake to see this as simply a film about cancer or scientist recruitment. Some viewers complained that the film was stronger as a piece of art than as an educational tool. And, indeed, the filmmakers saw themselves as much in conversation with the arts as with science. They played with surrealism, neoromanticism, and Renaissance anatomy, and conjured up (aurally and visually) genres of science fiction and, fleetingly, gothic films among other cultural references. In so doing, they mixed the scientific with the artistic, sometimes the fantastical, so that the lines between science and the arts could be very blurred—something that the filmmakers wanted, but that also drew criticism from some viewers, who grumbled that they could not distinguish what was real and what was imaginary. Such issues raised a problem for the sponsors, who wanted the film to present scientific facts as then understood. For the filmmakers, adherence to facts alone would make for a very dull film that would fail to inspire. Nor would cautious didacticism allow them full rein to develop the symbolic expression necessary to make a broader argument about the relationship of the body, cell, and cancer to science.

The chapters on the third project—*packaging*—focus on efforts to target the movie at different audiences, both internal and external. In regard to internal audiences, the book explores how public affairs specialists and filmmakers sought to keep scientists and physicians within the sponsoring agencies on board both during the production of the film and after; in regard to external audiences, the book explores efforts to shape the reception of the movie through distribution, "press handling," and by packaging the movie with other educational efforts, such as Lester Grant's book, the teaching guide, and various pamphlets, radio talks, and other media productions. This is a story of how cancer communications worked in the late 1940s and early 1950s. Neither Johnson nor Gilchrist believed that the film could promote itself, and they developed a strategy to recruit the media and educational organizations into their efforts. Both had backgrounds in newspaper reporting and exploited their connections with the press and their experience with what worked in different media.

It is at this moment that the story moves beyond the sponsoring bodies and the NFB and explores how Johnson and Gilchrist sought to manage the media and the broader public they sought to reach. At times the media and public responded as they wished, but often they did not, and Johnson and Gilchrist sometimes found themselves struggling to deal with the fallout. Part of the problem was that public criticism played into the hands of those within the involved organizations (especially the sponsoring organizations) who had opposed the film, disagreed with the way it was promoted, or had other axes to grind. For these reasons, Johnson and Gilchrist could feel vulnerable to adverse public or media responses. Their packaging was always in danger of coming apart, and because of the film's importance to their respective agencies, an unraveling could have had dire consequences for the role of health communications within their agencies. The scrapbook they compiled to provide guidance on how to run a successful health campaign seemed at risk of turning into an object lesson in failed logistics.

In many ways, the campaign around *Challenge* was unexceptional. Since their beginnings in the 1910s, health films had often been embedded within broader educational campaigns. These campaigns had been organized by a multitude of organizations—state and federal agencies, voluntary bodies, and commercial organizations such as pharmaceutical companies. Some campaigns developed within the sponsoring organization; others were farmed out to advertising, marketing, and other agencies or some combination of the two. Most had multiple stakeholders, including partnerships between state and voluntary organizations, advertisers and marketing corporations, educational and health bodies, and the many other organizations and individuals concerned with health and illness. These promotional initiatives had roots in the nineteenth century but came into their own in the twentieth, orchestrating a range of media to reach a mass audience: posters, pamphlets, exhibitions, lectures, theatrical performances, newspaper and magazine articles, lantern slides, and later film, radio, and television.[13]

Film was thus only one of a range of media technologies deployed in such campaigns. The scrapbook and other documentation for *Challenge* help to capture how such campaigns could work in the postwar period, their links to the development of federal governments' health communications, and perceptions of film's place within a broader media ecology, including the new technology of television. It also shows how viewers responded to the film, what they felt about the sponsors' goals, and how the filmmakers had interpreted them. Bert Hansen has argued that the period from the 1880s to the 1950s was a golden age for media representations of medical science, with growing public optimism about science and a high esteem afforded to medical researchers.[14] *Challenge* reinforces this notion, with government agencies offering up science as the remedy for the dread disease of cancer and seeking to reinforce popular faith in the social utility of science. Yet for some critics this inspirational role was undermined by the film itself, and even its supporters did not believe it could provide all they wanted from it.

So far, I have written as if each of the three projects was distinct. In fact, they blurred into one another, sponsoring into making, making into promoting, promoting into sponsoring, and other combinations besides. For example, there was no hard line between sponsoring and making the movie. Sponsorship did not stop with the signing of the memorandum of agreement between the Canadians and Americans. NCI and Canadian scientists and administrators were keen to review the film at various stages throughout production, and their public affairs officers supported them in this role, in part to secure their own (sometimes) tenuous positions within these agencies, in part to ensure that the film reflected current scientific practice or knowledge, and in part to promote their agencies' perspectives. But it turned out that it was quite unclear where the boundary between advice and interference lay, nor was it clear what should happen if there was disagreement among scientists or administrators. Scientists and administrators felt free to offer advice, but not all of it was consistent—some of it promoted themselves or their causes—and it sometimes strayed into areas that the filmmakers regarded as their own. At the same time, the filmmakers found themselves caught unawares, such as when it turned out that the scientific practices they had filmed on location were different from those of scientists who reviewed the film, which raised the question of whether any such film could be said to represent current scientific practice. Filmmakers were also concerned that scientific or administrative pressures from the sponsoring agencies would result in a cinematic disaster, albeit one that was scientifically or medically accurate and in tune with the sponsors' goals. At various times, the filmmakers would note, and occasionally plead with the sponsoring bodies, that what worked as science did not always work as film. It was at points such as these that the public affairs officers could despair. They were some of the strongest promoters of film within the sponsoring agencies, but they feared they could not control powerful scientists, physicians, and administrators within their own organizations, nor the outside filmmakers. At times they worried it could all turn out to be a fiasco.

David Kirby has argued that the science adviser in Hollywood films was part of a broader film system in which natural phenomena, scientists, and research spaces were portrayed in ways that made it difficult for audiences to separate fact from fiction, even as scientists themselves criticized films for confusing the two.[15] In this case, the sponsoring agencies adopted an institutional mechanism to address this confusion. They turned to an outside organization, the Medical Film Institute (MFI) of the American Association of Medical Colleges, which had been created after the war to help determine how to assess the value of films in medical training and public health education. Its original involvement with *Challenge* was as a convenient means by which the NCI could channel funds to the Canadian filmmakers, but it rapidly took on a broader role of mediating between the filmmakers and sponsors. Under its leader, the public health official David Ruhe, the MFI brought together physicians, public health officials, and scientists who also had experience and knowledge of film. They could speak to the scientists and physicians as fellow scientists and physicians, and to the filmmakers as experts in film, and so provided a means by which the tricky boundary between film and the worlds of science and medicine could be negotiated. Yet the science advisers themselves played a role in introducing what critics claimed were inaccuracies. An animation technique developed by one of the science advisers was a focus of such criticisms, and elsewhere the science advisers pleaded for the inclusion in the narration of phrases judged to be inaccurate. For the advisers this was in part to help create a sense of awe at the worlds of the cell and the work of science, to help the filmmakers produce something that would work as a film and keep audience interest, and to situate science and the natural world within a context and tone that would stimulate and inspire.

PART I

SPONSORING

CHAPTER I

The Americans

THE NCI'S DECISION TO commission *Challenge: Science Against Cancer* was the brainchild of Dallas Johnson (1912–2013), the first director of the institute's Cancer Reports Section, recently created to help the agency deal with growing public and press interest after World War II, and to fulfill a mandate to promote public education about cancer. Johnson had not begun her appointment at the NCI thinking of funding a film, and she adopted the idea only after being approached by a young novelist, Bernard V. Dryer (1918–95), who in July 1948 showed her a Canadian screenplay for a film about cancer research. Almost immediately she saw this as an opportunity to address one of the major problems facing the NCI in the 1940s: the shortfall in recruits to cancer research, which threatened to derail plans to expand research during this period. Johnson had earlier been tasked with developing educational materials that might tempt high school and college students to think of cancer research as a career. At first she had been unsure of a strategy to achieve this goal. The meeting with Dryer prompted her to think of using film to anchor a multimedia recruitment and education campaign.

Johnson had been hired in 1947 by Leonard Scheele (NCI director, 1947–48) as an information or public affairs specialist, and eventually as director of the Cancer Reports Section, the first office in the NCI to specialize in targeting a general audience, which would later become its Office of Communications and Public Liaison. The NCI had found itself overwhelmed: juggling countless requests for information from members of Congress, physicians, and the general public, as well as its existing efforts to produce public educational materials and to cultivate public support for the growth of federal support for cancer research after the war. By 1947, it was clear to the institute's administrators that they needed someone with special expertise in reaching a general, nonspecialist audience, but there was no one on staff who could do this. As a former journalist, writer, and educator, Johnson seemed to fit the bill, and she began her tenure seeking to address the flood of requests for information coming into the NCI and to develop public education materials which the NCI sorely lacked. However, a short while after her appointment she was given another task: not only to manage public interest in cancer but also to recruit scientists into the field. The beginning of cancer communications at the NCI was thus entwined in postwar efforts to fulfill a long-standing mandate to promote public education about cancer, to manage growing public interest in cancer after the war, and to expand federally supported cancer research.

The dramatic expansion of cancer research after the Second World War has been well documented, especially the roles played by some of those promoting these changes, notably the philanthropist Mary Lasker, but also some leading politicians, scientists, and administrators in various private and governmental agencies.[1] Yet there is remarkably little on the problems of recruitment that threatened the expansion, nor on the role of information officers in the broader efforts to transform this situation. As this chapter will document, Johnson's endeavors were part of a larger public relations effort to make cancer research a more attractive field to potential recruits by generating public support for expansion, justifying changes in the programs to facilitate it, and by tempting scientists away from more prestigious fields of research such as atomic physics or better-paid positions in industry, which drained the pool of available talent. As such, when Johnson was asked to figure out how to attract young scientists into cancer research, she and her newly minted section were thrust into the heart of efforts to solve one of the key problems facing the NCI in the 1940s. Her decision to make a film the center of her efforts meant that *Challenge* would be a key part of the NCI's recruitment campaign.

Dallas Johnson and the Cancer Reports Section

Leonard Scheele's decision to appoint Dallas Johnson to head the NCI's public information efforts came of a certain frustration. The deluge of public and media interest in cancer, and biomedical research more generally, left the institute struggling to keep its head above water and raised concerns that that the growing public visibility of research would generate unrealistic expectations of a cure. As Scheele put it: "Many people still refer to the speed with which we solved the problem of the atom bomb and wonder why, with vast spending of money, we cannot speed up research and solve the cancer problem on a similar fast time schedule."[2]

In Scheele's view, however, the "miracle"[3] of the bomb was not a good model for cancer. He argued that where the bomb had relied on advances in

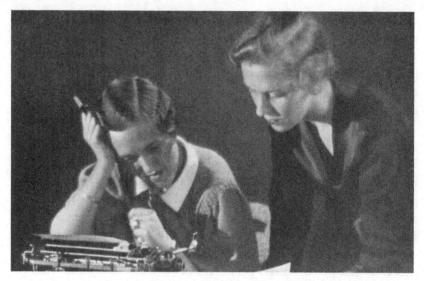

FIGURE 1.1. Helen Dallas/Dallas Johnson, right. Helen Dallas changed her name in the 1940s to Dallas Johnson, the result of a short marriage, with Dallas often substituting for Helen as her first name. Courtesy of Occidental College Special Collections and College Archives, *La Encina 1933*, p. 40.

developmental and applied science, advances in cancer would rely on basic research, which did not offer a solution in the short term. It could take many years, if not decades. So Scheele began to look for ways of calming such hopes, informing the public that the results of cancer research for patients were likely to come only in the long term, highlighting what was already known, and what, in the interim, could be done to combat this group of diseases. Johnson had the energy and background to take on the task.

Scheele wanted someone with experience of the media and education, and—like many information officers of the time in industry, government, and private campaigns such as the American Cancer Society[4]—Johnson checked both boxes. Her interest in journalism dated back to her education at Los Angeles Junior College and Occidental College, where the then Helen Dallas had been inspired by the charismatic president of Occidental, Remsen D. Bird (1888–1971), who persuaded her to edit Occidental's 1933 yearbook, *La Encina*. After college, Dallas (and after she married, Johnson) worked for the *San Francisco Examiner*; as a correspondent for the *New York Times*; an editor for the Institute for Consumer Education at Stephens College, Columbia, Missouri; a college educator and schoolteacher; and a writer of several educational

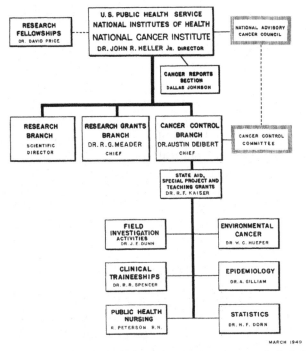

FIGURE 1.2. Organizational structure of NCI (March 1949), including the Cancer Reports Section, before the creation of Technical Services. Source: National Cancer Institute, *A Summary Progress Report*, 7.

pamphlets aimed at women and servicemen for the Public Affairs Committee of New York, a progressive public education organization. It was these skills that brought her to the attention of Scheele, who was looking for someone who understood and had connections with the media, knew how to present complicated ideas, and could advocate for the NCI to a general audience. Johnson began work following her appointment in 1947 answering directly to Scheele. The deluge of reporting on cancer, however, never seemed to stop, and despite all her energy and experience, Johnson alone was unable to keep up. Within a year her remit had expanded, and she now headed a small team in the new Cancer Reports Section.

The precise date of the creation of the section is unknown. The institute had no unit devoted to cancer education or information activities in 1946–7, which

tended to be spread across the various parts of the NCI prior to Johnson's appointment.[5] The first mention of the section is in 1948 under Scheele's successor
as NCI director, John Heller, apparently a stand-alone section at first (figure 1.2),
and then incorporated into a larger organizational unit called Technical Services, a staff office set up in the Office of the Director, NCI, in 1949.[6] Technical
services included three sections: biometrics (which undertook biometrical and
statistical activities concerned with cancer control and research); documentation
(acquiring, abstracting, and classifying scientific literature on cancer diagnosis
and related areas, especially cancer test information); and information (Johnson's Cancer Reports Section, concerned mainly with public and professional
education and outreach). In the official jargon, the Reports Section "collected,
interpreted, prepared and disseminated" information on both the cancer problem and the activities of the NCI to the public and professional groups concerned
with cancer. It served as the NCI's liaison office with other organizations, helped
to foster better understanding of NCI activities, and collaborated with the NCI's
cancer control program to promote efforts to control this group of diseases.

NCI and the ACS

One of the first tasks facing Johnson, as head of the Cancer Reports Section, was
to address the matter of the NCI's dependence on the American Cancer Society's
(ACS) educational materials and to reinvigorate collaboration between the two
agencies. The issue went back to the NCI's creation under the 1937 Cancer Act,
which had authorized the institute to cooperate with state health agencies in the
prevention, control, and eradication of cancer, a mandate it interpreted to include
efforts to educate the public about the disease.[7] The NCI had no educational materials of its own in 1937, so it worked out an arrangement whereby the American
Society for the Control of Cancer (ASCC, which became the ACS in 1944) allowed it to mimeograph its pamphlets, meaning that the NCI was almost entirely
dependent on the ASCC for educational materials in its early years. In time this
would change, and the two organizations began to collaborate to organize public
education programs and to publish education pamphlets and posters together,
using the former's unrivaled network of regional and state organizations, often
working in collaboration with local and state public health authorities.[8]

It was in this context that the NCI had first became involved in film. The
ASCC saw the NCI's interest in collaboration as an opportunity to relaunch efforts at producing educational films, which had stalled during the Depression. It
had limited funds for this purpose, and hoped that collaboration with the NCI

would allow it to produce motion pictures that it could not afford to produce independently, which could be used as part of broader public education efforts. During the early 1940s, the two organizations collaborated on two films aimed at persuading people to seek early detection and treatment of cancer. *Choose to Live* (1940) was a melodrama aimed at women, and *Enemy X* (1942) was in part a detective story, a film within the film, aimed at men.[9] But the cinematic collaboration between the NCI and the ASCC was short-lived. While the two organizations continued to work closely in cancer education, after *Enemy X* no joint NCI/ACS public educations films were produced until 1950, when a new coproduction, *Breast Self-Examination*, was released.[10]

The end of film collaboration was hastened by changes in the ASCC. In 1944, the old ASCC leadership was ousted by a small group of influential businesspeople and advertisers, who took over the organization and renamed it the American Cancer Society (ACS). Much more willing than their forebears to spend money to raise money, the new leaders had little patience for what they saw as a tightfisted old guard and introduced business models of fund-raising and education that involved substantial outlays of resources. The result was that funding increased dramatically for the new organization, its educational programs expanded significantly, and expensive communication technologies such as the movie became feasible: indeed, they became a key to cancer education programs and to efforts to generate political and financial support. Such financial independence allowed the new organization to distance itself from its former reliance on the NCI in the film component of its educational program, and the NCI, without a partner, abandoned filmmaking, releasing no new public education films before 1950. By contrast ACS film production soared. Its new film unit was headed from 1947 to 1951 by Adelaide Brewster, the original Betty Crocker, who oversaw an expanded film production schedule and the hiring of commercial film companies such as United Productions of America (UPA), John Sutherland, and Wexler Films to make its movies.[11]

Thus, by the time that the Cancer Reports Section was created, the film component of the educational programs of the NCI and the ACS had diverged, even as the NCI and the ACS continued to use each other's other educational materials.[12] Johnson's appointment did little to change things at first. She seems to have taken little interest in reviving collaboration over film but wanted to reinforce the other forms of collaboration between the two organizations, and to give more of an NCI imprint to the educational materials they both used. Her fear was that, without such collaboration, the messages of the NCI and the ACS might diverge, and that the existence of two cancer organizations with different messages about cancer would confuse the public, undermine NCI efforts to cultivate public support for increased federal funding for cancer, and harm public education. Scheele and Heller may not have needed much convincing, for the ACS was an ally in advocating for more federal funding for the NCI, and the NCI's cancer control program was already coordinating with the ACS. On her appointment, Johnson reinforced these efforts, beginning a series of co-publications with the ACS—pamphlets, leaflets, and books.[13]

Johnson's approach to educating people about cancer drew on her experience of consumer education, familiar from her time at the Institute for Consumer Education, and with the Public Affairs Committee. Johnson's publications on consumer education in the 1930s had portrayed systematic knowledge—clearly laid out for a public audience—as a basis of social action, and a means of overcoming the confusion of messages put out by interested groups on all sides of the consumer debate. Some of her publications edged toward a participatory imperative in which knowledge provided a basis for consumer protest, activism, and lobbying.[14] Others edged toward a technocratic imperative that asserted the leadership of consumer experts: the mass of consumers were seen as relatively passive, in need of expert leadership, and reliant on consumer organizations to critique business practices and to highlight cost-effective, quality goods and services.[15] Her public education work for the NCI tended to echo the latter approach: it urged the public to beware of quacks, and to actively inspect their bodies, but to trust physicians as the only experts who could identify the disease and treat it. Such knowledge claims provided a basis for asserting the leadership of physicians and scientists. The public, from this perspective, was largely ignorant of the disease and what could be done about it, and ignorant in that it often put trust in inexpert physicians, quacks, and purveyors of patent medicines. Ideally, from the NCI's perspective, the public should be active only insofar as it followed the recommendations of recognized physicians and the cancer agencies. It needed leadership, guidance from such physicians and agencies.

But Scheele and later Heller did not simply want Johnson to focus on cancer control. They wanted her to figure out ways of tempting high school and college students to think of cancer research as a career. Johnson herself saw this as an opportunity to demonstrate the value of her Cancer Reports Section to the research side of NCI, which was growing as never before, and eclipsing cancer control within the institute. She had a good relationship with the head of cancer control, Austin V. Deibert (figure 1.3 left), but she struggled to find acceptance among some on the research side, the phrase I will use to refer to both the Research Branch and the Research Grants Branch (see figure 1.1).[16] If her Reports

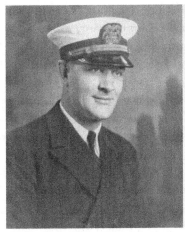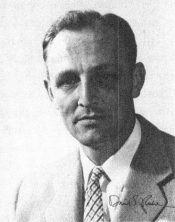

FIGURE 1.3. Left: Austin V. Deibert in PHS uniform and cap, 1932. Images from the History of Medicine, National Library of Medicine, NLM Record Unique ID 101413461; NLM Image ID, B06045. Right: David S. Ruhe, 1956. Images from the History of Medicine, National Library of Medicine, NLM Record Unique ID 101427569; Image ID B022672.

Section was to have a future at the NCI, she would have to show that it could help address some of the key issues facing researchers. However, it would also mean developing quite different ways of educating the public and, at first, she wasn't sure how to do this.

Recruitment

Recruitment problems were not new to the late 1940s. Indeed, they had been a major reason for the creation of the NCI in 1937. In arguing for the establishment of such an institute, cancer researchers characterized the field as one of immense technical difficulty combined with poor funding for research, and poor pay for cancer researchers—a young cancer researcher with two to five years' experience in 1937 could expect to earn the wage of a carpenter (US$1,500 to US$1,800 a year).[17] No wonder, they complained, that it was very difficult to attract people into the field when a man [*sic*] could make a name for himself much more easily in other scientific fields, and when pay was better in industry. For some practitioners, the hopelessness of the field reinforced the bonds between this self-styled beleaguered group: "There has been," one claimed,[18] "a singular friendship among cancer investigators owing to the quality of the research and the hopelessness of getting quick results." But others took a more pessimistic

view of the situation, such as the unnamed distinguished researcher who allegedly "tacked over his laboratory door the warning that Dante found at the
gate of Hell: 'Abandon hope, all ye who enter here.'"[19]

The problem of recruitment dogged the NCI throughout the 1940s and may
have worsened. Scheele lamented that "Potential scientists carried arms in World
War II instead of being trained as research workers and thus a generation of
scientists was lost."[20] In addition, the rapidly increasing need for scientists and
engineers to fight the World War and then to drive the Cold War arms race
produced what contemporaries called a "scientist gap" in the 1940s and 1950s;
a "gap" stretched further by the low birth rates of the 1930s Depression era.[21]
The NCI found itself competing for recruits from a dwindling pool, and just
at the time that funding for cancer research was beginning to explode, with
a consequent increase in demand for new young blood. Repeatedly, cancer researchers complained that young students were often more tempted by the better
prospects of work in industry. As one commentator noted, medical researchers
were the "POOREST PAID PROFESSIONALS."[22] "Small wonder," he noted in evidence to Congress in 1946,[23] "some of them do desert to industrial posts where
the pay is far better."

Dallas Johnson echoed the point about industrial competition the following
year.[24] But she also highlighted a new threat to cancer research from the growing
popularity of (especially atomic) physics as a career choice, then also attracting
substantial federal and private support.[25] The notion that physics was attracting
more than its fair share of recruits was not new. During the hearings that led up
to the creation of the NCI in 1937 the Memorial Hospital physicist Gioacchino
Failla noted that in general "students who have an analytic turn of mind, choose
for their careers physics or mathematics, but not medicine or allied sciences."[26]
In his view, physics in particular had an appeal that biology or medicine could
not match: "The spectacular advances made, for instance, in physics in the last
40 years have served to attract men with these qualifications to this field."[27]
Johnson expanded on this argument in the 1940s. In her view the extraordinary
triumph of the atomic bomb and the promise that atomic research held for the
future made physics an even more attractive field. "The climate of opinion," she
noted later,[28] "warmed by the atom, was drawing the best students into the physical sciences; the physical problems of man were being neglected." Her job, as she
saw it, was to develop a program of materials that would help to turn this around
and prompt students to think of cancer research as a career.

The need to do something about poor recruitment was particularly acute at
the time of Johnson's appointment. The 1944 Public Health Act had removed

a US$700,000 cap on the annual appropriations of the NCI, and its budget expanded dramatically. The US$2,500,000 allotment for grants for cancer research projects in fiscal year (FY) 1948 virtually doubled the total amount the Institute had had available for such grants in the preceding ten-year period 1937–47. Officials noted that this would permit support to cancer research in outside institutions on a much more extensive scale than had ever been possible before. Scheele looked optimistically toward an "increase in our research scientist pool, because there are now enough students in our colleges and universities to double our present pool within the next decade."[29] But the NCI also worried that the expansion of research would exacerbate the recruitment situation. They needed qualified people available to apply for the money.

In their efforts to attract qualified people, the NCI not only allocated more money to research, but also changed the ways it could be used. Until 1948, grants had been made only for specific projects that had to be outlined in some detail as to material, time, personnel, and funds. Scheele described this as a hand-to-mouth annual existence, and he urged reform. He wanted to provide surplus funds over and above immediate needs that could be banked against the future to ensure continuity in projects. He similarly advocated for the creation of block or institutional financing, which would allow institutions to select their research problems without interference from the groups providing the funds.[30]

Scheele had trained as a cancer fellow at Memorial Hospital from 1937 to 1939 and had had worked at NCI from 1939 to 1942 before leaving to serve in the European theater during World War II. He returned to the NCI and was appointed assistant director to Roscoe Spencer. The year he would spend in this post, before he succeeded Spencer as director of the NCI in 1947, would largely be devoted to coming up with new ideas for the reorganization and expansion of the Institute, including its grants program.[31]

Under Scheele's direction a new grants policy emerged that aimed to give research institutions greater freedom to determine their own activities and would allow scientists greater leeway in following research leads. Scheele intended such changes to permit the coordination of many different phases of cancer research in a single institution and make the field more enticing for qualified researchers. NCI researchers and administrators complained that one of the most serious deterrents to cancer research had been the lack of assured long-range support for projects, and they hoped Scheele's reforms would create a future in which grants could be given to research groups for at least two years ahead.

In addition, they also pointed to a new feature of the grant-in-aid program under Scheele, which was to give funds for the acquisition of land and the construction of laboratories and clinical research facilities.[32] The hope was that it would lead to the development of a small number of large cancer research centers in various parts of the United States, and that increased assistance could be given to support research beds and more clinical research in hospitals. All these developments would need staffing, and while officials hoped that brand new facilities would attract the right sort of people, they were not convinced that growth was sustainable given current recruitment patterns. As a 1949 report put it: "The current unprecedented expansion of research facilities, by both public and private institutions, has created a widening gap between the number of qualified workers needed to staff them and the supply."[33]

To help solve this problem the NCI expanded an existing program of research fellowships established in 1938 which made advanced training possible for qualified young men and women wishing to devote themselves to a career in science and needing financial assistance. With the enlarged appropriation for 1947–48 the program was stepped up. The fellowship program in 1938 had had twenty fellows, and fifty had passed through its programs by 1947. By 1948 there were more than 100 active fellows, and the NCI also sought to improve recruitment among women, traditionally better represented in medical and biological research than in the competing fields, especially physics.[34] Nevertheless, officials continued to worry about the long-term future, and it was for this reason that Scheele, and later Heller, turned to Johnson for help.[35] Her efforts to recruit budding scientists into cancer research was thus part of a broader reform of cancer research at the NCI, and it took her in a new direction—targeting students and young adults.

Children and young adults

In targeting children and young adults, Johnson at first turned for inspiration to cancer educational programs that began in the 1930s, mixing efforts to teach students the biology of cancer with efforts to persuade them to recruit their parents as patients into programs of early detection and treatment.[36] Among the first was one established by the Westchester Cancer Committee (founded c.1929), a component of the ASCC based in New York state, which came to be both a model of cancer educational efforts aimed at children, and a lesson in the problems of establishing such programs. In the view of the committee, children were a key to the future of cancer control because they were unlikely to share the prejudices of their parents about the disease—they did not generally regard it as incurable, nor did they exhibit the excessive fears of the disease and its treatment of their elders. Their minds were ripe for molding, impressed with positive messages about cancer.

Thus in 1936, it began working with school superintendents and science teachers to develop ways of teaching children about the biology of the disease, and four years later, in 1940, the committee published *Youth Looks at Cancer* for use in biology classes. It turned out, however, that educating students involved much more than handing out booklets. The problem was that many high school teachers did not feel qualified to teach the text *Youth Looks at Cancer*. So the committee arranged for physicians to talk to classes about cancer, and for a biology teacher from Memorial Hospital to offer school educators a short course of four lectures followed by a tour of Memorial Hospital. Fifty-six teachers accepted the invitation to attend the course in its first year.[37] Learning from such programs nine years later, Johnson began planning to recruit science teachers by commissioning a guide to help teachers make use of *Challenge* in the classroom.

Two years after publishing *Youth Looks at Cancer*, in 1942 the Westchester Cancer Committee expanded its efforts, broadening the focus of its campaign from educating children about the biology of cancer to recruiting them into programs of cancer control with the publication of a booklet, *Detectives Wanted!* "CALLING ALL BOYS AND GIRLS,"[38] the booklet began, the FBI ("the Family Bureau of Investigation"),[39] wanted children to be "G-men" to fight "Cancer the Gangster, one of the worst diseases in the world."[40] They were to learn the "CLUES FOR CANCER THE GANGSTER,"[41] to remind family members to be on guard for any of the clues ("grown-ups are careless about its earliest signs"[42]), to urge immediate examination by a doctor if they spotted any of the clues, and to root out and punish the gangster by surgery, x-rays or radium. "Remember! Cancer the Gangster may be at work in your home! Be on guard!"[43]

The booklet was published in early 1942 and by November more than 50,000 copies of *Detectives Wanted!* had been sent to schools, doctors, health officers, and others, part of a broader campaign in which over 100,000 pieces of other literature had been mailed to doctors and to the public.[44] And it also served as a complement to *Youth Looks at Cancer*, the latter teaching students about the biology of cancer, the other seeking to encourage them to persuade their parents to seek help. By October 1943, every high school and college in Westchester County had been supplied with copies of both booklets.[45] In 1946, local papers noted great things about the campaign: "Results show that the subject of cancer is losing its stigma, and that children are urging their parents to attend cancer clinics. They ask intelligent questions, they write essays on the disease, and they are learning that, caught in time, it is curable."[46]

Whatever the truth of such claims about the impact of the campaign, the ASCC/ACS (and by extension the NCI, still depended on the society for much of its educational material) continued to mix an approach that targeted children both as students of biology and as recruiters of parents. *Youth Looks at Cancer* was never out of print in the 1940s and 1950s, new editions were printed periodically, and copies circulated in schools across the United States. *Detectives Wanted!* was also widely distributed outside of Westchester County, and the two pamphlets came to form part of a broader effort by the ACS and NCI to get cancer teaching into schools.[47]

As part of these efforts, the ACS commissioned a film eventually called *From One Cell*, which, together with *Challenge*, was the first educational film about cancer aimed at school and college biology classes. In fourteen minutes, the movie traced the complex subjects of embryonic, regenerative, and degenerative cell behavior; and introduced the topic of the abnormal growth of cancer in part to clarify concepts of normal growth and in part to provoke interest in the as-yet unanswered questions of abnormal cell behavior. A pamphlet, *Teaching about Cancer: Thoughts for School Administrators* was mailed to 25,000 principals and 7,500 administrators of secondary schools.[48] "Students of biology are the doctors and research scientists of tomorrow," the ACS noted two years later,[49] "The Society's film *From One Cell* seeks to rouse their interest in cancer as a still unsolved biological and medical problem, as well as to teach facts about the disease." The ACS had begun to see film as a way of recruiting students into cancer research, at just about the time that Dallas Johnson also turned to film.[50]

What strategy?

Yet, when Scheele and Heller had asked Johnson to develop educational tools to recruit scientists into cancer research she had not immediately thought of film. It was clear to her that this task would require a different approach to that which she had already adopted for cancer control, itself borrowing from her earlier work in consumer education. Whereas public education efforts tended to encourage people to follow the advice of their physicians and to seek early detection and treatment, recruitment efforts meant persuading students to become involved in a different sort of activism, by becoming scientists themselves, and creating the knowledge upon which future medical practice would be based. The general public might have to follow the advice of physicians, but physicians, it was suggested, would in the future be guided by the scientists Johnson recruited, at least after suitable training.

A further problem concerned the place of cancer within the classroom. The NCI was already aware that some high school and college students undertook special projects on cancer, but recruitment efforts would, Johnson felt, require something much more than the occasional school or college project. So Johnson was faced with relying, once again, on the ACS's *Youth Looks at Cancer,* still in print and by far the best short introduction to the subject for the audience, along with the few biology textbooks that incorporated extensive discussions of cancer.[51] Given her desire to cooperate with the ACS, it seems likely that Johnson would have considered this possibility of relying on ACS publications, and she was also aware of moves to develop the ACS film that would become *From One Cell.* But she was also struggling to establish her new section within the NCI, to make it relevant to the research side of NCI, and to insert an NCI perspective into educational materials. Reliance on the ACS was not the best way to achieve these ends.

A more general problem concerned the changing aim of high school science education. Prior to the 1940s, the principal aim of high school science education was to show that science had something of value to offer students and the general public: its content or method provided tools that could be used in a variety of situations, often outside of institutional science.[52] This began to change with the growth of federal investment in scientific research and development during and after the war. Increasingly, a goal of sustaining the professional science community itself came to displace a goal of meeting the needs of the general public. Put another way, the goals of science education changed from improving the lives of students and citizens, to ensuring the success of the scientific enterprise itself. Such changes were a mixed blessing for Johnson, however. On the one hand, they provided an opportunity to turn science education to the benefit of the NCI, ensuring that it helped to draw young people into cancer research and biology. On the other, these changes also meant that the NCI found itself in competition with other areas of science for new recruits.

Johnson was thinking through all these issues in the first year or so of her appointment at the NCI, but there is little evidence that she had come up with a strategy to deal with them. It was at this point that in July 1948, she learned from Dryer that the Canadians were independently planning a film on cancer. Dryer had recently met with the National Film Board of Canada (NFB) in New York, where he had been given the script of a cancer movie which the NFB had in the works. The NFB was looking for a partner in making the film, and Dryer was enthusiastic enough to pass the script on to Johnson, who loved it and began to discuss the possibility of cooperation with the Canadians and how the script might be adapted to the needs of the NCI.[53] At last, Johnson had a project that would allow her to pursue her ambitions for the Cancer Reports Section, to place it at the heart of efforts to expand cancer research in the United States and indeed internationally, to put an NCI mark on cancer educational materials if the ACS decided to join in, and go on independently if the ACS decided not to come along.

Cooperation promised the possibility of pooling resources to make a movie more ambitious than the NCI alone could undertake. The Canadian funding was already in place, and an international coproduction had the advantage of giving the project a visibility that one financed solely by the NCI or with another American organization would not. It also had the advantage of allowing the NCI to draw on the resources of the National Film Board of Canada, which had developed a reputation as an innovative documentary filmmaker on a range of social and scientific issues.[54] Canadian reports noted that the US authorities specifically requested that the film be produced in Canada, because Canadian health education films—notably the *Mental Mechanisms* series sponsored by the Department of National Health and Welfare—had already made a strong impression in the United States.[55] American reports are unfortunately less revealing about their dependence on the Canadians.[56] Johnson later recalled that they were cheap.[57]

The Medical Film Institute

The Canadians might have been cheap, but Johnson's budget was small, and her Cancer Reports Section did not have enough to fund the NCI part of the collaboration. Johnson therefore tried to get the NFB to apply for a grant from the NCI, but the application came in too late, and some members of the National Advisory Cancer Council (NACC), the NCI's advisory body, doubted that a film could do the job of reaching potential research workers.[58] There were also concerns that a film on research might exacerbate the problem of unrealistic expectations, and undermine interest in cancer control; Johnson wanted to demonstrate her relevance to cancer research, but not to burn her boats with cancer control.[59] There was also the problem that because the NCI was a US government agency, bringing in the Canadians could mean a lot of bureaucratic red tape, and Johnson feared the involvement of the State Department. Her solution was to do an end-run around the State Department by persuading a US organization, the Medical Film Institute (MFI) of the Association of American Medical Colleges (AAMC) to apply to the NCI for a grant to make the movie, and for the MFI to make the arrangements with the Canadians.[60] The solution had the benefit for Johnson of financing the movie from the better-endowed NCI Cancer Control Branch under Deibert, rather than Johnson's depleted funds—the Cancer Reports Section was not authorized to issue grants—so also keeping an alliance with cancer control even as she reached out to the research side of NCI. It also had the advantage, Johnson believed, of allowing the AAMC to involve the Canadians without the fuss of the State Department. As will be discussed in later chapters, the NFB had acquired a reputation as a subversive agency among conservatives in the US and Canada, tainted with rumors of Communist infiltration, and staffed by people who espoused progressive causes. The State Department, she feared, could have created all sorts of problems for this collaboration.

Johnson's approach was a timely one from the point of the view of the AAMC. Movies had become increasingly important to medical education in the 1940s, notably after the federal government had produced medical and health education films during the war. The problem was that these movies were of variable quality, and there seemed to be little agreement as to what constituted a good educational film.[61] Thus in 1947 the AAMC established a Committee on Audiovisual Aids,[62] and in 1949 a Medical Film Institute (MFI), under David S. Ruhe (1913–2005) (figure 1.3 right). A United States Public Health Service (PHS) officer on a five-year leave from the service and a graduate of the Temple University School of Medicine in 1941, Ruhe had begun his medical career during World War II as a malaria researcher with the PHS before joining the MFI.[63] The MFI aimed to help in planning films, to create and foster high standards in film production regarding scientific content, educational value, and cinematic qualities. It did not generally make films but reviewed them for quality and effectiveness and acted as a consultative body during their production.[64] This last function was largely the role it undertook with *Challenge*, though unlike most of its other movies, *Challenge* was not a medical training movie, but one aimed at recruiting people to science.

The MFI thus emerged as much more than a convenient channel by which Dallas Johnson could direct money to the Canadians. It also provided a means of ensuring scientific oversight of the film. It helped in the appointment of the medical filmmaker and illustrator Vito F. Bazilauskas as a special consultant on the animation sections of the movie (Bazilauskas advised the animators on the scientific accuracy of their representations of the body and proposed a technical solution to the animator's problem of showing environmental threats to the cell). Bernard Dryer advised on the script and when the shooting was completed helped in the revisions to the narration. Both men—together with David Ruhe—were present at the showing of the rough cut and provided advice on how the final cut should be edited. Ruhe also worked closely with the NFB, acting at times as a second producer, monitoring costs, advising on location, helping with contacts with relevant scientists, and overseeing the animation. Yet their oversight was rarely seen as unwarranted. In interview, the film's director, Morten Parker, noted the light hand of the MFI: it understood the process of filmmaking, where to advise, and where to draw back.[65]

This last point highlights another role of the MFI. It not only provided advice to the movie makers on the scientific aspects of the movie, but also mediated between the movie makers and the cancer researchers. Many cancer researchers had strong feelings on what should be represented in the movie, but little understanding of filmmaking or public education according to the filmmakers and information specialists.[66] Such ignorance, however, did not stop some from telling the NFB how to do its job. For the NFB this was a one-off film, an important one, but nevertheless a one-off, and it may have been tempted to ignore some of these concerns, especially since—as will be discussed in chapter 5—the producer of the film feared the interference of sponsors too often led to bad films. But Johnson was in a different position, and if the filmmakers ignored the advice of powerful scientists within the NCI, it could undermine her work as an NCI information specialist. Hence the importance of the MFI as a mediator. As physicians and scientists, they had the ear of the scientists at NCI; as film experts they had the ear of the NFB.

But in 1948/9, this mediating role was still in the future. The first thing was to formalize an agreement to make the movie. In February/March 1949 a memorandum of agreement was drawn up between the NCI, the MFI, the National Film Board, and the Canadian Department of National Health and Welfare in which the NCI and the Canadian Department each agreed to contribute $20,000 for the Film Board to produce the movie. The NCI's $20,000 was in the form of a grant to the MFI which would be the responsible American agent in the production.[67]

CHAPTER 2

The Canadians

T HE AGREEMENT TO COPRODUCE a film was something of a coup
for the Canadians. Until then, Canadian health authorities had been
largely dependent on American educational films. Now for the first
time the Americans were to be dependent on a Canadian production. It was
a remarkable turnaround, but it also came with dangers for the Canadians.
Growing support for research in the United States threatened a hemorrhage of
Canadian scientific talent to American institutions. There was a risk that *Challenge* would hasten the departure of Canadians for richer American pastures.
How ironic that a Canadian gain in public health education films might turn
into a loss for Canadian science. Thus, for the Canadian health authorities the
dilemma of *Challenge* was how to collaborate with a potential competitor for
scientific talent.

The dilemma was particularly acute because one of the rationales for producing educational films was to promote Canadian values, needs, and identity.
In the years after the acquisition of political sovereignty from Britain in 1931,
several organizations had appeared with expressly nationalistic intent. Among
these was the Canadian Society for the Control of Cancer (CSCC)—the first
national campaign against cancer, founded in 1938, later known as the Canadian
Cancer Society (CCS)[1]—which attempted to bring order to the hodgepodge of
provincial efforts against the disease. The society came to see movies as a powerful means of indicating the peculiar nature of the threat that cancer posed
to Canada, and the distinctive ways Canadians responded or should respond
to it. For these reasons, it worried about Canadian dependence on American
productions, which it felt were not always suitable for Canadian audiences. A
uniquely Canadian campaign was needed, it claimed, that was quite different
from that carried out south of the international border. Its cancer movies thus
aimed to promote Canadian values and identity as much as to combat cancer.
It was unclear, however, how a movie like *Challenge* was to promote Canadian

values and identity, given the collaboration with the Americans and the threat that the United States posed to Canadian scientific ambitions.[2]

Yet, as this chapter will show, concerns about the dangers to Canadian cancer research of a film collaboration with the Americans only emerged in 1949 with the prospect of a contract with the NCI and MFI. Before then proposals for the film or films that would later mutate into *Challenge* imagined a quite different sort of production. Instead of a collaboration with the Americans, these proposals envisaged a film or films that would serve the goals of Canadian science, sometimes as a counter to American influence. Canadian cancer research, like that in the US, was expanding as never before during this period, and the goal of the film or films was to promote this expansion and protect it against the much larger and better funded American cancer effort, which tempted Canadian researchers to leave the country. As such it also marked a transformation in Canadian cancer education filmmaking that paradoxically mirrored changes in the United States in the new emphasis it gave to research.

Previously the few cancer education films produced in Canada—and the many more it imported—focused on control, encouraging Canadians, like their American counterparts, to undergo routine surveillance and to seek medical assistance the moment something that might be cancer was detected. In the 1940s, however, the focus of Canadian cancer campaigns began to change. While early detection and treatment remained important, they increasingly also focused on cancer research, funding for which—as in the US—increased substantially after the war, bolstered by new organizations founded to promote it and a new partnership between private cancer campaigns and the federal government. Such developments prompted a shift in the public education component of cancer campaigns, which now increasingly focused on research as well as cancer control. This, along with a new enthusiasm for film as a tool of public education in the Department of National Health and Welfare (DNHW) and among nongovernment Canadian cancer organizations, eventually led to funding for the film that would become *Challenge*. It began life as part of an effort to buttress Canadian research and control against American threats, and later—when the Americans came on board—to focus more on international endeavors.

Americans and Canadians

Before the mid-1940s, Canadian cancer organizations had taken little interest in producing motion pictures for public educational purposes. A handful of Canadian films were in circulation, generally targeted at provincial rather than national audiences, but these were dwarfed by American productions spilling across the border. When in 1945 the Canadian Cancer Society (CCS) surveyed the use of films in cancer, it found that very few were available, most of which were American.[3] As F. G. Butterfield, the provincial secretary of the Saskatchewan branch of the CCS, noted in 1947: "So far as motion pictures are concerned, I think we have missed the boat, most definitely, because we have not utilized moving pictures or the moving picture industry in getting our story across to the public. That is one place we have fallen down badly."[4]

Canadian reliance on American cancer education films went back to the 1920s, when the first movies produced by the American Society for the Control of Cancer (ASCC) had been distributed north of the US/Canadian border.[5] American dominance faded slightly in the 1930s, when ASCC production slumped because of the Depression, and two short documentary films—*Rays of Hope* (1937) and *That They May Live* (1942)—were released by the Saskatchewan Cancer Commission.[6] But with the exception of a few film trailers, these were the only Canadian public cancer education movies produced before 1947, though a number of provinces produced technical or semi-technical movies for specialist audiences, some of which also may have been screened for general audiences[7] (table 2.1). Thus, as American cancer movie production picked up in the late 1930s and early 1940s, American-produced movies such as *Choose to Live* (1940) and *Enemy X* (1942) once again came to dominate Canadian public cancer education.[8]

At first sight, Canadian reliance on American movies might not seem much of a problem. All were focused on cancer control, which in Canada, as in the United States, meant early detection and treatment.[17] From this perspective, the key object of control was to identify and treat (mainly by surgery and/or radiation) cancers as earlier in their natural development as possible, before they grew too large to be successfully treated, or metastasized elsewhere in the body. To achieve this meant persuading Canadians to go to their physicians at the first signs of what might be cancer. Yet Canadian health organizations—like those in the United States—worried that people might delay seeking help out of ignorance or a paralyzing fear of the disease or its treatment. In their view, cancer education movies provided a powerful means of educating the public about cancer and of countering the fears that Canadians might have of the disease or interventions against it.

Despite these common interests, the CCS and other Canadian health organizations were concerned about their reliance on US movies. The CCS reported that movies such as *Choose to Live* and *Enemy X* were well received, but "Their

TABLE 2.1. Canadian-Produced Cancer Education Movies, 1937–1947

Date	Title	Produced by/for	Notes
1937	*Rays of Hope*[9]	Saskatchewan Cancer Commission	
c.1941	*A Nurse Looks at Radiology*[10]	Produced by Claribel McCorquodale, Supervisor of Nurses in the Department of Radiology of the Toronto General Hospital	Silent picture, but McCorquodale had speaking equipment, attended all screenings, and showed the film on request. Using a series of animations, it illustrated what the radiologist sees by means of X-ray, the various duties of the nurse in this department, and the treatment of cancer by means of radium. The film was aimed at nurses but may also have been used for general audiences.
1942	*That They May Live*[11]	Saskatchewan Cancer Commission	
1942–43	Unknown title (Trailer)[12]	Unknown	100 ft. 35-mm trailer shown in 75 rural theatres in Manitoba. (Not stated if this is a Canadian production)
1946 (April)	Unknown title (Trailer)[13]	CCS	1-minute trailer
1947	Unknown title (Film)[14]	London unit of the CCS	
1947	Unknown title (Film)[15]	J. Ernest Ayres	Stolen after its screening and returned 48 hours later by a man who bought the projector from the thief. This may be a professional rather than a health education film.
1947	*The Cancer Crusaders*[16]	British Columbia branch of the Canadian Cancer Society	

greatest criticism is that they give American Statistics, and information pertinent to their own Facilities."[18] In addition, in the view of the CCS, American campaigns were overly aggressive about the dangers of cancer, and risked undermining Canadian cancer control efforts by generating excessive fear of the disease or its treatment in audiences. Canadians, the CCS believed, did not respond well to the sorts of emotional appeals that might work for Americans, even though the ASCC/ACS also worried about generating excessive fear of the disease or its treatment and had monitored and modified their films to avoid this. In the view of the CCS, films targeted at such audiences not only had to provide information of direct relevance to Canadians, but also had to be of a different emotional tone than those produced south of the border. Such concerns about tone and emphasis made it difficult to adapt American cancer movies for a Canadian audience—"Canadianized"[19] as the CCS described it—and helped to make a case for homegrown films, or for adopting alternative methods of getting a message across. Much Canadianization involved little more than "cutting off their [ACS] trailers and putting on some of our own, with their permission."[20] "Surely Canadians have the right to be presented with the Canadian picture as far as our work is concerned,"[21] one cancer society official suggested.

At first, Canadian campaigns tended to focus on other methods of getting their message across. Newspapers, magazines, radio, and countless pamphlets, posters, slides, and lectures were cheaper to use, and more adaptable to local and Canadian circumstances. American campaigns had found that these methods allowed them to target a variety of different audiences, often more effectively and cheaply than movies, which were not always adaptable to the specific concerns of different audiences. Canadians found that in addition they were well tailored to the decentralized, often fragmented, campaigns in different provinces. But Canadian cancer organizations continued to hope that film might yet be turned to their advantage. Like the Americans, many came to see movies as having a power to persuade mass audiences that other communication technologies lacked, and they continued to plan or hope to promote a distinctive Canadian movie that could enhance programs of cancer control. From 1944 such plans to create an "all Canadian film"[22] gained new impetus, though it could be difficult to get them into cinemas, especially the longer ones. "The importance of keeping these films short has been forced in upon us, by the experience we have had in trying to interest theatre managers in accepting films," noted one public health nurse,[23] "Anything longer than a single reel trailer, which takes about 9 minutes, is frowned upon."

Producing a distinctively Canadian movie was not only about the practicalities of getting them into the cinemas. It was also about developing a distinctively *national* campaign, one that united the various provincial cancer campaigns. As Charles Hayter notes, until the creation of the Canadian Society for the Control of Cancer in 1938, Canadian cancer campaigns had been organized at the level of the province.[24] The CSCC hoped to change this, and to bring the disparate provincial efforts together. However, its head office was relatively weak, and the provincial branches of the society retained substantial autonomy. Fund-raising was locally organized, cancer treatment remained a provincial jurisdiction, and cancer education tended to be undertaken by the provincial branches. The growing interest of the CSCC in movies provided it with an opportunity to assert leadership over the provinces. Busy with fund-raising and education, provincial branches would be only too happy, the CSCC central office believed, to take advantage of any films it produced, and so would allow headquarters a means of influencing provincial cancer education efforts—this despite the fact that most Canadian cancer education films to date had been provincial productions.

More broadly, movies also offered an opportunity to project a distinctively Canadian approach to the problem of cancer, and a distinctive image of Canadian physicians and patients. Not only were Canadian statistics and facilities to be included in these movies, but the films were also to portray science and medicine as crucial to the health of postwar Canadians. American anti-cancer campaigns, however, seemed to undermine these goals. To the CSCC, their penchant for emotive appeals to fear or hope threatened to disturb the reserve, as the CSCC saw it, of Canadians, and hence to weaken efforts to get Canadians to their doctors and to trust in science and medicine. For all these reasons the Canadian authorities wanted to produce their own films.

First proposals

The CSCC first considered producing a movie in 1944, but the cost for the small organization with a small budget was prohibitive. Thus, in the fall of that year it attempted to persuade the Department of National Health and Welfare to cover the costs of production.[25] The suggestion was that the department might cooperate with the National Film Board of Canada to produce films for use by the CSCC. The first tentative approaches to the DNHW were followed in July 1945 by a formal letter from the CSCC to propose such an arrangement, primarily to produce films for cancer control.[26]

The timing seemed auspicious to propose a collaboration. First, as in the United States, Canadian enthusiasm for film as a tool of propaganda had blossomed during the war. In both countries, propaganda movies had gained a new mass audience of military men and women, schoolchildren, theatergoers, and community groups. Film budgets had grown, and some propaganda movies began to employ well-known actors, producers, directors, and animators, and to employ film techniques developed in entertainment films over the previous decade or so. In the United States, government agencies tended to import individuals and organizations from commercial cinema to make propaganda movies, and to contract out efforts to assess the impact of film on various audiences. In Canada, by contrast, homegrown production was dominated by the National Film Board, funded by the federal government, which drew largely on its own stock of talent.[27] While the NFB's wartime propaganda films were increasingly criticized in the postwar years, it had an enviable record as a producer of documentary films and came to be a partner to the DNHW and other Canadian agencies involved in health education.

The second reason things seemed auspicious was that the DNHW was then reorganizing and film seemed likely to be a key part of its future information efforts.[28] The DHNW's predecessor agency, the Department of Health, had been created in 1919, with a mandate to develop a broad public health education program. But early public health education efforts had fallen victim to the vagaries of party politics, economic policy, and underfunding. A Division of Publicity and Statistics was discontinued in 1921, only two years after it was created, and for the next fifteen years publicity and education would be distributed among various divisions within the department. Then in 1938 publicity and education were centralized under a new Division of Publicity and Health Education, which was restructured in 1945 when the health functions of the Department of Pensions and National Health were taken over by the creation of the Department of National Health and Welfare. It was in the context of this reorganization that CSCC approached the DNHW.

The third reason things seemed auspicious was the involvement of the DNHW in the social welfare reforms that followed the June 1945 election of the new minority Liberal government under William Lyon Mackenzie King.[29] A month after the election, the government proposed a universal pension program for Canadians sixty-five and older, an extension of federal responsibility for the unemployed to include all those who could be employed, generous federal subsidies for provincial public works, and a universal and nationwide health insurance program. In the end the government pared down its reforms. However, as part of its efforts to cultivate public support for the government's ever-changing policies toward health care provision, the DNHW began to increase its promotional and educational activities. The Division of Publicity and Education was reorganized and renamed the Information Services Division (ISD), its staff and budget were increased, and it began to reevaluate its earlier public education materials, including the use of film.[30]

The moment thus seemed propitious in July 1945 for a formal appeal by CSCC to the DNHW. Not only was the DNHW reviewing the use of film, but there were many others calling for homegrown health education films. Christian Smith (Department of Health, Saskatchewan) claimed that "There is a desperate need of good Canadian films,"[31] "As much as possible," he echoed the sentiments of the CSCC,[32] "the health pictures produced in Canada must reflect the Canadian scene, and Canadian conditions must be met." The point was repeated by other writers, who like the CSCC argued that Canadians would respond much more readily to films that reflected their own experiences than those produced elsewhere. With this endorsement of the need for Canadian-made educational films and the prospect of a better-funded public education effort by the department, the CSCC was hopeful of securing government funding. But in the short term it was not to be. The department responded to the proposal of cooperation by suggesting that the King George the Fifth Silver Jubilee Cancer Fund for Canada—a philanthropic fund established in 1935[33]—might fund the project. It estimated the costs at CAN$25,000 for a color movie to be made by the NFB.[34]

The involvement of the King George the Fifth Silver Jubilee Cancer Fund for Canada highlights the specificities of developing a Canadian national cancer campaign. As the name suggests the fund had been established to celebrate the silver jubilee of George V, and gave a particular imperial twist to efforts to promote Canadian national identity around cancer.[35] The nation might have acquired political sovereignty from Britain in 1931, but the king remained king of Canada, and voluntary organizations like the fund (established by the governor general, appointed by the monarch) promoted the sovereign as a source of national and imperial unity. The fund had been a major source of funding for the CSCC when it was created in 1938,[36] and its potential involvement in financing film production for the CSCC in 1945 promised to cement the imperial links at the very time that the NFB was beginning to hire native-born Canadian filmmakers rather than imported British ones, and to focus more on Canadian issues.

It is unknown whether the CSCC took the Department of Health and Welfare's advice to go to the King George V Fund for a film. It received other monies, but quite insufficient for film production. As one CCS official put it, referring to hopes of including 35- and 16-millimeter films in a broader educational program costing CAN$85,000: "How can we, who received $25,000 last year from the King George V fund to inaugurate a national program, think in terms of visual education costing $85,000?"[37] The only cancer movie made before *Challenge* was *The Cancer Crusaders* (c.1947), a 16-mm motion picture released by the British Columbia Branch of the Canadian Cancer Society, though as table 2.1 suggests some other shorter films were also available that year, along with some technical films aimed at professional audiences that may also have gained a public viewership. The branch erroneously believed this to be the first Canadian movie devoted to public education and information.[38] The Saskatchewan movies *Rays of Hope* (1937) and *That They May Live* (1942) were apparently forgotten or unknown in British Columbia.

The 1947 proposals

After the aborted effort to persuade the DNHW to fund a film, things remained quiet for a couple of years. Then, in 1947, the Canadian Cancer Society (the former CSCC) raised the issue again with the DNHW, taking advantage of new cancer control initiatives within the department—part of broader efforts at health reform by the new Minister of Health, Paul Martin, that eventually became a federal system of health grants, including for cancer control. To set the policy ball rolling, the department organized a conference in January 1947 to coordinate the growing number of cancer organizations in the country and to promote research.[39] Sensing an opportunity, advocates of federal involvement in cancer mobilized anxieties about what they saw as the dearth of federal funding for this disease. For example, they noted that in 1947 cancer ranked as the second highest cause of death in Canadian mortality records, dwarfing the numbers of Canadian casualties in the Second World War.[40] Yet the expenditure on cancer did not reflect this discrepancy. While the war had cost Canada close to CAN$19,000,000,000, the amount spent on cancer control for the same period amounted to not more than CAN$5,000,000. The conference aimed to change all that. "Our Canadian attack on cancer has been in the nature of guerrilla skirmishing,"[41] a report on the meeting noted. What was needed was "total mobilization," which would involve "not only funds but also educational effort, research workers, and diagnostic and treatment facilities organized into a superb striking force under a united command."[42]

In its proposal to this conference, the CCS urged the DNHW to support cancer films, as part of a proposed comprehensive educational campaign with the prevention of cancer as its theme.[43] The campaign aimed to build on what the CCS proposal described as the rapid public acceptance of past campaigns against smallpox and diphtheria, which, it claimed, had demonstrated the success of medical science in combating disease. It wanted to reach the largest practical percentage of the total Canadian population in twelve months, and movies were to be at the core of the campaign.[44] Motion pictures, the CCS proposal noted, had a "dramatic, direct, quick impact"[45] on the public that would help combat the appeal of quacks.[46]

The CCS therefore recommended a general movie campaign that would involve the production of three different films. The first was to be a theatrical movie, tentatively titled *Power Also for Good*—a black-and-white two-reeler for distribution to commercial outlets that would deal in dramatic terms with the mobilization of science against cancer focusing on radium and atomic energy. The second was to be a technical movie, tentatively titled *Report on Cancer*—a color movie for distribution to every Canadian university and every provincial cancer association, dealing exclusively with the technical aspects of cancer research, especially "that end of it in which Canadian endeavour has shone."[47] The use of color, it argued, would particularly appeal to this audience: "By doing it in color we believe that the benefits derived from true-to-live depiction will be tremendous for those personnel whose work it is to study cancer in all its forms."[48] Finally, the CCS proposed to produce an educational movie, targeted at schools and clubs, and tentatively titled *Human Document*. The movie would revolve around a central heroic figure. "This person would be someone whose work has been chosen to be the central character but we feel sure there is someone whose great scientific ability can fire the imagination of the audience in much the same manner that Ehrlich—Pasteur—Curie and Banting have."[49] Versions in 35 mm and 16 mm would be made for distribution.

In addition to the three movies, the CCS report also recommended continuing Canadianizing foreign cancer movies and incorporating the latest scientific developments into them. It also proposed to create theatrical trailers (1½ minutes) for use in commercial outlets across Canada. And finally, it also considered the venues in which movies might be released. Of these the most important were (movie) theaters, which—with an average weekly audience of four million Canadians—ranked with radio and the press in importance for mass educational campaigns targeted at what the proposal called the "unorganized public." Next were the organized 16-mm circuits, especially the industrial and rural circuits, and special 16-mm showings in schools, to organizations and special audiences (perhaps the *organized* public?). Finally, it proposed to develop filmstrips for schools and industrial and special groups that would use them in addition to motion pictures or alone, because they were not equipped to show motion pictures.[50]

Against fear and boredom

In its efforts to devise a movie campaign the CCS was careful to distance its approach from that of the American Cancer Society (ACS, the successor to the ASCC). In the 1940s, the ACS had begun to organize aggressive public education campaigns that drew criticism for exacerbating public fear of the disease.[51] Without mentioning the ACS by name, the authors of the 1947 CCS report set out an alternative vision of public education. They argued that all films would use a positive approach: the idea of cancer as a scourge would not be used "to club the audience over the head with resulting fear and repugnance."[52] Rather movies would show that headway was being made in the fight and that treatment was not altogether quite as hopeless as they believed some people thought. "It cannot be stressed too much that the success of any such campaign depends entirely on making your audience feel free to discuss cancer and not in making them shudder and want to shy away from talk about it. They must be left with a definite feeling of HOPE."[53]

If the CCS sought to distance itself from the aggressive approach associated with the ACS, it also sought to distance itself from the sorts of propaganda movies that the NFB had put out during the war, commonly criticized for their hectoring tone.[54] The CCS proposals warned that audience reactions in film theaters showed a "public weariness"[55] of documentary film, and in particular the sort of film produced during the war: "The type of film shown in recent seasons has obviously worn out its welcome."[56] The authors of the report argued, however, that the public was not bored by films based on fact or dealing in fact, provided they were of good quality, which many documentaries were not. Therefore, films for the theater audience "required guaranteed entertainment merit as their most important characteristic!"[57]

Worried about both fear and boredom, the CCS wanted to entertain their audiences—a move that ironically took them closer to the Americans than they may have wished to acknowledge. American cancer education movies had long sought to entertain as much as to educate, and indeed this tendency to entertain had been strengthened in the 1940s due to the influx of Hollywood talent into propaganda movie production, the difficulty of getting educational movies into cinemas, and because the American promoters of cancer education programs also wanted to counteract the fear and anxiety that postwar campaigns generated about cancer.[58] The ACS wanted people to fear cancer, but not to fear it so much as to create a fatalistic paralysis about the disease that undermined the message of early detection and treatment.[59] Paradoxically, for all their concerns about American movies, this is also what the CCS wanted; they just differed over what constituted a good balanced between hope and fear. The CCS tended to regard most American films as leaning too much toward fear, even when the ACS felt that a balance had been achieved. The irony is that the Americans sometimes felt much the same about the Canadian films. Thus, when *That They May Live* was screened in the US, one commentator noted that "its approach was so clinical that audiences became quite frightened and could not stand it."[60] If the Canadians saw American films as inducing paralytic fear, Americans could see Canadians films as doing much the same.

Lieutenant Colonel Gilchrist

The cost for a Canadian film was substantial—estimated at between CAN$75,000 and CAN$95,000—and while the department was unable to provide this level of funding, the CCS found a much more receptive audience about the idea of a film than it had received in 1944/45. Much of this was because of the new director of the DNHW's Information Services Division, Lt. Col. C. Whitney Gilchrist (appointed 1946), an enthusiast for film as an educational tool, who would play a key role in transforming the proposals by the CCS into the film that would become *Challenge*. He was to be the Canadian counterpart to Dallas Johnson at the NCI. [61]

Gilchrist had come to the Information Services Division—like Dallas Johnson at the NCI—with a background in journalism. Before the war, he had worked as a newspaperman in St. John, New Brunswick, and held an appointment as a staff member of the Canadian Broadcasting Corporation; in 1942 he began an Army career in public affairs.[62] (He was promoted to lieutenant colonel in 1944, a rank that he retained in civilian life, sometimes abbreviated to colonel.) On his appointment to the DNHW, he set about expanding the role of the division, facilitated in part by the appointment of Paul Martin as minister a few months later. According to his biographer, Martin valued good publicity as a means of achieving his political goals, and with his appointment as minister

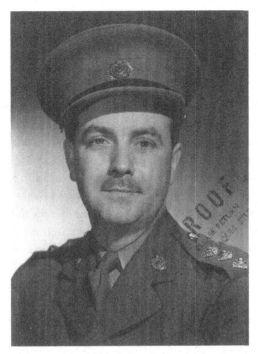

FIGURE 2.1. Captain (later Lt. Col.) C. W. Gilchrist. mid-1940s.
Source: 8th Hussars Museum, Sussex, New Brunswick. Fonds
13.55: C. W. Gilchrist. Reference code CA HM 13.55.

he now had the necessary administrative machinery to realize his ambitions. Gilchrist and Martin do not seem to have had the easiest of relations. Nevertheless, it was under Martin that the staff and activities of Gilchrist's division expanded, Gilchrist balancing promoting health with promoting Martin.

Film was to be a central part of this expansion. In 1947 Gilchrist noted that during the last year or two his department had devoted a sizable slice of its education and information budget to film. Not only had it produced seventeen films and filmstrips, but it had a further thirteen in production or in the scripting stage. The division had also collaborated with the National Film Board to create four film libraries: a Public Health Library with 150 titles, a Biological and Medical Library for professional use with a like number of prints, a Physical Fitness and Recreation Film Library, and a Welfare Library, the last newly organized. The department also evaluated numerous films from Canada, the United States, Britain, and many other countries, and made prints available to government departments, organizations, or individuals on a low-cost rental basis. It was under

Gilchrist that the department commissioned one of its most famous series: *Mental Mechanisms* (1947–50), the widely acclaimed series of three dramatized films about mental health made by the NFB, and which Canadians would suggest later helped to entice the Americans into coproducing *Challenge*.[63]

Over the next decade, the NFB would produce about 140 French and English films for the DNHW, most of which incorporated identifying symbols of Canadian nationalism—snowy landscapes and winter sports, children singing French and Maritime folk songs, federal and provincial flags, the scarlet coated RCMP officer, the parliament buildings, Niagara Falls, the Rocky Mountains, the Canadian Pacific Railway, French habitants, and Atlantic fishing villages.[64] There were concerns that NFB's vision of the national identity did not reflect regional diversity or the specificity of local health problems, but the focus on Canadian national identity provided a means by which the government could project a vision of Canada recognizable to Canadians in its health education films. As we shall see later in this book this was to be something that the NFB would incorporate into early versions of the script that would become *Challenge*—though not the Canada of snowy landscapes and scarlet RCMP uniforms. Instead, it sought to make an appeal for Canadians to support Canadian cancer research, and to stop the drain of talent from Canada to the richer waters of American cancer research.

Canadian cancer research

The idea that the film should focus on research went back to the CCS's proposals at the January 1947 meeting organized by the DNHW. In the early 1940s American commentators had worried that an emphasis on cancer research in public education movies could work against cancer control by suggesting that scientists and physicians did not know as much as they claimed about cancer.[65] Canadian discussions make no mention of such concerns, and the emphasis on Canadian scientific endeavors allowed them to appeal to nationalist sentiment, in two different ways. One was an appeal to an explicitly Canadian identity, distinct from that of the United States and Britain. The other was an appeal to an identity that transcended Canadian provincial politics and concerns. Unlike cancer control and treatment, research tended to be more a national than a provincial jurisdiction.[66]

The growing interest in supporting research was signaled after the January 1947 conference, when a National Cancer Institute of Canada (NCIC)—a joint initiative of the CCS and the DNHW—was established and began plans for a national campaign against cancer. Early reports suggested that the NCIC would "co-ordinate all Canadian cancer control work into a concerted, well-financed attack on the disease from every aspect."[67] However, in time the CCS and the NCIC came to divide their activities; the CCS was to promote cancer education and lay activities in the cancer field, and to be the fund-raising body for the NCIC; the NCIC's main function was to be research. Treatment remained a provincial jurisdiction, with the society giving leadership and financial support through local branches.[68]

The CCS's 1947 film proposal must be seen in this context. Although it began life as the CCS's contribution to the January 1947 conference, in time it became part of the society's efforts to promote cancer education and lay activities, and also to raise funds for the NCIC. Having been broadly endorsed by the conference, the proposal landed on Gilchrist's desk as part of planning for a national campaign against cancer. There followed a few months of negotiations, but with the DNHW now committed to the campaign, Martin pressing for health care reform, and Gilchrist an enthusiast for film, the department finally agreed to finance an educational motion picture about cancer: one film, not the three proposed at the meeting, and the estimates of CAN$75,000 and CAN$95,000 had also been whittled away. On November 19, 1947, the DNHW was authorized by Order in Council No. 4194 to spend CAN$20,000 on the project.[69]

If there was disappointment at the diminished funds and films, it is not recorded. However, the authorization came at a good time for the NCIC, which was then working to stimulate and accelerate research and the "mobilization of talent"[70] to "interest men in the field of cancer research."[71] To this end it wanted—much like the Americans—to improve compensation for scientists, offer grants-in-aid of research, provide training fellowships, and build well-designed and fully equipped research centers.[72] But all this would take money. The NCIC hoped the film would help attract private donations through the CCS, now responsible for fund-raising, and cultivate public support for greater federal government funding, which until then had been quite anemic. Reports suggested that from 1935-45 the federal government had spent less than CAN$5,000 through the National Research Council on efforts to find the cause and cure of cancer. The NCIC wanted to turn this situation around. The film would, the NCIC hoped, form part of a coordinated appeal by the government and the CCS.[73]

At first the department seemed torn between producing a campaign (money-raising) film or an educational/recruitment film about cancer research and treatment.[74] In 1948, a recommendation by the NCIC to the Department of

National Health and Welfare resulted in Martin authorizing a special film depicting the problem of cancer research and control. The board of directors of the NCIC agreed to have the film screened for scientific accuracy and held that the finished product should be ready in time for the Federated Cancer Campaign in April 1949.[75] (In February 1948, the CCS had proposed to conduct a United National Campaign in 1949, which would also generate support and funding for the institute.[76]) According to Norman Chamberlin of the National Film Board, the new script that was then being prepared would be a first-class presentation, designed to educate the public in the matter of research, and to be ready for public distribution in April 1949.[77]

Two months later, in July 1948, Dallas Johnson heard about the Canadian preparations. By this stage, the CCS had given up its earlier doubts about the NFB. The positive reception of the first films in the *Mental Mechanisms* series seemed to dim its concerns about the tone of NFB wartime propaganda movies, as did the growing enthusiasm of the Department of National Health and Welfare for NFB films. The NFB had produced a film script for the cancer film, and Johnson was enthusiastic. For the first time the Americans were interested in using a Canadian rather than an American production company. And how quickly things had changed. If in 1947 Butterfield had argued that the Canadians had missed the educational film boat as regards cancer, by 1948 things were quite different. This new film promised to turn around years of domination by the Americans in the cancer education film field.

There were, however, dangers for the Canadians in this collaboration. Cancer research was dominated by the Americans, and the US seemed to be tempting some of the best Canadian scientists to leave the country. Collaborating with them risked the danger that Canadian scientists would flee the relatively impoverished research opportunities in Canada to staff the expanding research facilities in the United States, and so undermine the NCIC's efforts to grow research in Canada. Indeed, the NFB script included an oblique appeal to keep Canadian scientists from migrating to better paid positions, or to places with more and better equipment or better conditions of work.[78]

Such concerns, however, did little to weaken NCIC support for a joint film venture with the Americans. Canadian scientists were beginning to obtain grants from the NCI to undertake research in Canada, and if the film helped to promote cancer research more generally, there was the prospect of more money.[79] Moreover, American scientists were also coming north to learn techniques such as tissue culture (a course at the Connaught Laboratories in Toronto, where some of the scenes of *Challenge* would eventually be shot).[80] Given that the film was to be produced by a Canadian film production company, there was also the chance that Canadian scientists and facilities would figure prominently in the film. And besides, the Canadians faced the same problem as the Americans in that young scientists were choosing careers in industry and physics rather than cancer research. A well-financed film with American and Canadian money might stem the trend to the benefit of both.

It was against this backdrop of concerns that in February or March 1949 the Canadian Department of National Health and Welfare signed the memorandum of agreement with the NCI, the Medical Film Institute, and the National Film Board to finance the movie.[81] There are suggestions that by then the department was thinking of producing two films (though offering no more money), and the first was to be the research film.[82] The next step would be to begin production.

PART 2

MAKING

CHAPTER 3

Baiting the Hook

T HE NFB HAD BEGUN work on the film before the Americans got involved, commissioning a script from Maurice Constant, a member of its staff, soon after the Canadian Department of National Health and Welfare had allocated CAN$20,000 to the project. The involvement of the Americans changed everything. Suddenly the picture's budget jumped to $40,000, and the NFB had a new partner (the Medical Film Institute of the AAMC), and a new sponsor (the US National Cancer Institute) in addition to its existing sponsor, the Canadian Department of National Health and Welfare. Constant's script was central to this transformation, for it was the bait with which the NFB caught and reeled in the NCI. The July 1948 meeting where Bernard Dryer showed the script to Dallas Johnson at the NCI was no accident. Dryer was doing the bidding of the NFB, a fishing exercise to tempt the Americans to cosponsor the film, and so help the board address the difficult financial and political position it faced after the war.

There was, however, no guarantee that the Americans would come in, so when he started Constant was faced with two competing demands. He had to produce a script that might appeal to the Americans, but—if that did not happen—he also had to produce a script that would address Canadian concerns, including the problem of Canadian scientists abandoning the country. The two demands were an uneasy fit, for the Americans were unlikely to sponsor something that that addressed Canadians' national concern about the threat to their cancer research posed by the United States, while the Canadian sponsors were keen to ensure that such a message come across should the film be a solely Canadian production. Constant's script might have been the bait to tempt the Americans to support it, but it also had to ensure that the Canadians remained on the hook.

Ralph Foster and Maurice Constant

A key individual in the commissioning the script was Ralph Foster (1911–95), the Deputy Commissioner of the NFB.[1] As second in command, Foster would

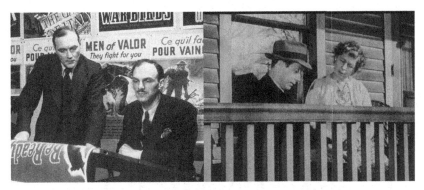

FIGURE 3.1. Left: John Grierson (left) and Ralph Foster (right), 1944.
Source: National Film Board of Canada, reproduced courtesy of the
NFB. Right: Maurice Constant (left) and an unknown actor in a
scene from *Challenge*. Source: Frame grab from *Challenge*.

take an important role in guiding the movie through production, and it was
he who would appoint Maurice Constant to draft the first script. So far in this
book, I have emphasized the roles of American and Canadian health and cancer
agencies in promoting this film. It is possible, however, that they would never
have come together without Foster, and Foster had different agendas than either
the Canadian or American health agencies. His goals were to encourage better
cooperation between the NFB and the United States, to fend off allegations of
Communist subversion within the NFB (see chapter 4), and to develop NFB
coproduction efforts. The decision by the Canadian Department of National
Health and Welfare to put CAN$20,000 into a cancer film provided an oppor-
tunity to push all these agendas.

Born in Toronto, the son of a wholesale grocery merchant, Foster had a career
in newspapers before he joined the NFB, including taking charge of the illustrations for the *Star Weekly*. With this on-the-job training in design, in 1942 he was
hired by the NFB first as Director of Creative Skills, and then from September 1,
1943, as Chief of Graphics. He took his first venture into film production when
he directed the newsreel and photographic recording of the First Quebec Conference held August 1943 between Winston Churchill and Franklin D. Roosevelt, and hosted by the Canadian Prime Minister, Mackenzie King. Then in
June 1944 he moved to London as war correspondent for the NFB, in charge of
newsreels, and was the NFB liaison officer with the Canadian armed forces. The
following year he was loaned to Australia to help the government there establish
a film board modeled on the NFB.[2]

TABLE 3.1. The Structure of Maurice Constant's June 1948 script

Sequence	Brief description of action	Live action / Animation
1 Doctor's office	1. Off-camera woman is examined for cancer. 2. Husband [?] of woman walks to the window and stares at the starry sky	Live action
2 Historical sequence	1. Camera moves into interstellar space, traveling slowly among the galaxies, nebulae, constellations, and celestial bodies.	Animation/ Live action
	2. The celestial bodies turn into a Zoroastrian sky, then emerge depictions of the worlds of ancient Egypt and Greece and the Middle Ages, before the camera spins down to a map of the American continent as misunderstood by early geographers and the "mists and phantasms of the past," all sequences interspersed with (live-action?) scenes illustrating the state of medicine during these periods.	
	3. Now a microscope is seen in closeup, seemingly aimed into space before a burst of white light wipes everything else off the screen. The eyepiece forms a circle that narrows to a frame within which microscopic structures in movement come into focus. (The effect intended suggests the idea of the microcosm against the macrocosm.)	
	4. Something white fills the screen. The camera backs away to medium distance to reveal a lab-coated scientist bent over something that turns out to be a microscope.	
3 The cell-as-universe/ Normal and abnormal growth	1. Framed within a circle is a stylized and highly idealized version of a living cell suggestive of celestial bodies moving in interstellar space.	Animation/ Live action
	2. Animation sequence of conception, embryonic growth, cell division, and abnormal cancerous growth concluding with a white sheet drawn over a body.	

4	The work of science	1. The scientist asks what is this thing called cancer; an aberration of life itself. 2. Scenes that illustrate the deadly consequences of cancer in humans, its antiquity, and the various organisms affected by it. 3. The hope that science can solve the problem, and the "billion (?)" dollars put toward this goal annually. 4. Various illustrations of science's approaches to the cancer problem: experiments on mice, tumors grown in eggs, tar on a rabbit's ear, and the work of chemistry, biochemistry, bacteriology, genetics, physics. 5. Conclusion: "We are delving into a problem [as] complex as life itself."	Live action
5	Doctor's office/research into diagnosis treatment and prevention	1. What can doctors do for those with cancer? 2. Research to find a reliable test for cancer. 3. Statistical research. 4. Discussion of how current knowledge about the cancer cell has led to research/interventions against cancer 5. Costs of research/the need for funds to solve the cancer problem	Live action
6	Concluding sequence	1. Scientist: "As you can see, this is not a matter only of satisfying a philosophic or scientific curiosity. It is a matter of life and death!"	Live action

Foster returned to Canada in 1947 as Deputy Film Commissioner, supervising the production and distribution of NFB films and visual aids. He became involved with the Canadian Cooperation Project, a plan to increase the flow of American dollars into the country by informing the American public though film and other means of Canada's need.[3] He also began to develop the NFB's approach to international coproduction. The NFB's founder and first commissioner, John Grierson, claimed that the NFB was among the first documentary film producers to provide an international approach to peacetime themes, working with the United Nations (UN) and UNESCO among other bodies.[4] International coproduction was a mechanism by which international projects could be developed; since *Challenge* was among the early coproductions that Foster was involved in, he used it to work out how an international coproduction approach with the Americans might work more generally.[5] During his involvement with the film, Foster would cooperate closely with the various interested parties, and it is clear from the tone of some of his letters that he developed personal friendships with some of his American collaborators, especially Dallas Johnson (with whom he shared an interest in issues of publicity and graphic design) and David Ruhe at the MFI (with whom he exchanged concerned husband notes, since both their wives were pregnant at the time).[6]

But in 1948 much of this was yet to come. The beginning of an arrangement with the Department of National Health and Welfare was emerging, and with the Canadian cancer organizations. These bodies wanted the projected film (or films) for specifically Canadian purposes: to promote Canadian (cancer/biological) research, and to correct the dependence of Canadian cancer campaigns on American educational films. Foster, however, had a different agenda. He saw the film or films as an opportunity to further his internationalist efforts, and the commission from the Canadian health agencies would provide a way of doing this. Specifically, he realized that the Canadian commission provided an opportunity to develop a treatment/script that could then be used to entice the Americans. It is probably for this reason that he assigned Maurice Constant to write what became the June 1948 treatment, hoping to use it as a means of opening discussions with potential American collaborators.

Maurice Constant had only recently joined the NFB and was not an obvious choice for scriptwriter given his lack of experience.[7] Following an education at the University of Toronto, Constant (1914–2002) had had a varied career: he joined the Canadian Officer Training Corps, the Socialist Zionist organization, Hashomer Hatzair, and the Communist Party, fought in the Spanish Civil War, and flew for the Royal Canadian Airforce during World War II. When the war ended, Constant returned to the University of Toronto, graduating with a Bachelor of Arts degree on June 6, 1947. After graduation he claims he had two job offers, one to head the Biochemistry Division of the Ontario Science Foundation, and the other from the NFB. He joined the film board on November 27, 1947, eight days after the Department of National Health and Welfare was authorized to spend CAN$20,000 on a cancer film. *Cancer Research* (as *Challenge* was first called) was one of his first scripts. He would remain at the NFB until September 24, 1957.

Constant's appointment to the NFB coincided—and was perhaps the result of—a growing feeling on the production side of the NFB that the film board should put more emphasis on science in their films.[8] *Challenge/Cancer Research* was among the early efforts in this direction, and Constant's background in science (albeit limited: he had taken science courses during his first stint at the University of Toronto) perhaps partly explains why Foster selected him as the scriptwriter for this production, given the technical issues involved. But doubts remained about whether he had the experience necessary to write the sort of script that was needed either for the filmmakers to work with, or for Foster's political purposes. Such concerns seem to have grown over the next year, even after Constant produced the first version of the script for what would become *Challenge*. Thus, when Bernard V. Dryer gained an impression of him as "a combat veteran on the film front,"[9] Foster was prompted to issue a corrective: "I wonder what he said to you to make him sound like a combat veteran on the film front. It must be the grim experience he underwent in the research field, because in these parts he qualifies as a youthful zealot with no calluses."[10]

Constant was a problematic appointment as scriptwriter for *Cancer Research/Challenge*. He had a scientific background, but not the experience of scriptwriting to do the sort of job that would work for all the agendas behind this film. By June 1948 he had given a copy of the treatment to Foster (actually, a detailed *script*, which is the term I shall use for it: a treatment can be a detailed scene-by-scene breakdown as this is, or a shorter prose piece written before the first draft of the script), who was beginning to plan to use it to attract American cosponsors. But it was not a perfect script for this purpose. Perhaps Foster had not informed Constant of his ultimate goals, or perhaps it was the inexperience of a "youthful zealot." Whatever the cause, Constant's script gave little attention to cancer research as an international endeavor that included both Americans and Canadians. On the contrary, it tended to reflect the national fears that Canadian scientists were being tempted abroad by better pay and facilities. The message would work well for the Canadian sponsors as they initially imagined the film. It would not, however, help Foster in his ambitions for international collaboration, unless the national sentiments were ditched, and other themes given more emphasis.

The June 1948 script

Constant's 1948 script (table 3.1) opens in a doctor's office at night. A well-dressed man is listening to voices coming from behind a white screen over which is thrown a stethoscope. He is tense. A woman's voice—perhaps his wife's—is heard from behind the screen "It's only a lump, Doctor. There is no pain. But it kept getting bigger and bigger. . . . It doesn't hurt, Doctor. Is it dangerous? (Pause) Is it a tumor? Is it cancer?"[11] The doctor's disembodied voice recommends a biopsy.

The man gets up, walks to the window, and stares out at a starry sky. The camera slowly moves up to the window. The sky fills the window, and the camera moves through the window into the sky and eventually into interstellar space. It travels slowly among the celestial bodies—galaxies, nebulae, and constellations—which, the script informs us, become the motif for a historical journey of attempts to answer the woman's question: "Just what is it, Doctor? What is this thing?"[12] We move through treatments of Babylonian, ancient Greek, medieval and Renaissance efforts to answer the question. The stars initially form a Zoroastrian sky—an astrologer's vision of the heavens. The stars appear linked by the outlines of the mythological figures that peopled the skies during the Babylonian period. They then reconfigure to show ancient Greek figures, then a Gothic arrangement of heavenly lights, and then we return to interstellar space before spinning down to the American continent, depicted at first as "misunderstood"[13] by early geographers, before the image resolves and the outline of the geographical shape of the continent as depicted in the 1940s emerges.

Each of the preceding starry images accompanies a historical account of changing understandings and interventions against cancer. Each starry sky dissolves into a world view—the Egyptian world with pyramids, priestly incantations, and amulets against disease; the Greek world with ancient surgical instruments; the world of the Middle Ages with an unsanitary old hospital, and dirty, bloody hands thrusting the crude surgical instruments of the period toward the patient. All these worlds are blurry, symbolic of ignorance and darkness. The Egyptian world is flat, its edges fading to darkness; the Greek world is Homeric, flat, surrounded by dark waters which fade to nothingness; the medieval world is also flat, reminiscent of a three-dimensional model of a medieval geographer's chart with wondrous creatures filling in the geographical blanks. This imagery, the script informs us, is intended to draw a parallel between geographical ignorance and ignorance of the body and disease culminating in the rectified map of the American continent mentioned above.

Eventually the screen is filled with a montage, a mass of material representing what the script calls the mists and phantasms of the past (astrological charts, incense, ancient medical instruments) against a background of a microscope signifying the beginnings of modern science. We look into the microscope and a burst of white light blasts everything on the screen away, and microscopic structures come into focus, surrounded by the night sky. The sky, which once signified the ignorance of the past, is now juxtaposed against the microscopic world— the effect intended, the script tells us, is the microcosm against the macrocosm, drawing a parallel between the inner world of the cell and the outer world of interstellar space. Something else white appears and fills the screen. The camera backs away to reveal a white-coated scientist who at the climax of the historical sequence looks up from the microscope and says, "This piece of cancer tissue is made up of living cells."[14] We have returned to the biopsy the doctor recommended in the opening scene, and the significance of the scientist's statement is punctuated by a succession of triumphant, enthusiastic chords. Triumphant not because the woman has cancer, but because it is now understood by science.

Now we shift from live action back to animation. Framed within a circle the viewer sees something suggestive of celestial bodies moving in interstellar space. The scene, the script tells us, reminds us of the starry skies that have driven the film's story so far. This is not interstellar space, however. Instead, it is a stylized and highly idealized version of a living cell and its contents. Whereas the earlier imagery of the stars emphasized the ignorance of the pre-scientific world, the image of the cell-as-universe is used both to show modern medical knowledge of the inner workings of this world, and the huge scale of the problem of cancer, as the narrator notes "Look at these vast spaces! This is not a universe of stars and planets, but the universe within a single living cell. It takes 10,000 of these to make the end of your finger."[15] The film shows us parts of this universe— the nucleus, the mitochondria—before shifting to a growth theme—beginning with sperm and egg and cell division, differentiation, and the emergence of organs—until we see the normal body and its parts working harmoniously. The music, the script tells us, is to comment on and mimic the development theme. Its rhapsodic tone evoking joyous, healthy normal life. As each organ is mentioned, a rhythm peculiar to it is to be heard in the music (blood, heartbeat; nerve, staccato tingling.)

The mood now changes. "Ominous discordant chords; a harsh, sinister im-placable, perversion of the 'growth' rhythm—representing the uncontrolled malignant growth of the cancer cells. They build up tension with increasing drum-beat tempo."[16] We now view abnormal growth until finally the body is killed in a climax of rhythm and cacophony. Eventually there is silence, except for the cancer rhythm, and then complete silence: the rhythms specific to each organ stop one at a time. The music resolves into the music of the spheres, and we see a shot of a white sheet as it is drawn over the body. The scientist now asks a more precise version of the woman's question: what causes normal cells to go wild, out of control? The woman's voice returns with the human anxieties be-hind the story "Is it dangerous, Doctor?"[17] "Is it cancer, Doctor?"[18] "The tone of her question is paralleled and imitated in the whining and howling of a dog,"[19] a segue into a discussion of cancer in animals.

Next the mood shifts to one of hope: the solution to the cancer problem through the scientific method, a sequence accompanied by a montage of technical civilization and an example of the scientific method. The music begins a "quest" rhythm, "suggesting a hunt ('detective story' type of thing),"[20] as the script puts it. We approach a group of men in white coats clustered around something that is hidden from us. Suddenly—with shock effect—we are given a closeup of a tumor, and the camera moves back to reveal the person who has the tumor. (The instruc-tion is: "Use a tumor which is typical but not too horrible to demonstrate."[21]) We now see another tumor, this time on a mouse. There follows a demonstration of how cells removed from the mouse can be kept alive in tissue culture or trans-planted into other animals for research purposes. Then there are discussions of agents such as tars and other chemicals that can be used to cause cancers in animals, of chronic irritation as a cause of the disease; studies of radiation and biochemistry to understand the cancer cell; the role of genetics and research on heredity, mutation, and the effects of the atomic bomb; and the role of viruses revealed by the electron microscope and investigations on the milk factor: a ref-erence to the 1936 discovery that a cancer-causing agent, called a "milk factor,"[22] could be transmitted by mouse mothers with cancer to young mice while nurs-ing. This section ends with a shot of a stormy sky and the commentator noting, "We are delving into a problem [as] complex as life itself."[23]

We return to the original opening scene of the doctor's office—the music now signifies "suffering humanity".[24] The woman's voice asks "Doctor, what can you do for me?"[25] and the focus of the narrative moves to research on cures. The music shifts to an "Energetic 'hunt' music, quick, alert, tense; suggestive of hounds fol-lowing a spoor."[26] The narrative focuses on the need for a simple, cheap reliable test for cancer; on the use of statistics in identifying causes of cancer; and on efforts to find an agent that will selectively attack cancer cells and leave normal ones unaffected. There is discussion of the possible uses of hormones, radiation, and chemicals in therapy, all of which evolves into an account of the huge scale of the effort against cancer—conferences, journals, dollars—and an appeal that echoed the concerns of the National Cancer Institute of Canada:

> It's no use fooling ourselves. If we are to keep our young scientists—one of our country's greatest assets—from migrating to better paid positions, from going to places where they can find more and better equipment to work with, where they can find better conditions of work, then we must provide them with proper equipment, security, and a reasonable standard of life. This is <u>also</u> our job and yours. . . .[27]

By "yours," Constant meant the audience's job.

Constant also provides an alternative conclusion that focuses on the humanitarian value of cancer research rather than on concerns that Canada was in danger of losing the best scientists.[28] A coda develops this theme, reprising the human and intellectual concerns about cancer with the scientist concluding, "this is not a matter only of satisfying a philosophic or scientific curiosity. It is a matter of life and death!"[29]

Quests

It should be clear from this description that the film is much more than a plea for greater resources for Canadian cancer research. It sought to evoke the triumphs of modern science more generally, the threat posed by cancer, and the role that modern science might play in its defeat by making the body, cell, and cancer subject to its interventions. It will be recalled (chapter 2) that the Department of National Health and Welfare was torn between making a film about cancer research and treatment and one that was intended to raise money. The script included both themes. It focused on research but concluded with an appeal to the audience for support (though the nature of the support is not spelled out, nor whether it should come through philanthropic donations or taxes or both). It is also different from the sorts of cancer education films that had been made prior to this. There is little or no reference to early detection and treatment, the staple of previous anti-cancer films. Instead, it subordinates the treatment story to that of research.

The script's narrative thread is framed by the human consequences of cancer: It starts with a melodramatic recreation of a diagnosis of cancer at the beginning and ends with an account of the human costs of cancer. In between, the story is a progressivist tale from dark days of human ignorance and superstition to the light of modern science and how it has been applied to cancer. The story aims to portray cancer as a field of urgent humanitarian need and great intellectual excitement, and to evoke wonder at the complexity of the body and nature, admiration for the ingenious ways in which scientists and physicians attempt to understand and combat the disease, and amazement at the vast scale of the problem.

The film is organized around several quest narratives. One quest is the interstellar journey from ignorance to a materialist scientific world view (something that Constant advocated as a socialist and scientist). A second quest is the practice of science itself (something the scriptwriter imagined would be evoked by hunt themes in the music), which, the script suggests, provides the way to understand and defeat cancer. A third quest is the journey within the normal cell, with its vast spaces akin to the interstellar journey shown earlier in the movie. Finally, there is the quest of the woman, from her discovery of the lump through the biopsy to hope. The scientific quest (together with the emergence of a scientific materialist world view) is crucial to all the others: it is central to the quest for the cure for cancer, to the woman's journey through cancer to hope, and to the knowledge necessary to travel through the cell. Note also the significance of music and sound to these quests: the music moves from ominous discordant chords (signifying cancer), to the hopeful "quest" rhythm, and to the hunt music signifying science and medicine's quests to understand cancer and to find a cure.

Constant's narrative is marked by a play on popular interest in space fantasies with its parallels between interstellar and intracellular space.[30] Many space fantasies in the 1940s alluded to Cold War anxieties about Communism, a subject that Constant as a Communist or former Communist avoided, even as the NFB sought to distance itself from accusations of Communist infiltration. He also made only the briefest of references to Cold War concerns about atomic annihilation, with a fleeting mention of the effects of the atomic bomb. Instead, much as advocates sought to turn American and Canadian enthusiasm for space fantasies into something that promoted an American space program, so Constant sought to turn this enthusiasm into something that would promote cancer research, turning the viewer (and more clearly in later versions of the script, the scientist as well) into a space-age explorer, travelling through the cell as if it were outer space, with constellations of cytosomes and centrosomes passing by. As in space-age fantasies, Constant took the viewer places that were then impossible (for most viewers, in the case of this film) to visit in real life, both inside the body and in outer space. This imagery would also give a visual indication of the vast size of the cancer problem, and also of the opportunities available to the viewer/cancer

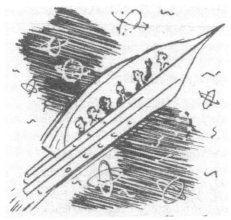

FIGURE 3.2. Traveling in outer space or the inner world of the cell: an illustration that accompanied a public announcement of the release of the film. Source: *Cancer Control Letter*, no. 28 (April 28, 1950): 1.

researcher who is intrepid enough to venture into this strange world, both of which would be echoed in some of the publicity around the film (figure 3.2).

The script also reveals Constant's struggle to balance hope with shock or disgust. It will be recalled that the Canadian cancer societies were concerned about the extent to which fear was used in American-produced educational films, worried that it was not appropriate for Canadian audiences, and wanted an approach that would emphasize hope. Constant's script seeks to promote hope, and science as the means to this hope, but the narrative drive is also created by the anxiety and fear of the woman patient, her animal-like whine, and the shock of viewing a tumor. But recall the note in the script: "Use a tumor which is typical but not too horrible to demonstrate." Constant wanted to shock, but not to shock so much that people would turn away from the film, an old concern that had shaped cancer education films since the 1920s.[31] Here shock was to act as a narrative gateway to the sequences that depict scientific approaches/ solutions to the cancer problem, signaled by the transition from human tumor to mouse tumor. The danger was that the shock or disgust evoked by the tumor might overwhelm the hope evoked by such solutions and approaches—hence the instruction about gauging the horribleness of the growth.

Constant's narrative was also marked by a play on older associations between women and nature as when the tone of the woman's anxious question "parallels and imitates" the whining and howling of a dog. But where anti-vivisection propaganda could identify women with animals abused by male science, in this script animal experimentation is to save women with cancer. No place here for those critics who wanted to promote feeling rather than the scientific method as a guide to understanding, nor for the assertion that women's special affinity to the world of nature allowed them to critique the experimental method. Experimentation, including on animals, in this version of the script, would lead to the solution to the cancer problem.[32]

The story would change quite dramatically after the Americans got involved. Foster would no doubt have expected such changes, since he wanted Constant's script to open discussions about coproduction, which would mean that others would have a say in the message the movie was to promote and how it would be told. In addition, his doubts about Constant's skills as a scriptwriter would only grow over the next few months, and others would be brought in to refashion the script (though Constant retained the title of scenarist). Later scripts would therefore drop some of the themes in the June 1948 Constant script and transform others: The "ignorance of the past" theme would disappear, and with it the progressivist history of the emergence of a materialist scientific world view; the growth theme and its cancerous/malignant perversion would remain, but the cancer no longer killed the body and the sequence in which a white sheet was passed over a body was abandoned, or perhaps transformed into the white sheets of a hospital bed, and the hope they embodied; the links between maps, geography and the cell-scape or body-scape remained in some of the later iterations of the script, but do not appear in the final version of the script/film; the cell-as-universe theme survived, though the filmmakers struggled to figure out whether to hammer the home the parallel with space travel by including an explicit treatment of outer space in the film alongside the inner space of the cell; the human story of cancer was retained in different versions of the script but changed significantly, and lost the melodrama of the opening scene in Constant's script; the patient's quest theme would also be transformed, as would the "interstellar space theme" and the woman's fear of cancer—indeed the central patient herself was transformed into a man. New writers and new sponsors meant that the script was malleable, constantly changing with changing interests and agendas.

CHAPTER 4

Mr. Foster Goes Fishing

W ITH THE FIRST SCRIPT complete, Foster now started to look for an American sponsor, and—as second in command at the NFB— he did this for institutional reasons as much as filmic ones. The commissioning of the film in 1948 came at a challenging time for the NFB. Its first commissioner, John Grierson, had resigned in 1945, ushering in an unsettled period for the board.[1] Under pressure from Ottawa, the new commissioner, Ross McLean, cut staff, and critics on all sides of the political spectrum attacked the board—for some it was propaganda for the party in power, for others it was a lair of left-wing subversives, if not Communists.[2] Then in 1945, Grierson and his secretary were linked to the spy circle revealed by the Soviet defector Igor Gouzenko.[3] The result was that the NFB became the object of several investigations, including one by the Royal Canadian Mounted Police (RCMP) that began an inquiry into allegations of Communist infiltration of the board in 1948.[4] The controversy, combined with reports of NFB wasteful spending, and pressure from the private film industry opposed to a public film agency, eventually resulted in McLean leaving the NFB, in early 1950, the appointment of Arthur Irwin as film commissioner, sweeping changes in the structure of the NFB, and a New National Film Act.[5]

As McLean struggled with these problems in 1948, the prospect of a contract with the Americans for the cancer film became welcome. Not only did it promise more money at a time of financial cutbacks, but it may also have helped to counter the perception of Communist infiltration, and revive the NFB's hopes of an internationalist outlook for its documentaries. Internationalism had become a major focus of Canadian cultural life in the early Cold War, but it was a source of controversy for the NFB, which sometimes pushed internationalist agendas that did not fit government agendas.[6] For example, in the 1940s, the NFB had produced three controversial documentaries, including one that had attracted government criticism for its provocative suggestion that two governments existed in China, one favored by the West under Chiang Kai-shek, the other a Communist regime under Mao Tse-tung (now also Mao Zedong).[7] *Challenge* provided an opportunity to develop a different internationalist perspective, one that was more congenial to the government and the Americans.[8]

Challenge also provided an opportunity for the NFB to promote two other new initiatives in the 1940s. One was to develop a program to use film to encourage American public support for Canada: a revised script could do this by highlighting Canada's role in cancer research. The other was to find new sources of funding by developing international coproduction efforts in which the NFB joined with non-Canadian sponsoring organizations to make a movie. The NFB had long used coproduction approaches within Canada and, as noted in the previous chapter, had worked, for example, with the Department of National Health and Welfare and other government agencies on several films. But international coproduction was something new. *Challenge* was one of the NFB's early international coproduction projects, and a key venture by which the board worked out the issues involved in this approach.

Coproduction (national or international) was complex process that involved keeping many different groups and individuals onboard, all of which had their own interests and agendas that had to be addressed and reconciled. It should thus come as no surprise that the film was a constantly evolving production, adapted and readapted to the concerns of those involved in the film. In this context, Constant's emphasis on fears that Canadian scientists were being tempted elsewhere by better pay and facilities disappeared from later versions of script. The latter tended to portray the fight against cancer as an international fight, driven by research centers across the world, from any one of which clues as to the nature and treatment of cancer could emerge. This vision of scientific internationalism meshed well with the efforts by the NFB to reduce the political heat it was experiencing, as well the concerns of both the American and Canadian sponsors, who as collaborators no longer wanted a film that trumpeted national scientific achievements or goals at the expense of the other.

Casting a line in American waters

In July 1948, Foster met Adelaide Brewster (the Motion Picture Director in the Publicity Department of the American Cancer Society [ACS]) and Bernard V. Dryer at the NFB's offices in New York City. Foster gave both copies of the script. Brewster showed it to Charles Cameron—the ACS's Medical and Scientific Director—who enthused about the script but did not see how the ACS could make it that year. (It already had a full public education program, and would release five public education films in 1948/9, including *From One Cell,* targeted, like *Challenge,* at biology students.[9]) Brewster hoped that they might be able to do it the following year, but the ACS does not seem to have pursued the matter, and it soon dropped out of the collaboration.

Foster's fears about the suitability of the script for American sponsors were likely assuaged by the ACS's initial reaction and were further calmed by the NCI's response. This came about when Dryer showed the script to Dallas Johnson. Johnson noted that she "really thought the mood and tone excellent"[10] and passed it on to the directors of the NCI's cancer research branches for comment.[11] Johnson was about to go on vacation for seven weeks and expected to respond when she returned on September 10. Dryer also wrote in August 1948 reiterating the enthusiasm both he and Johnson had for the script: "whatever minor unwieldiness it had technically there was no doubting the comparative rarity of its sincere approach and its even more rare quality of a lofty unified concept."[12] He too wanted to discuss the script with Foster and Constant when Johnson returned in September.

On September 13—three days after Johnson had been due to return from vacation—Foster wrote to Dryer to renew contact, suggesting that he would likely be in New York in September—he later changed this to November 8.[13] Constant, he noted, was delighted at the possibility of collaboration with the NCI (and the ACS, which was still a potential collaborator at this time). In other correspondence, he noted that the Canadian Department of National Health and Welfare was leaning toward the production of two films, one based on Constant's cancer research script, to be directed mainly toward non-theatrical distribution, the other a one-reel theatrical subject emphasizing the sociological and human-interest values in the cancer program. He thought that they would consider both films as a project to be jointly cosponsored by the NFB and the Canadian and US governments, and they were prepared to put up $20,000 immediately if the US government agency was willing to do the same, with the NFB contributing a further $10,000.[14]

Foster's letter prompted a quick response from Dryer.[15] He noted that the NCI—and John Heller, its chief—were interested in the collaboration, and he wanted to discuss this further. Two days later Lt. Col. Gilchrist at the DNHW wrote to confirm the arrangements.[16] He reminded Foster that under Order in Council No. 4194 dated November 19, 1947, it was already authorized to spend CAN$20,000 on a cancer film. It would not spend any more and would like to see the US Public Health Service and the NFB come in for similar amounts. It wanted to see things as far ahead as possible by March 31, 1949. (Recall that the board of directors of the NCIC wanted the film ready for the film circuit in time for the Federated Cancer Campaign in April 1949.) It was at this point that Johnson asked the NFB to apply for matching funds from the NACC, and as we have already noted in chapter 1 this application failed, because it came in too late for consideration, NACC members had doubts about the film, and Johnson admitted she was not on the ball, swamped with other duties.[17] She recommended that they try again for the March meeting of the NACC. The deadline for the release of the film set by the Canadian Department of National Health and Welfare began to slip. Gilchrist had hoped that things would be much further advanced by March 1949.

Thus, by early 1949 it was still unclear where the American funding was to come from. Moreover, the Department of National Health and Welfare was also concerned that the Constant script was still being considered for the joint project. The department's concerns about the script are not known, but they prompted letters from the Foster apologizing for what looked like an apparent lack of consultation and noting that they had also agreed with the Americans about some changes in the story. Constant's script would have to be revised, he noted, but the Americans agreed "that thematically the script provided direction and a useful beginning."[18]

For its part, the Canadian Cancer Society also seems to have had doubts about whether a suitable script existed that would engage audiences. As one CCS officer put it in February, "we should not embark upon a matter of this kind unless we are quite sure that we have an appealing and dynamic story to tell and that effective means must be undertaken to secure such a story as a basis for the script."[19] To complicate issues further, the CCS may still have been still considering a film focused on cancer control as much as research, perhaps picking up on the earlier idea of two films, one targeted at research, the other at control. This official had recently watched *That They May Live*, the 1942 cancer control film made in Saskatchewan. Echoing earlier American concerns discussed in chapter 2, he doubted it could provide a good model for the sort of film they wanted. "To my mind," he wrote,[20] "it might be shown to employees in industrial plants, but certainly not to audiences of women . . . the film is not one that can be shown to popular audiences across the country in keeping with the views we held concerning the type of film desired."

By March, the funding arrangements on the American side seem to have been resolved, and the CCS's hope of a control movie seems to have disappeared. Instead of renewing their application to the NACC, the NCI now received funding via the Association of American Medical Colleges, which had successfully applied for a grant to the NCI. An agreement was signed in March/ April 1949—the Canadian Department of National Health and Welfare and the United States Public Health Service (responsible for the NCI) each providing $20,000—a total of $40,000. The NFB was a party to the agreement but did not commit itself to any money, as Gilchrist had hoped. The first monies were to be transferred by April 15; and the transfer was to be completed by June 15.[21]

The following schedule was agreed on:

Production analysis	March 11–14, 1949
Treatment	May 1, 1949
Storyboard	June 13–15, 1949
Advance rough-cut	September 1, 1949
Interlock	December 1, 1949.[22]

Interlock was the last point at which changes could be made to a film inexpensively. It involved the screening of the fine cut (the stage after rough cut, a preliminary piecing together of the film by the editor) with all the picture and sound in place. Following approval at interlock, the NFB would cut the camera original film, mix the sound, and have a print made. Any changes after that point would be expensive. The schedule was tight, and while the treatments were produced more or less on time, other production deadlines would be missed.

Revising the script

With the agreement in place, Constant began to revise and rethink his original script/treatment. By now Foster had appointed a producer and a director for the movie—Guy Glover and Morten Parker respectively, of whom more in the next chapter—and it is likely that they closely supervised the revision, and perhaps wrote some of it. In an interview Parker echoed some of Foster's anxieties about Constant's limitations as a scriptwriter. He thought that Constant was too didactic and academic for this sort of film, anxious to get every fact across to the public, sometimes at the expense of what Parker thought would work as a film.[23] Parker's recollection is that Constant was quietly moved into more of a research than a writing role. Thus, while one of the early treatments (May 12, 1949) lists Constant's name as author, the narrative has a different feel than other versions, and the writing style is different. Yet as mentioned earlier, Constant retained the title of scenarist, and his new cowriters did not abandon all his ideas. Some were incorporated into the new narrative almost without change; others (such as the starry sky and the quest narratives) were transformed and introduced in different ways.

By May 1949, Constant and his collaborators had produced several story outlines for the film of which three survive, two dated May 5;[24] and the other, slightly longer, dated May 12.[25] So far, the production was running according to the schedule agreed to back in April. The May 1949 treatments—not scripts but outlines of the story—are all slightly different, and the two dated May 5 are full of scribbled edits that capture something of how the writers were thinking and rethinking how to tell the story. Of the two dated May 5, the one that begins with the title page "Outline of structure"[26] is likely the earlier draft since the other is very similar to the May 12 treatment. The May 12 treatment is not preserved on paper, but on the stencil that would have been used in the mimeograph process, when it would be wrapped around an ink-filled drum for printing. It is a fragile document, and difficult to read in places.

Although the May treatments were constantly being modified, they share some differences from the older June 1948 script. With the Americans now involved, the oblique reference to desires to keep Canadian scientists in the country had disappeared. There is also no appeal for public support of the sort that had concluded the June 1948 script. Instead, all the May 1949 treatments regard cancer research as a vast international endeavor and the individual scientist as a small part this endeavor rather than someone in danger of being poached by foreign countries. The internationalist theme fitted the agendas of both sponsors, and Foster's desire to promote coproduction efforts, as well as the broader agenda of encouraging American public support for Canada, at least insofar as the motion picture promoted Canadian research as part of the international endeavor.

Ditching nationalist sentiments also allowed the filmmakers to modify the representation of the character of the scientist. Here the scientist becomes someone who is almost immune to material reward. The point is best made in the earlier of the two May 5 scripts—the "Outline"—where a scientist is challenged by a reporter who has heard of a new "cure" for cancer. The writers of this treatment show that as the facts of cancer (and the absence of an easy cure) are made clear to the reporter, his attitude changes. It passes from "indignant disappointment to thoughtful (if somewhat cynical) admiration." [27] "What keeps you people plugging away?" he asks, [28] "With this kind of ability . . . you could be doing a lot better for yourself elsewhere, where the rewards—and the results—are a little greater? . . ." "Well . . . it certainly isn't the money. . . ."[29]

It is in scenes such as this that the treatments begin to reinvent the character of the scientist. The problem with the June 1948 appeal to nationalist sentiments was the implication that a young scientist seeking to start a career and a family might find a more secure life elsewhere than Canada or cancer research. The internationalist perspective that emerged with the coproduction allowed the scriptwriters to sidestep this problem. No longer a scarce national resource to be kept in the country at all costs, the scientist now emerges as a relatively selfless figure—unimpressed by material concerns, part of a vast international effort against the disease, inspired by a fascination with the unknown, a pioneer on the cutting edge, a twentieth-century St. George fighting the dragon of disease. He or she would also be motivated by the thrill of a publication that makes him or her "a member in full standing of the world community of scientists,"[30] and by the excitement and intellectual gratification of announcing at a conference the successful culmination of years of experiment. How rewarding to hear the comments of a professional colleague, whispering in the audience: "a nice piece of scientific investigation."[31] Such was the character of the scientist as it emerged in the first of the three May 1949 treatments.

Yet even this character was not without its problems. The scientist might be immune to material reward, but not to professional recognition and perhaps vanity. The reporter sequence, for example, suggests that scientists could be motivated as much by the search for professional recognition as by a desire to extend knowledge and fight cancer. The point is made by the "nice piece of scientific investigation" comment. After basking in the glory of professional recognition, the scientist stops himself suddenly (according to the treatment) and quickly goes on to talk about the positive findings in the field of applied cancer research (therapeutics). The sudden stop gives the temptation of self-seeking away, and the entire sequence was cut from the two later versions of the treatment. All three May treatments portray the scientist as motivated by the excitement and rewards of science and the humanitarian desire to do something for those afflicted by the disease. But by abandoning the reporter sequence, and the "nice piece of scientific investigation" episode, the later May treatments also quietly discarded the suggestion that the temptation of professional ambition might outweigh humanitarian impulse.

Another characteristic of the scientist also emerges in these May treatments, related to a portrayal of science as a slow, uncertain worldwide enterprise that involves years of patient research. This was the scientist's humility in the face of the immensity and complexity of the cancer problem. No longer motivated by the promise of material reward or by the search for professional recognition, the scientist in this iteration of his/her character is driven by the desire for knowledge and the promise of being an explorer in strange new worlds, a small part of a vast international research enterprise. The world of the cell was a universe of its own, and the scientist like an interstellar traveler, an explorer in this universe, trying to figure out its workings and why it sometimes went wrong.

In these ways, the scriptwriters struggled to define the character of the scientist, which changed from one iteration of the treatment to another. The character now had to fit with the international nature of the production, and allow the sponsors to recruit scientists without the promise of vastly greater material resources, or salaries that might compete with industry, and yet also served to conjure up something of the prestige of a career in atomic physics. The character of the scientist—as selfless, relatively uninterested in material reward or professional recognition, humbled by the scale of the cancer problem, yet excited by the opportunities beginning to open up—addressed some of these problems. They would continue to refine this character in the scripts that followed, but its core features seem to have been worked out in May 1949.

There are other differences between the May 1949 treatments and the June 1948 script. The new treatments give much less emphasis to the human consequences of cancer, and the revisions suggest that the writers were struggling to figure out how the humanitarian impulse might be harnessed: in the earliest version of the treatment someone has written "Something missing here"[32] in the margins, and later treatments add a section on the human consequences of cancer missing from the first treatment. The story now opens not with the diagnosis of the woman's cancer, but the wonder of interstellar space, an echo of the starry sky in Constant's earlier script. And like the earlier script the new treatments also draw parallels between the macrocosm of outer space and the microcosm of the cell. But the quest narratives of the earlier Constant script are missing or changed. The story of progress from the dark days of ignorance to modern light is much shortened. The story of the patient's quest for a cure is also abbreviated, as are efforts to use shock and fear to focus the humanitarian impulse. Also gone is the earlier script's effort to evoke an association between women and nature. The woman's question—what is it, Doctor?—is buried in the middle of the movie, and given to a man, and he does not whine like a dog.

In the May 1949 treatments, the story of science's quest to understand and combat cancer is given center stage and presented as an invitation to young scientists to enter the field. In the earliest version of the treatment, this is done quite explicitly. Using a flashback technique, we see the scientist as a student ("in civvies"[33] —i.e., without his lab coat) in a tissue culture laboratory discussing with an older man his desire to get into cancer research, which becomes an opening to sequences that explore how the young man might approach it and the various branches of science that he might consider. The other two May treatments do not use this technique. Instead, they seek to draw the viewer into the film by drawing a parallel between the interstellar travel and the journey through the cell-as-universe.

In the June 1948 script the starry sky served to evoke the phantasms of the past, but the May 1949 treatments suggest that the writers are still figuring out what to do with the motif of starry sky, and whether it should invoke the older misconceptions about cancer, the body, and healing. The earliest of the three May treatments abandons the use of the starry sky to evoke the phantasms of the past (historical misconceptions are evoked in other ways, see below). This association returns in the second version when a telescope is depicted "sweeping across the sky (and wiping the absurdities of the past off the screen....):"[34] amulets, votive gods, charms, crude ancient instruments and so on. And then it disappears again in the May 12 version. In general, the cell-as-universe sequences—and the "starry" skies within the cell—serve the different purpose of highlighting both the current ignorance of science about cancer, the huge scale of the problem, and the great opportunities open to scientists.

The May 5, 1949, treatments

A comparison of the two May 5 treatments (table 4.1) gives a snapshot of the fluidity of the film at this point. It shows the filmmakers, over one day, trying to figure out how best to organize the movie, and the symbolic characters of the scientist and patient within it. Scenes are moved around, reordered, details added or removed, and sequences merged or separated, as the filmmakers try to work out how to organize the themes of the film, what to emphasize, and how to do this cinematically. Sometimes the topics are dealt with didactically (recall Parker's concerns about Constant's academic bent), at other times symbolically (such as a flask glowing as if there is life in it, perhaps a reference to tissue culture), and at other times scientific themes are mixed in with others, such as the character of the scientist. At this stage of production, it would be relatively cheap to make changes—just some more paper, ink, and time in the script room.

Both of the May 5, 1949, treatments begin in the same way. They open (table 4.1, sequence 1) with a crashing chord, and a huge sphere zooms toward us out of darkness and rushes past the viewer to one side. We are moving through interstellar space.... We see stars twinkling in the distance, followed by an imposing parade of heavenly bodies, the blaze of a comet, the twinkle of thousands of galaxies, the vortex of a nebula, and the slow passage of a constellation. The commentator, "a cool, incisive voice, riding on the music and the rhythm of the visual procession,"[35] announces "THIS JOURNEY... IS FOR THE YOUNG IN MIND... FOR THE CURIOUS...FOR THOSE TO WHOM THE UNKNOWN IS A CHALLENGE!"[36] And then: "ON A DEAD PLANET, SPINNING OUT [OF] ITS PRESCRIBED ORBIT A MILLION LIGHT

TABLE 4.1. Comparison of the Two May 5, 1949, Treatments

The following is a précis of the sequence structure and the subjects/approach of each sequence derived from the two treatments.

	"Outline of Structure"	"Treatment for Film on Cancer Research"
1	**Introduction and Titles** - Sound of a crashing musical chord. A huge sphere zooms toward us and rushes past to one side. We are moving through interstellar space. Commentator: This journey is for the young in mind. For the curious. For those to whom the unknown is a challenge! - Scientist at work at night. Commentator: There are thousands like him trying to save human lives, to solve the mystery in the flask. - Titles here or superimposed over the earlier movement through space. - Scientist puts out the light, leaves. A ray of light from the window makes the flask glow as if it had a life of its own.	**Introduction and Titles** - Sound of a crashing musical chord. A huge sphere zooms toward us and rushes past to one side. We are moving through interstellar space. Commentator: This journey is for the young in mind. For the curious. For those to whom the unknown is a challenge! - Scientist at work at night. Commentator: There are thousands like him trying to save human lives, to solve the mystery in the flask. - Titles superimposed over the movement through space, which fade and mix to churning storm clouds of Earth atmosphere. - Discussion of man's control of nature, which leads to the application of human intelligence to understand the secret of growth— "Cabbage or King" quote.
2	**The cell; normal growth; abnormal growth.** - A sequence, mainly animation, to briefly explain the fundamentals necessary to understand the cancer problem: the cell, normal growth, abnormal growth. - End of the sequence: Commentator uses the "dreaded word" for the first time: "This is cancer."	**The cell; normal growth; abnormal growth.** - An expanded version of the description in "Outline of Structure." - Mainly in realistic, three-dimensional animation, we get a vivid picture of the cell-as-a-universe. There follow descriptions of various themes regarding the cell, body, normal and abnormal growth. - At the end of the sequence the commentator uses the word cancer for the first time: "This is cancer."

3	**Cancer as a menace to human life.**	**Cancer as a menace to human life.**
	- Cancer: more than an object of scientific curiosity. Its meaning in terms of human lives and misery. One in eight deaths will be caused by cancer. It respects no age, but heaviest toll is from the middle-aged and elderly.	- We zoom back from an extreme closeup. We are looking at a small ulcer on the hand of a man. Man: It doesn't hurt. Commentator: If it hadn't been caught in time it would have killed him. Man: What is it, Doctor?
	- A sequence of two or three shots: cancer attacks all forms of life.	
4	**The failure and despair of past approaches to cancer.**	**The failure and despair of past approaches to cancer.**
	- Introductory comment: Cancer is an age-old affliction. Short historical sequence to indicate the disease's antiquity, the hopelessness of an approach based on ignorance and superstition, the vestiges of which are still with us.	- Short historical sequence (animation and actuality shots) of crude, ancient instruments, amulets, votive gods, charms, etc., to illustrate the antiquity of the disease and the futility of an approach based on ignorance and superstition.
5	**The attack on cancer. The hope of the present. Its record of successes.**	**The attack on cancer. The hope of the present. Its record of successes.**
	- Hopes for success against cancer are based on the scientific method	- Sequence of a telescope removing the absurdities of the past from the sky, an aerial view of distant lakes and forests that mixes to a pan of a photomicrograph, and a cut to scientist looking into a microscope.
	- Cite the record of the method's past successes as a cause for long-term optimism regarding cancer	- A list of scientific successes against other diseases
	- Brief and simple definition of the meaning of the scientific method. (What have we got that the ancient Greeks and Babylonians didn't have?)	

(Cont.)

	"Outline of Structure"	"Treatment for Film on Cancer Research"
6	**The scientist against cancer and, in general, how he is approaching it.** - Symbol of the flask (opening scene) begins sequence on the human side of the scientist and explains how every field of science is related to cancer. - Flashback technique: the scientist as a student discussing with an older man his desire to get into cancer research. - He is told the problem is essentially one of growth. But how does he want to approach it? Does he want to be a biochemist, geneticist, bacteriologist, or physicist? - As each branch of science is mentioned we can introduce the setting typical for it. Later, when we go into each field in greater detail, we will begin each section with this previously introduced "habitat," and with the "filter" voice of the scientist.	**Carcinogens: The work and contribution of the chemist** - Chemists have isolated various cancer-producing agents found in daily work such as lubricating oils in cotton mills, radioactive ores, luminous paints - These may be preventable causes of cancer - But for the chemist the question is how and why do these carcinogens act? - Visual analogy of a button that starts a machine. It is known that certain agents start a cancer; they press a button. Little is known about the cancer process itself; what goes on inside the cell.
7	**Tissue culture as a primary tool of cancer research. (A continuation of sequence 6)** - Two points: (1) living tissue, cancerous and healthy, can be cut out of a living animal, and kept alive indefinitely; (2) the cut-out cancer tissue will, if injected into a healthy animal, continue to grow there until it kills its new host. - The two characters of the young and older scientist. The scientist sums up the purpose of all this: Try out the effects of chemicals on cancer tissue or see what makes a bit of normal tissue become cancerous. He holds up a tissue culture flask: "Interesting possibilities, aren't there?"	**Tissue culture as a primary tool of cancer research.** - Extreme closeup of cell mixes to a closeup of a flask. Pull away to reveal hundreds of such flasks in a tissue-culture laboratory - With proper care the tissue in these flasks will live and grow indefinitely. We learn how tissue is cultured in eggs, glass, and animals and its significance for research. - Now scientists can observe under the microscope the growth and behavior of individual cancer cells, including by means of time-lapse photography.

- The flashback above is over. Back in the lab we saw at the beginning, the younger scientist now older regards the flask and repeats: "Very interesting possibilities...."

8 Carcinogens: The work and contribution of the chemist (Perhaps incorporated into the above flashback)

- Commentator: Use of tar by two Japanese scientists in 1918 to produce tumors in rabbit ears. "This is where the Chemist comes in."
- Kind of work involved in isolation of the hundreds of substances capable of producing tumors. Its importance for the protection of workers in contact with chemicals.
- Knowing how to "start" a cancer is not the same as understanding the "cause" of cancer. It is known that certain agents start the cancer process. Less is known about the cancer process itself.
- Hormones have a structural similarity to substances known to cause cancer. What does this mean, if anything?
- The chemist's weapons include tagging components of food with isotopes that are then followed through the body (visuals: Geiger counter/ mass spectrometer) to study patterns characteristic of health and disease. (The contribution of the physicist).
- Reiterate the interrelationship of the great number of scientific disciplines involved in cancer research. The contributions made by each: illustrated where possible with their particular apparatus, paraphernalia and technique.

- "From a little piece of tumour we can obtain a large harvest of material for experimentation. You can watch it, study its growth and behaviour, try chemicals on it, smash it, filter it, try it hot, try it cold, put it under the xray[sic] machine, or the microscope."

Genetics – Heredity and cancer. The important role played by mice as a tool.

- Poster of a two-headed cow/sounds of a carnival barker rounding up an audience.
- Mix and extreme closeup of the wire netting of a mouse cage in animal room of a genetics department. Commentator: Anomalies such as that above are not as interesting as the fact that a cow always produces a calf, not another animal.
- View of animal room and geneticists from the mouse- eye view of the cage. Visuals of the ever-active animals, and the techniques used for maintaining and breeding them. The importance of pure breeds in genetic studies regarding cancer, and of mice as a tool in cancer research.
- Visual: Single division of a cell. Commentator: Radiation can artificially alter the chromosomes to cause mutations to be born. Does something affect the chromosomes of the normal cell to cause it to produce cancerous offspring?

(Cont.)

"Outline of Structure"	"Treatment for Film on Cancer Research"
9 **Genetics – Heredity and cancer. The important role played by mice as a tool.** - Poster of a two-headed cow/sounds of a carnival barker rounding up an audience - View of animal room and geneticists from the mouse-eye view of the cage. What determines inheritance? What determines what one generation passes on to the other? What does this have to do with cancer? - Importance of pure breeds in genetic studies regarding cancer, and of mice as the lowly heroes of the piece, and why they are used in genetics research. - What is the mechanism of inheritance? What happens? What does it have to do with cancer? Chromosome as a way of understanding the secret of heredity. In them lie the factors that determine the character of the adult that will grow from this cell. Visuals (animation or actuality): A single division, the chromosomes, the phases, etc. - Various means such as X-rays can artificially alter the chromosomes to cause mutations to be born, whose characteristics pass to succeeding generations. Scientists are waiting to see whether children of atom-bombed Japanese parents will show the effects of radiation. Is cancer due to a mutation? Does something affect the chromosomes of the normal cell to cause it to produce cancerous offspring? - Story of young geneticist who interrupts the family's Sunday drive (brings them into the lab) to maintain the rigid, uninterruptable schedule of the experiment.	**Virus studies: The work of the bacteriologist. Mention of the electron microscope and the complexities typical of the cancer problem. Milk Factor as an example.** - Extreme close up of cell. Commentator: Does some microbe cause cancer? Use of comparative animation to show the difference in size between microbes and viruses. - Story of the "milk factor": An example of how the scientist goes about his job. Illustrated by Dr. [Samuel] Graff's "Mouse Dairy." After "milking" the mice, the use of various techniques (ultracentrifuge, electrophoresis, etc.) to separate out the active fraction builds to a climax with the isolation of the virus and a view of what it looks like as seen by the electron microscope. Commentator: This has only been proven in mice, not men, and is only a first step. What is the chemical composition of the virus? And (returning to the extreme closeup of the cell) what does the virus do to the cell?

10 **Virus studies: The work of the bacteriologist. Mention of the electron microscope.**

- Is cancer contagious? Not due to a microbe, but some (animal not human) cancers are due to a virus. A virus is not a microbe; it is much smaller. It is a minute living particle too small to be seen with the most powerful microscope. But with the electron microscope, physics has opened this world of matter that lies on the borderline between the living and the non-living. In the case of some cancer tissue, you can grind it up, and make an emulsion of it and pass it through porcelain filters. Some agent (no microbe could pass through) does pass through with the clear liquid, because if you inject this liquid into a healthy animal you get exactly the same kind of tumor as the one from which you made the emulsion.

- As yet there is no evidence that a virus causes any human cancer. Do viruses just start cancer? Or are they involved in the cancer process itself? Is there a virus in every cell waiting for some factor to stimulate it?

Cell as Industry/Factory: The work of the biochemist.
- Extreme closeup of cell: Idea of cell as chemical industry on a vast scale.
- Role of biochemist in cancer research. Animation shows thousands of feet of "factory space" available in the cell because of the smallness of the particles with it. Actuality shots from industry used to maintain analogy between cell processes and those in factory production and maintenance.
- The biochemist compares the constituents of normal and cancer cells and looks for differences in chemical reactions (rate of breathing, utilization of foodstuffs, accumulation of breakdown products). What goes on in the cancer cell that is different from the normal cell
- End on single cell ... dissolve to next scene.

(Cont.)

	"Outline of Structure"	"Treatment for Film on Cancer Research"
11	**The complexities typical of the cancer problem. Milk Factor as an example.** - Milk Factor: An example of the multiplicity of factors that may be involved in cancer research. - Mammary tumors in mice are passed on by the female. How? We do not yet know. Then it is shown that the cancer "factor" is passed on to the young by something in the mother's milk.… The bacteriologists, therefore, believe it may be a virus. But the biochemists show that—even though the "factor" may be a virus passed on in the mother's milk—the presence of hormones affects the results. - And then further research brings out the importance of the effects on "Milk Factor" of diet, age. - And finally, all these results are for mice, not men.…	**Applied research. Where the object is not understanding but cure.** - Interior of hospital: Nurses, interns, patients. Dissolve to operating room, biopsy in progress. The surgeon: "I need a simple test for cancer." - Speeding up the tempo with shots and staccato treatment, the film deals with the following items to build up a feeling of overwhelming and constant activity: - hormones against cancer of prostate and breast - radioisotope to "burn out" cancer of organs that soak up specific elements - radium and bigger X-ray machines - cell poisons to kill or inhibit cancer cells but not normal cells.
12	**Applied research. Where the object is not understanding but cure.** - List some of the most immediate needs. - Story told by a scientist harried by a reporter regarding a new "cure" for cancer. Reporter passes from indignant disappointment to thoughtful (if somewhat cynical) admiration. - Partly flashback: The scientist/commentator explains what keeps him in the game: fascination of the unknown, the feeling of pioneering on the edge of knowledge, of playing the twentieth-century St. George against the Dragon of disease. - Visuals: Perhaps an interesting composition with shadows on the wall—using microscopes, flasks, etc.—as symbolic background for this part of the speech.	**The whole picture. Cancer research is coordinated. It is international in scale** - The work does not go on in isolation … shot of a conference in which the nameplates of all countries seem in evidence testifies to the international character of cancer research. - 17,000 journals a year report on progress being made.

- Scientist: Then, the thrill of seeing months of labor neatly summarized in a paper that makes you a member in full standing of the world community of scientists. Then, the excitement and intellectual tussle of announcing at a conference the successful culmination of years of experiment; to hear the comments of the profession, "a nice piece of scientific investigation"; he stops himself abruptly and goes on to tell about positive findings in the field of applied cancer research.

- Commentator: The nature of the work going on in these fields, and some positive results.

-The treatment of this part of the film will produce a feeling of overwhelming and constant activity, the atmosphere and excitement of a hunt. The items will be kept very short and the pace fast and staccato.

- Items needed: 1) A cheap, reliable test for cancer. 2) Chemical examination of the waste products of cancer patients and healthy people. 3) Studies of the specific requirements of cancer cells. So that we may "starve" them out. 4) Statistics and their usefulness in indicating new avenues of investigation. 5) Hormones to fight cancer of the sex organs. 6) Radioactive isotopes to "burn out" cancers of organs that soak up elements of a particular kind. 7) Cell poisons that kill or inhibit cancer cells but not normal cells.

(Cont.)

"Outline of Structure"	"Treatment for Film on Cancer Research"
13 The whole picture. Cancer research is coordinated. It is international in scale. - The work does not go on in isolation. Research is by its very nature international in character, transcending—as an exercise of the human intelligence—the bounds of language, geography, or politics. Its work is organized in conferences, committees and institutes, and its progress reported in 17,000 journals a year.	**Conclusion** - Avalanche of 17,000 journals a year in every language and topic mixed to the opening sequence of the journey though interstellar space. - Commentator: Sums up the sense of the film. Music begins its peroration. - The celestial world fades and grows pale. Mix to wispy cloud in the pale early morning sky. Tilt down to reveal the exterior of the lab building and the scientist of sequence 1 hurrying along, exchanging greetings with the milkman. Enters the lab, pulls up the shades, and stands gazing at the flasks glowing in the morning light. - Commentator: In this flask lies the answer to a mystery - Scientist rolls up his sleeves: Maybe this time
14 Conclusion - Avalanche of 17,000 journals a year in every language and topic mixed to the opening sequence of the journey though interstellar space. - Commentator: Sums up the sense of the film. Music begins its peroration. - The celestial world fades and grows pale. Mix to wispy cloud in the pale early morning sky. Tilt down to reveal the exterior of the lab building and the scientist of sequence 1 hurrying along, exchanging greetings with the milkman. Enters the lab, pulls up the shades, and stands gazing at the flasks glowing in the morning light. - Commentator: In this flask lies the answer to a mystery - Scientist rolls up his sleeves: Maybe this time.	

YEARS AWAY...MAN HAS GONE SO FAR IN ADJUSTING HIMSELF TO HIS ENVIRIONMENT [*sic*] THAT NOW ... HE IS EXAMINING THE MYSTERY OF LIFE ITSELF."[37] An astral body fills the screen.

The next scene is of a scientist hunched over his work or a face reflected in a large flask.[38] The scientist gets up, moves to the window (like the man/husband in the earlier script) and looks out at the night scene of the sleeping city. He starts to close up shop, and the commentator notes that there are thousands of men like this working into the night trying to save human lives by solving the mystery of growth—the title of the movie fades in, superimposed over the movement through interstellar space—*The Mystery (or Riddle) of Rampant Growth*, though the earlier of the two treatments also suggests it might be superimposed over the movement through space earlier in the sequence.[39]

The first significant divergence between the two treatments occurs at this point. In the earlier May 5 version, sequence 1 ends with the scientist switching off a light and the sunlight glinting off a flask to make it seemingly glow with life. Then we move to an animation sequence (2) that briefly explains the fundamentals of understanding of the cancer problem—the cell, normal growth, and abnormal growth—which concludes with the commentator stating, "This is cancer." (The "Something missing here"[40] comment appears among the marginalia at this point, where the treatment explains that we are now ready for the sections that follow.) Having established cancer as a disease of cells and abnormal growth, the treatment then goes on to explore the importance of cancer as a menace to human life (3), the hopeless approaches to cancer of the past (not represented by a starry sky) (4), the hope offered by present-day approaches (5), and the character of the scientist: the flashback scene of a young scientist in civvies (6). There follow sequences on tissue culture (7), carcinogenic substances: the work of the chemist (8), genetics: heralded by a circus scene and a two-headed cow (9), viral approaches to cancer including electron microscopy (10), the complexities of the cancer problem (11), applied research: research on therapeutics and diagnosis (12), and "The Whole picture," (also "THE BROAD PICTURE")[41] where the coordinated, international scale of cancer research is considered (13). A concluding sequence (14) returns us to the flask motif of the beginning.

As table 4.1 illustrates, however, the second May 5 treatment diverges from this structure. In this later version, sequence 1 does not end with the titles but continues with a very brief account of human progress (that includes an unattributed reference to the C. S. Lewis poem "The Walrus and the Carpenter" missing from the earlier version: "cabbage or a king, the growth process is the same."[42]) that ends with a closeup of a face on a glass flask (an echo of the flask in the earlier

treatment, but without the glow, now with a commentary on tissue culture research, and the idea that it involves an almost miraculous ability to keep cells alive
outside the body forever).[43] The narrator repeats the comments about thousands
of men like this working into the night to solve the problem in this flask, a living
cell. It is only now that we move to a "realistic, three-dimensional animation"[44]
(sequence 2) of the cell as a universe, carrying out all the basic functions necessary
to life. We see cell growth, and differentiation, the development of the human
body, demonstrating processes of normal growth, followed by a sequence on abnormal growth that ends with the commentator stating, "This is cancer."[45]

We are now at the point in the treatment where the unknown scribbler had
written "something missing here" in the earlier version—the missing bit seems
to be the human consequences of cancer. While sequence 3 in both treatments
focus on the theme of cancer as a menace to human life, the sequence in the
earlier May 5 version focuses on statistics and the fact that cancer attacks all
forms of life, while the sequence in the later May 5 version focuses on the human
consequences of the disease. The camera in this later May 5 version pulls back to
reveal a small ulcer on the hand of a man (the ulcer being, perhaps, the resolution of Constant's concern in the 1948 script not to use a horrible tumor). The
commentator reassures us that it has been caught in time. It is the man with the
ulcer who asks the question the woman asked in the June 1948 script: "What is
it, Doctor?"[46]

There follows in both May 5 versions a sequence (4) on the history of cancer
(the antiquity of the problem, and the futility of approaches based on ignorance
and superstition). In the later treatment, this sequence is followed by an animated sequence (5) derived from Constant's 1948 script where a telescope wipes
the sky clear of the phantasms of the past, followed by a scene focusing on the
renewal of "Man's"[47] interest in the material world, and the beginnings of exploration: an aerial view of distant lakes and forests that mixes to the camera
panning over a photomicrograph of a section of tissue, which looks much the
same as the preceding landscape (none of which is present in the earlier May 5
version, but which reintroduce themes from Constant's 1948 script). The link
between the exploration of geographical landscape and of the body-scape has
been established. We see a scientist looking through a microscope, and the commentator highlights the successes of the scientific method—antibiotics, immu-
nization, surgery, and the replacement of vital deficiencies—as reasonable cause
for optimism in the struggle to understand abnormal growth.

In the earlier May 5 version, sequence (5) is quite different, however. There is
no telescope wiper blade, no parallel with geography, no scientist looking into

the microscope. Instead of visually illustrating how science wipes away older approaches, it focuses more didactically on the scientific method, its definition, the hopes vested in it, and its differences from earlier approaches to cancer and knowledge; a focus absent from the later treatment. Thus, while both focus on scientific successes against other diseases, the earlier version attributes this much more systematically to the methodology of science.

Such variations illustrate how, over the course of May 5, 1949, Constant, Parker and Glover sought to work out how to tell their story. I will not discuss all the differences here (for fuller details see table 4.1), but some of the major variations can be mentioned. The next sequence (6) in the earlier May 5 treatment focuses on the human side of the scientist and how he [*sic*] approaches the problem of cancer, while sequence 6 in the later May 5 treatment ignores this topic and jumps into the issue of carcinogens. Both treatments then come together (sequence 7 in both) to look at tissue culture research (the earlier version a continuation of themes in the previous section focusing on the character and approach of the scientist; the later version, absent the scientist's character, a more factual treatment of why tissue culture is an important technique and what scientists can do with it.) Now the two treatments diverge again, the earlier version belatedly taking up the question of carcinogens (and going beyond the sequence in the later May 5 treatment to look at the work of the chemist more generally), the later treatment taking up the topic of genetics and the role of mice in such research.

From there on the sequences in both treatments are out of sync, and each equivalent sequence also covers different topics and approaches them differently. Sequence 8 in the earlier treatment is on carcinogens, while in the later version it is on genetics. Sequence 9 (early version) is on genetics (a more detailed version than the one in the later May 5 treatment), in the later version it is on virus studies and the complexities of the cancer problem. The earlier May 5 treatment only gets to virus studies (minus the complexities issue) in sequence 10, while sequence 10 in the later treatment is on the cell as industry or factory (a sequence/theme missing from the earlier version). So it goes on: the early treatment gets to the complexities of the cancer problem in sequence 11 (part of sequence 9 in the later version); while sequence 11 in the later version is on applied research (sequence 12 in the earlier version), followed by sequence 12 the whole picture (sequence 13 in the earlier version) followed by the conclusion sequence 13 (sequence 14 in the earlier version).

Both treatments end with the international character of science and a return to the scientist we met at the beginning. The later treatment, for example, concludes with an avalanche of 17,000 journals a year in every language and on every topic, which mixes to a recapitulation of the opening sequence of the journey through interstellar space. The celestial world begins to fade and grow pale, and mixes to a wispy cloud trailing across the early morning sky. Now the camera tilts down to reveal the exterior of the laboratory building and the scientist we saw at the beginning of the picture hurrying along deep in thought, passing a moment to exchange greetings with the milkman. The night has passed. He enters the laboratory, pulls up the shades and stands gazing at the flasks, glowing in the morning light. The scientist takes off his coat and rolls up his sleeves. "MAYBE THIS TIME...."[48]

May 12, 1949, treatment

We know little about the response to the May 5 treatments, except that a further treatment was produced on May 12. This largely followed the ideas developed in the two May 5 treatments with some further juggling of sequences, expansions and contractions, ideas on cinematic presentation. The text is difficult to read in the stencil of the May 12 version, but the crashing chord of music does not seem to appear in the opening sequence, nor does the huge sphere make an appearance.[49] Instead a starry sky resolves into a new title—*The Scientist versus Cancer. The Mystery of the Rampant Growth*, after which the treatment follows a trajectory that is only slightly different to the second of the May 5 versions, and ending with the "MAYBE THIS TIME...."[50]

The June 1949 shooting script (table 4.2)

Sometime between May 12 and June 1949 the treatments mutated into a shooting script; the version of the screenplay that was intended to be used in the production of the film. The title had changed again—now the movie was called *Man Against Cancer*—as had the narrative; indeed, the narrative would continue to change up to the time that filming began. Even then the filmmakers would continue to adjust the script to fit the contingencies of filmmaking. Consequently, there are several iterations of this final version of the script, and the one used for shooting the film seems to have been rewritten, probably during the filming, and likely printed shortly after. We begin with the first iteration of the shooting script from June 1949, which was the one used and annotated by the director, Morten Parker, during the live-action shoots.[51]

TABLE 4.2. Shooting Script (June 1949)
Script in bold refers to differences with the final version of the film

	Sequence title	Brief description of action	Live action/ Animation
1	Clinic and Titles	Version 1: **Begins with the making of a film within a film. Then, the film itself starts with a hospital waiting room.** Mr. Davis enters. Then as for version 2. Version 2: Starts with a hospital waiting room. Mr. Davis enters, and is taken to see a physician and two scientists.	Live action
2	Normal and Abnormal Growth	Mr. Davis becomes an outline, and a cell emerges that grows into an embryo and then a man, before the scene changes to the story of abnormal growth (cancer)	Animation
3	The Physician's Conference Room (labeled here the Pathologist's Laboratory)	We return to Mr. Davis, who is reassured by the physician that his cancer—**now revealed as on the lip**—is a curable type, and is sent on his way. The physician is left alone looking at a slide of a (tumor?) cell, with a question: Why is the cancer problem so difficult?	Live action
4	Cell-as-Universe	The physician walks into the slide, shrinks, and disappears. We are traveling through the cell as if it were outer space, with constellations of cytosomes, centrosomes, and other parts of the cell passing by.	Animation
5	Tissue Culture	The animation dissolves to an animal **(rabbit?)** in a cage, which becomes the starting point of a sequence on the use of cells grown outside the body in cancer research.	Live action
6	Cell-as-Universe (Genetics)	We are traveling through the cell again, this time to watch cell division and chromosome separation.	Animation
7	Genetics	A man, woman, and child are in a laboratory. **There is a family resemblance between them.** They are looking at a mouse—the hero of research—that becomes the starting point of a sequence on the role of mice, fruit flies, and **other unspecified animals** in genetics research.	Live action
			(Cont.)

	Sequence title	Brief description of action	Live action/ Animation
8	Cell-as-Universe	We return to the cell surrounded and sometime overlain with swirling images. Here the cell is supposed to be an industrial organism, breathing, feeding, transporting, converting, manufacturing, etc	Animation
9	Biochemistry	A sequence on research into biochemistry, the life processes of the cell, which merges into a tea-bag scene, in which scientists discuss the latest finding over lunch, designed to show the character of the scientist.	Live Action
10	Cell-as-Universe (Environmental Cancer)	A view of the cell surrounded by a swirling mist to denote environmental threats.	Animation
11a	Environmental Cancer	A sequence on various environmental and occupational causes of cancer, how they are studied through field investigations, statistics, and laboratory research, and the importance of prevention.	Live action
11b	**Cell-as-Universe (Environmental Cancer)**	**Brief transition sequence to between environment and clinic.**	**Animation**
12	Clinic	We now explore the use of radiation in cancer, a sequence in which Mr. Davis arrives in the rain at a clinic, where he is treated with **radium**. We then move to a section on those who are not as lucky as Davis to have a treatable cancer, to research to find a test for cancer, and the hope that science offers those with cancer.	Live Action
13	**International**	Begins with a sequence showing an **international meeting**, after which we see a sequence with a scientist in the office late at night talking with his wife, which returns us to an account of the character of the scientist, the long time period needed to train a scientist, and the vast international scope of the scientific endeavor against cancer. The sequence then follows with students listening to a lecture on cancer and watching a cell on the screen. The sequence and the film end with a **shot of a scientist in heroic composition, at a micromanipulator, making adjustments.**	Live action

The June 1949 script was quite different from the Constant script of a year before. Of the four quests only three remained—the historical quest from ignorance to knowledge had disappeared—and the remaining quests are all modified. The patient's quest for a cure has returned (an expanded role for the male patient who briefly appeared in a May 1949 treatment, replacing the woman patient of June 1948): Mr. Davis, the symbolic patient, has a treatable cancer, and the film follows his diagnosis and treatment (though, curiously, not his recovery, which would later be covered in the theatrical version of the film). The quest of science continues, which—as in the June 1948 script—provides a way to understand and defeat cancer, albeit in the future. And the journey through the cell-as-universe persists, with its huge size akin to outer space now symbolic of the vast scale of the cancer problem.

The cell-as-universe sequences not only help to conjure up the vast scale and complexity of the problem of cancer but are also used to structure the script by providing biological context for the live-action sequences: the animation illustrating a biological subject followed by a live-action sequence that illustrates how science is tackling the subjects of the preceding animation, a structure that would be maintained in the final version of the film (see table 4.3). Thus an animated sequence in which the viewer travels through the cell as if through outer space is followed by a sequence on tissue culture research; an animated sequence on chromosomal separation is followed by live-action sequences of the science of heredity; an animation of the cell as a vast chemical industry is followed by live-action sequences on biochemical approaches to cancer; and an animated sequence on the external threats to the cell is followed by one on environmental causes of cancer. This structure of animation followed by live action forms the central core of the film and is bookended by the opening sequences (a film within a film sequence, the entry of Mr. Davis, and an animation of what has gone wrong with him) and the final ten minutes of the film, which is mainly live action. The human story of cancer is also reintroduced with an expanded version of the patient's narrative that appeared back in May: the story of Mr. Davis whose cancer causes him anxiety but is ultimately curable. The caution about gauging the horribleness of the cancer is no longer mentioned in this version of the script. However, Mr. Davis's cancer provides an opportunity to explore (in animation) the themes of normal and abnormal (cancerous) growth.

The theme of the character of the cancer scientist emerges with renewed emphasis in this script, as someone who is uninterested in material reward, driven by intellectual curiosity and humanitarian concern, completely involved in his or her research, a small part in a vast international effort against the disease. No

TABLE 4.3. The Final Structure of *Challenge* as Released in 1950

	Sequence title	Brief description of action	Live action/ Animation
1	Clinic and Titles	A hospital waiting room. Mr. Davis enters, and is taken to see a physician and two scientists concerning a tumor on his cheek.	Live action
2	Normal and Abnormal Growth	Mr. Davis becomes an outline, and a cell emerges that grows into an embryo and then a man, before the scene changes to the story of abnormal growth (cancer).	Animation
3	The Physician's Conference Room	We return to Mr. Davis, who is reassured by the physician that his cancer is a curable type, and is sent on his way. The physician is left alone looking at a slide of a (tumor?) cell, with the question: Why is the cancer problem so difficult?	Live action
4	Cell-as-Universe	The physician walks into the slide, shrinks, and disappears. We are traveling through the cell as if it were outer space, with constellations of cytosomes, centrosomes, and other parts of the cell.	Animation
5	Tissue Culture	The animation dissolves to a mouse in a cage, which becomes the starting point of a sequence on the use of cells grown outside the body in cancer research.	Live action
6	Cell-as-Universe (Genetics)	We are traveling through the cell again, this time to watch cell division and chromosome separation.	Animation
7	Genetics	A man, woman and child are in a laboratory, looking at a mouse —the hero of research—that becomes the starting point of a sequence on the role of mice and fruit flies in genetics research.	Live action
8	Cell-as-Universe	Next we return to the cell surrounded and sometime overlain with swirling images. Here the cell is supposed to be an industrial organism, breathing, feeding, transporting, converting, manufacturing, etc.	Animation

	Sequence title	Brief description of action	Live action/ Animation
9	Biochemistry	A sequence on research into biochemistry, the life processes of the cell, which merges into a tea-bag scene, in which scientists discuss the latest finding over lunch, designed to show the character of the scientist.	Live Action
10	Cell-as-Universe (Environmental Cancer)	A view of the cell surrounded by a swirling mist to denote environmental threats.	Animation
11	Environmental Cancer	A sequence on various environmental and occupational causes of cancer, how they are studied through field investigations, statistics, and laboratory research, and the importance of prevention.	Live action
12	Clinic	We now explore the use of radiation in cancer, a sequence in which Mr. Davis arrives in the rain at a clinic, where he is treated with X-rays. We then move to a section on those who are not as lucky as Davis to have a treatable cancer, to research to find a test for cancer, and the hope that science offers those with cancer.	Live Action
13	Scientists	A scientist in the office late at night talking with his wife, which returns us to an account of the character of the scientist, the long time period needed to train a scientist, and the vast international scope of the scientific endeavor against cancer. The sequence ends with students listening to a lecture on cancer, and watching what becomes the closing credits sequence	Live action
14	Closing credits	Cell-as-universe theme (echo of sequence 4), as the closing titles roll.	Animation

place here for those who might be tempted by the better pay and prospects of industry or (for Canadians) the United States. No place either for those whose goal is professional recognition. Now the filmmakers build on the character of the scientist developed in the earlier treatments, encouraging their intended audience to become research biologists or cancer researchers without offering more pay or better working conditions, or even the prospect of professional recognition. The internationalist theme is also emphasized here with the introduction of "foreigners" in different parts of the film, stressing the vast international effort against cancer, though some of these "foreigners" may have been French speakers, doubling as a nod to French Canadians.

The June 1949 script begins with a film-within-the-film.[52] The opening scene starts with a medium close shot of a symbolic photo mural or bas-relief of an unspecified scientific subject. The camera dollies back to reveal an assistant cameraman on a ladder adjusting a 750 (a light producing 750 foot-candle intensity). He is looking toward the cameraman (called Mitchell) as we continue to dolly back. The scene is a clinic waiting room. There are patients in chairs watching the proceedings. Film paraphernalia is scattered all about. There is considerable activity: simultaneous conversations, an electrician rolls in a light, a "Script girl"[53] at the rear of the scene, nurses around. At the end of the dolly, to one side of the frame, we see the director, a couple of nurses, an intern, a man in a business suit (the doctor), all watching the preparations.

The director and the doctor are talking. The former explains the aims of the movie (to illuminate the hope in cancer provided by science and research) and the doctor mentions the triumphs of modern medicine.[54] He looks around the assembled patients and points to examples of patients who have benefited from research on insulin in diabetes, penicillin, and the work of Ehrlich, Jenner, and Pasteur. Then someone calls out. "Action," and the film begins again with a repeat of the medium close shot of a symbolic photograph of a scientific subject, now accompanied by a triumphant chord of music, which continues, punctuating each successive title. A patient—Mr. Davis—enters the shot and is taken by a nurse to meet three scientists—one a doctor called Doug and the others, Drs. Ron Farrell and Peter McVicor. Davis is asked to remove his coat, and the three scientists begin a discussion of a paper by "Jennings" on growth.

We now transition to the first animated section of the movie—normal and abnormal growth. Mr. Davis becomes an outline, which reverts through embryo to egg. The animation then follows the normal growth, division, and differentiation of the cell and body organs until—using a time-lapse technique the embryo becomes a child that then becomes an adult man. The section on normal growth is accompanied by a musical "growth theme,"[55] which comes to a gradual stop with the adult man, and then suggests order and harmony, while the visuals build up an image of the intricate, complex structure of the body and of a multiplicity of purposeful and harmonious activities. The purpose of this section, the script tells us, is to emphasize the wonder of the human body as a purposeful, planned, and smooth-functioning machine to provide a contrast to the uncontrolled, disruptive, purposeless activity of the cancer cells. The narrator notes that sometimes the cells do not stop and start growing again. We now move to "abnormal growth"—the opening chord of the "cancer theme" "a strident, malignant, somewhat demonic perversion of the 'growth theme.'"[56] We watch a tumor form on the lip, pressing on neighboring tissues, and invading other parts of the body to form deadly new colonies. Eventually we return to the original lip site. The cells are still dividing, and they fill the screen. The narrator notes: "This is cancer!"[57] The scene is reminiscent of one in Constant's 1948 script, except the body is not killed.

We now return to Mr. Davis, who has a cancer of the lip. Doug the doctor, McVicor, and Farrell examine him and reassure him that the chances are ninety out of one hundred that that he can be cured. Davis lets out an audible sigh of relief—instruction: but not a broad one (perhaps an indication of the Canadian patient's self-restraint?)—and leaves after being told that he can begin treatment with his own doctor. Farrell and McVicor also head back to the lab and offer Davis a lift, which he refuses. Doug is alone in the room. He picks up a slide, inserts it in the projector, and then walks toward it. His shadow is cast onto the screen. The narrator asks why cancer is such a difficult problem.

We now transition to the second animated sequence: "Cell-as-Universe." Doug the doctor is walking into the picture, disappearing as he shrinks, "like an explorer who has vanished into a new world."[58] We begin a journey through the living cell, which is treated in terms of size and time as if it were indeed a universe; a tiny unit of life 1/2000th of an inch in size, but a world in itself. "Because of the scale used, it should give the effect of a journey through interstellar space. We pass strange bodies in motion in different planes, backs of vapours [*sic*], flowing strands of viscous liquid, etc." [59] "Look at these vast spaces!" notes the narrator,[60] "This is not a universe of stars and planets, but the universe within a single living cell." The vast scale of the imagery conjures up the vast scale of the research problem, for within the single living cell is "the answer to the riddle of cancer, tied up inextricably with the mystery of life itself." [61]

The next sequence is live action and begins the story of how science is seeking to understand the problems of life and of cancer. It focuses on tissue culture research, and how tissue can be kept alive indefinitely once removed from an animal. The visuals show an animal (the script asks: "rabbit?" [62]) asleep in a cage that stirs when approached by a scientist, before we move to a view of the scientist and his assistant manipulating tissue cultures. We see cancers grown in glass, transferred to egg yolks, and cultivated in animals. Those in tissue cultures are poisoned, their growth is measured, among other operations.

We then move to the third animated sequence, also labeled "Cell-as-Universe," in which we "wander through the cell (as universe) slowly approaching, as though it were a distant moon, the nucleus. As we approach, and while yet distant from the center of action, the nucleus goes from metaphase to telaphase."[63] Something amazing is about to happen. "From here on," the shooting script notes,[64] "the total effect is that of an infinitesimal and quite innocent spectator who finds himself caught up in some cosmic revolution. We see an inside 'virus-eyeview' of a single mitotic division." We have slowly zoomed into the center of a division. There follows a cut or mix to an exterior view of the daughter cells separating as the music climaxes. This serves as a lead in to the next live-action sequence on genetics, which involves three individuals, a boy (David), his mother and Uncle Frank. There is an obvious family resemblance, highlighting the theme of heredity. All three are looking at something with extreme interest—it could be the previous animation, but it is not. It is a mouse. We now are introduced to mouse genetics and its relevance to cancer, and later the genetics of the fruit fly.

The next animated sequence, another "Cell-as-Universe," focuses on the biochemical processes of the cell. The camera travels through the higher reaches of this realm, looking down on countless activities below. Interspersed are closer views of process: conversion, breakdowns, changes of form and of quantity, solids to gases and, conversely, gases to solids. The script tells us that it is "like a tour through a series of vast factories in full production, in which no foreman or recognizable goods are in evidence, yet which achieve an overwhelming feeling of ordered process, of planned and ceaseless activity."[65] The narrator meanwhile tells us that the cell breathes, feeds, transports, converts, manufactures, breaks down, and builds up. "The cell is not just a single factory, it is [a] tremendous complex of chemical industries. These are the processes we associate with life."[66] And the question is how the processes of the normal cell differ from those of the cancer cell. This serves as prelude to the next live-action sequence on biochemistry.

The biochemistry live-action sequence begins with a Warburg apparatus measuring the difference in respiration between cancer and normal cells. But then the film veers in another direction to focus on the scientist him/herself. The next shot is of a teabag, and a doctor lifts a beaker off the stand with tongs. It is lunchtime and the instructions tell us that the purpose of this scene is "to capture a little of the character of the scientist and his co-workers... their complete absorption in their work."[67] The lunch table is in the middle of the laboratory, and the camera is to capture the scientific apparatus there. Margaret is invited to lunch, but she is finishing her research. The commentator intones "Time, persistence, patience.... There is no royal road to facts, to knowledge, to understanding... to an answer to the eternal question... 'What happens inside the cell to start the cancer process?'"[68] Someone has penciled into the margins of the script "foreign accent?"[69]—next to the scientist's lunchtime chat—suggesting that perhaps this scene may also have been intended to illustrate the international character of science.

We now move to the next animated sequence—another cell-as-universe—that briefly explores environmental cancers. A single cell seen against a background of swirling mist. This is followed by live-action sequences that explore different environmental causes of cancer—the sun, cosmic rays, work (occupational hazards including chemicals, radiation, tar), and the importance of statistics to the identification of these causes—and the dismissal of race as a decisive factor. We see a test tube inverted and a liquid pour out and down into a shiny container. We then transition to an animated cell-as-universe sequence, so that it seems briefly as if the contents of the test tube in the live action sequence are pouring into the cell in the animation sequence. The commentator asks what this chemical does to the cell. How does it start the cancer?

At this point, the structure of an animated sequence followed by a live-action sequence gives way to a series of live-action sequences, absent any animation. We start with a sequence on therapeutics: Mr. Davis is going for treatment, radiotherapy, and the film delivers a message that mixes optimism about Mr. Davis and patients like him with concern for those for whom such hope does not (yet) exist. Much more can be done now than a few years ago, the script tells us, yet many cancers cannot be identified until they have grown so much that they cannot be treated effectively (the message of early detection and treatment that dominated both American and Canadian educational campaigns against the disease). There follows a plea for a cheap reliable test for cancer, before we move to another sequence that stresses the international character of the research endeavor against cancer—we see a conference auditorium with scientists, some in conversation in a corridor: "One or two recognizable as foreigners."[70]

The next (live-action) sequence returns to the theme of the character of the scientist. Here a scientist is talking on the phone late at night to his wife about their son Jimmy, and bills to be paid—domestic stuff. He is in his office; it is late at night. He is tired but relaxed. The camera examines the desk, bookshelves, and office: "The visuals here and in succeeding shots in office will be of carefully selected and illustrative materials and equipment revealing nature of office and character of scientist."[71] The narrator meanwhile tells us how long it takes to train a scientist—twenty years, plus "a better-than-average share of intelligence and imagination,"[72] and echoing the concerns of the NCI and NCIC the narration noted: "These are qualities that are much in demand . . . in industry for instance . . . where salaries are higher and working conditions better."[73]

The man finishes his conversation and leaves the office. We see him walking out of the lab at night, while the narrator tells us about his character with a series of questions. What keeps them in research? The fascination of the problem? A natural, dogged, persistent curiosity? There is a brief account of progress, a sideswipe at quacks and ignoramuses, and then a series of questions about what may cause cancer. The scientist reappears—the next day, in morning light—and talks with students. Students enter a lecture theater, and the lecturer tells us and them that science is converging on the mystery of life. The movie closes with a shot of a scientist in heroic composition, in deep concentration, at a micro-manipulator, delicately making his adjustments. The narrator or lecturer concludes with a ghost of the June 1948 plea for better funding, now stripped of its nationalist undertones: "Final understanding will be no happy accident, it will be the result of applied intelligence, of time, money and unceasing effort . . . above all, unceasing effort."[74]

June-November 1949

Sometime between June and August, Constant and his collaborators scrapped the opening film-within-a-film sequence and the symbolic photograph and replaced it with another hospital waiting-room scene—this new scene opens with a high-angle long shot of the waiting room filled with patients sitting on long wooden benches—the effect, a new script tells us, is vault-like and echoey. This script is labeled a shooting script, but it seems to have been produced during or after the shooting of the live-action sequences, perhaps to guide the editor; a cleaned-up version of the annotated June 1949 shooting script used by Parker while on location.[75]

In the new script, the camera scans various patients while the narrator intones a list of past medical triumphs against diabetes, tetanus, bacterial endocarditis, and other diseases. This list provides an opportunity to set out the international flavor of science because the research that led the defeat of these diseases came from Canada, Japan, England, and elsewhere. It also provides the introduction to the challenge of cancer. The narrator notes that today the resources of science are targeted at this disease, symbolized by Mr. Davis, who enters the picture and approaches a nurse who takes him to see Doctor Doug and Doctors Farrell and McVicor.

The introduction of the list of scientific greats may have come from the sponsoring agencies themselves. Not only did they want to portray the effort against cancer as an international effort, but they were also keen to recognize the achievements of the other cosponsor. Thus, the NCI tissue culturist, Wilton R. Earle (1902–64), suggested that the Canadians Frederick Banting and Charles Best (famed for their discovery of insulin) be mentioned in the opening scene listing scientific greats.[76] They were included, as were Americans, George Hoyt Whipple, George Richards Minot, and William Parry Murphy (famed for their discoveries concerning liver therapy in cases of anemia). A synopsis prepared for the Canadian premiere noted that the scientists listed in the opening scene were "working all over the world."[77]

The scene with the three scientists—Dr. Doug and his colleagues—is also changed: the discussion of Jennings' paper is gone, and the chit-chat between Davis and the doctors is also shortened. Now we get to the point quickly, as Doug the doctor informs Davis, introducing Farrell and McVicor: "These gentlemen are research scientists. Just put your coat over there. (He winks broadly). As soon as they find the answer your worries are over."[78] This serves as an introduction to the first animation scene—normal and abnormal growth—which is unchanged, as is the next scene (Mr. Davis' diagnosis), and the rest of the movie

At this point Constant might have thought the writing was over, but it was not. Foster reported at the end of August that "Constant had produced a script which he regarded as final but Glover has pushed his nose back into the trough for further development."[79] Indeed, Constant's work did not end until much of the live-action shooting was over. Constant traveled with the film crew on location, and he seems to have spent time on the set writing and rewriting, adapting the script to the contingencies of the shoot, as well as acting a minor part in the film (figure 3.1). The script thus continued to evolve.

Sometime between August and October/November 1949, the character of Doug—one of the three men who review Mr. Davis's case—changed into Ross, and that of McVicor into Dr. Ramm, a South Asian figure played by a Sikh actor, Jerneja Singh "Jerry" Hundal (figure 7.2).[80] (Race here is perhaps symbolic of the international character of science, though Hundal had lived for years in

Canada). The name McVicor was given to Farrell's character. The international theme was also enhanced by the addition of a black female student and some French-speaking scientists, as much the "foreign accent" mentioned in the June shooting script as a gesture to the French-Canadian audience.

There were some other changes. The ending was modified so that the film concludes not with the scientist in heroic mode, but with a scene in a lecture theatre, the lecturer ending the film with words adapted from Constant's June 1948 script: "we are dealing here with an enormous problem . . . the problem of life itself"; [81] and the sequence on an international meeting about cancer was cut, and likely mutated into the concluding student lecture sequence (table 4.3). But some these changes seem to have happened as the film itself begun production, and the filmmakers sought to adapt the script to the contingencies of filmmaking. The script had served its purpose of bringing in the Americans and had been changed to meet the needs and agendas of the new sponsors, the concerns about Constant's limitations as a scriptwriter, and the scriptwriters' struggle to get the major themes across in ways that they thought would work visually and aurally. It would continue to change as the filmmaking proper got underway. Text and paper were to become sound and image.

CHAPTER 5

Producing and Directing

O NCE THE AGREEMENT WAS signed with the Americans in Febru-
ary/March 1949, Foster faced two urgent tasks. One was to revise the
June 1948 script (the subject of the last chapter); the other was to put
together a film crew. To that end, he assigned two NFB employees to oversee
the movie: Guy Glover, newly returned from the United States, would be its
producer; and the thirty-year-old Morten Parker would be director. Together
Glover and Parker set out to recruit a team to make the movie. Parker recalls
meeting with Glover to figure out who in the NFB was available and who they
wanted, and then arranged for them to be assigned to the project.[1]

Glover's and Parker's approach to the film—and the sponsors' demands—was
informed by their long experience of working at the NFB, and especially by the
ideas of the founder of the NFB, the documentary filmmaker John Grierson
(figure 3.1). Grierson believed that the goal of documentary film was not to capture the phenomenal—the mess of events that paraded before a camera—but
to use the phenomenal to reach a more abstract or generalizable reality. To this
end, he advocated what he called "the creative treatment of actuality,"[2] the use,
for example, of dramatic recreations and animation to tell a story about something much bigger than the details that the camera captured. Thus, the goal of
documentary filmmaking to Grierson was not to record every detail of a subject,
but to present a broader argument, which meant, when the idea was extended
to *Challenge*, the presentation of an argument for making the body, cancer, and
the cell objects of science, subject to its interventions, and for enticing audiences
to think of cancer as a possible scientific career.

This approach to filmmaking had been there in embryo in the narratives outlined in the shooting script. This was to be a film that would use symbols to
evoke the character of the patient and scientist, the wonder of the body and cell,
the excitement of the opportunities open to investigators, the vast scale of the
cancer problem for science, and the hope the latter offered—all to show how
science approached the body, cell, and cancer, the potential of future research,

and to tempt people into studying cancer. Glover and Parker had been involved in the development of this script, but once written their task was to turn paper into celluloid, and this meant bringing in other technologies of filmmaking—cameras, animation, ambient sound, narration, music, special effects, and editing—to conjure up these themes. Guided by the script, Glover and Parker would seek to coordinate these technologies to present the film's argument through the creative treatment of actuality. The sponsor's hopes of using this film to tempt new young scientists into cancer research would be framed by the hand of Grierson and those who followed him.

Glover and Parker

That Glover and Parker interpreted this commission through the lens of the NFB's filmmaking culture and practices should come as little surprise. Both had long worked for the NFB, including for Grierson before he left in 1945. Thus, when Foster assigned them to this film, he was appointing people steeped in the filmmaking culture of the NFB. He was also appointing people whose skills complemented one another. Glover had a background in animation, about which Parker was less knowledgeable, so he oversaw much of the animation work. Glover's roles thus blurred the boundary between producer and director, especially in the animation sequences, while Parker was to concentrate on shooting the live-action sequences, before joining with Glover to oversee how the two—animation and live action—should be stitched together in the editing room, along with the musical score and the narration.

(Herbert) Guy Glover (1909–88)[3] had joined the NFB in 1942 as the production assistant to Norman McLaren (also his life partner), one of the first hires in McLaren's new animation unit, before he moved on to directing and producing at the NFB[4] (figure 6.1). After a time away from the NFB (1946–49), he returned as producer in Unit A, one of four NFB production units (A, B, C, and D), each run by an executive producer. *Challenge* was his first production after his return. The specific reasons for his assignment to the film are unknown, but he had two skills that were particularly useful to this movie: like Constant he had had an early training in biology; he also had a background in animation.

As producer of *Challenge*, Glover's role was to bring the film in on budget and on time, as well as overseeing the writing, directing, editing, sound and musical composition. He may also have consulted with Foster over who to hire as director, alongside his work of figuring out who else to hire for the film. Thus, Glover was also involved in the rewrites of the script that Constant, Parker and others made after June 1949; he contributed to the live-action scenes when he got involved in selecting locations for the filming (though he does not seem to have traveled to the shoots); and later he had input into the editing of the movie, its sound effects, and its music. All these roles were part of his task of keeping *Challenge* to schedule and to budget (though the schedule set out in the 1949 agreement slipped, and he failed to control costs when the animation budget spiraled up, and the NFB had to ask the Americans for more money). In this last task, he was answerable to Ralph Foster, who kept a close eye on the movie until he left the NFB in January 1950.

Glover's involvement, then was much more than as someone who coordinated and kept an eye on the books and the clock. He had an important creative role, especially in the animation sequences of the movie. Indeed, according to Colin Low, one of the two animators on *Challenge*, Glover was *the* cohesive artistic figure behind the movie. Part of the reason he said this was probably Glover's background in animation. Glover himself emphasized this, and in later years claimed that he brought an animator's perspective to live-action films. Where the non-animator viewed the shot, he noted, the animator drew the frame, and so learned a lot about the nature of cinematographically synthesized motion, and therefore also about relative speeds, pacing, rhythm and about what the camera does to the material it captures. The animator's perspective was thus not simply about animation, but an approach to filmmaking more generally.

The animator's perspective, to Glover, informed filmmaking in several ways. Glover claimed that the animator's need to give life to his drawings—to create a "film organism,"[5] as he described it—meant that when he turned to live action, he or she was acutely aware that film was so much more that what was seen through the camera. Thus, Glover claimed that the animator knew better than most that great care had to be taken with the planning of the live-action shoots to ensure that it worked as a film when it came time to put all the sequences together. Filmmaking—including documentary and educational filmmaking—was a creative process, not simply a faithful reproduction of what the camera recorded, he claimed, echoing Grierson. The animator recognized—perhaps more than other filmmakers, according to Glover—that it was crucial to avoid what he called "the most treacherous artifice of all—the artifice which maintains that to 'bring 'em back alive' is gospel truth."[6] Put another way, what the camera brought back, imprinted on film, was only the beginning of the creative process, and not everything needed to be brought back.

Such comments about the animator's perspective on filmmaking helped to rationalize Glover's involvement in the live action as well as the animation. I

have noted that he was involved in planning the locations for the live-action sequences of *Challenge*. He also saw a role for himself in overseeing the scripting
and shooting of the live action that Morten Parker was to direct. For Glover,
such oversight alongside careful planning would also facilitate later parts of the
film's production—the editing and special effects necessary, for example, to the
transitions between live action and animation. Thus, he inserted his views on how
the film should be directed and shot as part of his role as producer, helping Parker
figure out what was financially feasible and how to get it done on time. Crucially
for a producer concerned about costs, Glover claimed that the nature of their
work taught animators to be concise, and having learned brevity, they carried this
perspective into situations where conciseness was not so necessary. Brevity and
planning would be essential to controlling the costs of a film, and they also gave
the producer a reason for interjecting his ideas on how the film should be made.

     This animator's perspective on filmmaking was no doubt congenial to Low,
but there were also other reasons he might have seen Glover as the creative force.
As part of his effort to keep *Challenge* on schedule and within budget, Glover
had to pull the various aspects of the movie together. He was involved in recruiting people to the film, including Low and his co-animator, Evelyn Lambart.
His efforts to oversee the budget and schedule gave him many opportunities to
talk to all those involved in production about issues beyond his formal remit.
Given his long experience and interest in the imaginative aspects of filmmaking
it was almost inevitable that these discussions blurred into creative issues, more
formally the province of the director. Perhaps with different people or circumstances this blurring of the boundaries between producer and director could
have been a problem. But Glover and Parker seem to have had a good working
relationship, and if this blurring of their roles raised any tensions between them,
they do not surface in the archives or the recollections of those I interviewed.[7]

     Low's perception of Glover's role may, however, overstate the case, for the an-
imation was carried out quite separately from the rest of the movie. Buried away
in the animation studios on Sparks Street in Ottawa, some distance from the
main NFB buildings on St. John Street, Low would have been unaware of much
else going on with the film.[8] He had close connections with Glover, who had
considerable interest in and experience with animation, and who provided Low
and Lambart with suggestions as to the style of animating the body and cell they
adopted. By contrast the director, Morten Parker, had relatively little knowledge
of the technicalities of animation.[9] Before the animators set to work, he talked
to them about the subjects that needed to be animated and the length of each
sequence. But then he left them to get on with it, except for periodic consultations

and progress reports. His focus was on the live-action and location work, which Low would have been only dimly aware of. Parker would turn his attention to the animation again when the location shots were done, and it was time for the editor, Douglas Tunstell, to piece the live action and animation into a coherent narrative.

Morten Parker (1919–2014) was born in Winnipeg, Manitoba (figure 7.1). He graduated from the University of Manitoba, worked as a journalist on the *Winnipeg Tribune*, wrote for radio, and published an entertainment paper in Winnipeg before joining the NFB on June 5, 1943.[10] In an interview, Parker recalled that he moved to Ottawa because Gudrun, his wife, had obtained a job at the NFB, one of several women filmmakers recruited to the NFB during the war, along with Evelyn Spice Cherry (1906–90), who had made the Saskatchewan Cancer Commission's *That They May Live* in 1942.[11] At the NFB, he learned the art of filmmaking on the job, and within a few years was writing and directing NFB movies, including *Maps We Live By*, 1947 (co-writer with Gudrun Parker), *The Postman*, 1947 (director), *The Home Town Paper*, 1948 (director), and *Family Circles*, 1949 (director; co-writer with Gudrun Parker), before being assigned to *Challenge*. For Parker, *Challenge* was simply another assignment: he had no prior interest in subject as a filmmaker, though he noted that his father had recently died from cancer.[12] Within the NFB he had a growing reputation as a safe pair of hands and, because of the American connection, *Challenge* needed a safe pair of hands. This was to be one of the big NFB productions of the year.

The Hand of Grierson

Given Glover's and Parker's training within the NFB, it should be no surprise that *Challenge* drew on NFB approaches to filmmaking in the late 1940s and early 1950s. Its mix of live action and animation was strung together with the voice-of-god commentary that many NFB documentaries used to pull together the narrative. It used dramatic recreations and animation to tell its story, Grierson's "creative treatment of actuality." And it sought to target a relatively well-educated, technically skilled group of people; individuals whom NFB leaders felt might be expected to play a significant social or political role, in this case through cancer research. These approaches—albeit first applied to documentary film—had been embodied in Maurice Constant's June 1948 script before Parker and Glover became involved, and they remained in the rewrites of 1949.

Both Parker and Glover had trained and worked under John Grierson until his resignation in 1945, and the film contains inflections of Grierson's filmmaking philosophy. The first has already been mentioned—the creative treatment of actuality. As Ian Aitken notes, the roots of this approach can be traced to Grierson's interest in philosophical idealism, and its impact on his vision of film as an instrument of social persuasion.[13] For Grierson, an idealist approach to filmmaking meant that naturalistic representation had to be subordinated to symbolic expression. The task of the filmmaker was not to represent the particular and superficial phenomena of empirical reality, but to use the phenomena to reach a more abstract, generalized reality, the essence of the age, its underlying historical forces: a view that meshed well with Glover's animator's perspective of documentary filmmaking as a creative process, not simply a faithful presentation of what the camera recorded. This meant that there was no necessary contradiction between documentary and drama—drama could reveal the essence of the age, more than a focus on documenting what Grierson called the "bank holiday of frenzied events,"[14] the mess of details that might appear before the camera.

Dramatic recreations were thus central to Grierson's vision of the documentary film, and found an inflection—albeit, perhaps, stripped of its philosophical idealism—in *Challenge*, which used dramatic recreations and animation to represent the nature of research, the character of the scientist, the scale of the scientific problem, and the wonder of nature. Thus, Mr. Davis is described as a "symbolic patient." [15] "He is symbolic of hundreds of thousands of patients with a disease that presents one of the most baffling problems of science—the challenge of cancer."[16] So too, scientists and physicians such as Dr. McVicor were symbolic of the many scientists and physicians working on cancer, with their selflessness, lack of interest in material reward, and commitment to research. As Brian Winston argues regarding documentary film, individuals within the movie stand both for themselves and the group of persons of their type; the part stands for the class.[17]

But symbolism was not simply asserted in the script or the pamphlets that publicized the film. It was also created in the course of the making of the film by the actors who served the roles of symbolic scientists and patients; by the editing that helped determine the rhythm of the movie (for example, slow unhurried pacing to symbolize hope; faster cuts to symbolize urgency or concern); by the camera work and lighting (such as high-angle shot and bright lighting in the opening sequence [see table 4.3, sequence 1] used to emphasize the calm and hope of the symbolic "houses of healing" [18] or the low-angle shots that help to emphasize the threat posed by cancer to Mr. Davis when he first enters as the symbolic patient [sequence 1]); and through the soundtrack and music (as when the noise of scientific equipment represents the unceasing work of science [sequence 9], or the music seeks to depict normal and abnormal growth [sequence 2]). Attempts to use sound to create symbolic meaning had been part of scripts from the very beginning (recall the woman's whine in Constant's June 1948 script, when it transforms into the sound of an animal) and they remained (even without the animal whine) in later iterations of the script and in the filming itself.

The second example of Griersonian philosophy in *Challenge* concerns his suspicion of the capacity of mass communications to reform the public. As Aitken shows, in the 1920s Grierson's engagement with the Chicago School of Sociology and the work of Walter Lippmann made him skeptical about the capacity of the "rational citizen," of democracy itself, and of mass communications to offset what he saw as the inadequacies of mass society.[19] While he saw film as a tool of social action (a view echoed by Parker[20]), he also was influenced by contemporary beliefs that society must be governed and guided by elites. In his view, documentary films were most effective when directed to the middle classes, the educated, who might, in his view, play a significant role in democratic processes. He distinguished between a "rational" and "mature" citizenry, the latter of which could be created by informing audiences of the significant generative forces in a society, and achieved through mass communications practices aimed at an intuitive, nonintellectual level. *Challenge* was consonant with such a view. Its target audiences were not the masses, but the small group of science students who might one day become cancer researchers, and as a secondary audience, the educated public who might be persuaded to support cancer research, and the film used practices such as dramatic recreations that aimed as much at the nonintellectual level as the rational. Its aim was to create a cadre of scientists who might one day lead the fight against cancer, much as Dallas Johnson had imagined consumer organizations as leaders of a relatively passive public, and Grierson imagined the middle classes as leaders by virtue of their involvement in the democratic process. From all these perspectives, the less-educated public (as consumer, politically active, or concerned about cancer) was imagined as relatively docile or (if active) unreliable, and in need of expert leadership, which in the case of the film would be provided in part by the voice-of-god narrator who explained to the viewer what was going on in the screen.

Third, *Challenge* also reflected Grierson's vision of the social as superior to the personal and individual.[21] Grierson saw the state as a positive force, the highest level of the social, a view that would have been congenial to the founder of the state-financed NFB, who saw a trend away from laissez-faire toward government planning, coordination, and leadership of national social and economic life, and a consequent need for state involvement in public education to support these activities.[22] In the narrative of *Challenge*, the state has no role, except for the mention of the government sponsors of the film in the titling, the supporters of most research. Instead, individual scientists—as they emerged in the narratives of later iterations of the scripts—are subordinate to another social organization, the broader international community of scientists. They were part of a vast international scientific effort to understand and defeat cancer, each scientist contributing day-by-day, hour-by-mind-numbing-hour small pieces of knowledge to the emerging picture of this group of diseases. They were ciphers in a vast war being waged against these diseases, but paradoxically also persons of special character—people so absorbed in their work, so committed to solving the scientific conundrum of cancer that they revealed a selfless quality. They were uninterested in material reward, willing to subordinate themselves to a higher, humanitarian goal of defeating cancer, and to play their small part in the enormous effort.

These inflections of Grierson's philosophy were present in all of *Challenge*'s many scripts, though Parker and Glover sometimes saw other factors than Grierson as shaping the film. Thus when, for example, I write that dramatic recreation in *Challenge* was "perhaps, stripped of its philosophical idealism," it was because while the filmmakers used dramatic recreation, they generally did not appeal to such a philosophy, and they sometimes invoked other explanations for its use. Parker, for example, explained the turn to dramatic recreation in the 1940s and 1950s not in terms of philosophical idealism but because many documentary filmmakers wanted to move into narrative cinema. Grierson's idea of the creative treatment of actuality provided a useful justification for incorporating such narrative techniques into their films.[23] Glover, as I have mentioned, saw dramatic recreation from the animator's perspective.

Glover himself later noted that the "creative interpretation of reality"[24] as he put it, was central to a Canadian approach to short films that emerged after 1946, which at its best also involved the orderly exposition of the film material, neat and economical cutting, and exacting technical standards. And he, retrospectively, included *Challenge* among these types of film, its combination of elaborate animation and conventional live action a contrast to the workaday "simple film idioms"[25] of the majority of the NFB's informational, instructional, and educational movies. Many Canadian short films had serious faults, he complained, echoing and expanding on the concerns of the Canadian Cancer Society about the quality of wartime films. Subjects were not well researched, "the main cause of a superficiality of treatment and a distressing lack of humility before the facts."[26] He also complained of the tendency of the films of the NFB to add a partial or safe view of controversial material; for the commentary in a film to overinflate the importance of the material; and he noted "even when over-writing was absent, lack-lustre verbal material often weighed down the visuals." [27] Few directors, he claimed, showed strong instinct for pure cinematic treatment, a situation not helped by the dependence of many films on sponsors who felt impelled to interfere so that most films suffered from an indifferent handling of the subject in terms of planned or "choreographed"[28] movement, and from imposed forms which seemed, he noted, to be accidental. "Little grasp was demonstrated of the principle of the pacing," he claimed,[29] "either of action within the frame or of cutting (the control of the rhythm in which the shot or scene is changed). The rhythmic structure, therefore, was often slack and arbitrary." In addition, he complained about poor dramatic writing and direction of actors.

It should be noted that these criticisms—surprisingly (for an NFB insider) made in public—were published in 1958, well after *Challenge* was released, but Glover had been mulling them for some time, and they are suggestive of the concerns that he brought to this film. While Grierson's notion of "creative treatment of actuality/reality" was praised, the institution that he created—the NFB—had produced countless films that had not lived up to the ideal, and the risk was that *Challenge* would succumb to such problems. Given the resources thrown at it, this was not a film that would suffer from a lack of research. But the filmmakers had to struggle against the board's tendency to play it safe and for sponsors to interfere—this in addition to all the other problems that Glover noted. These may have been the consequence of filmmaking culture at the NFB as much as the fault of the filmmakers themselves. *Challenge*, for Glover, was not only about the challenge of cancer, but also the challenge of making a quality film within the constraints imposed by the culture of the NFB and its filmmakers.

Finally, it is likely that Glover would have had problems with elements of the moral perspective through which Grierson viewed the underlying historical forces, the essence of the age. As Aitken shows, Grierson defined positive ethical values (strength, simplicity, energy, directness, hardness, decency, courage, duty, and upstanding power—some of which were part of the character of the scientist in *Challenge*) and negative ones (sophistication, sentimentality, lounge-lizards, excessive sexuality, homosexuality, nostalgia, bohemianism, status-seeking and social climbing—none of which appear in the character of the scientist in *Challenge*).[30] It is, however, likely that Glover would have rejected Grierson's definition of negative values. Both he and McLaren were guarded about their sexual preferences, but they were well known as a couple within the small world of the NFB, discreet if open.[31] By 1949, they were living together in a flock-wallpapered apartment in Ottawa, where they held regular parties attended by many senior NFB people, including Ross McLean, the commissioner of the NFB. (Colin

Low, then quite junior, recalls some of these parties, with Louis Applebaum, the composer on *Challenge*, playing the piano.[32]) He also continued a love affair with ballet, the theater, and other arts. Grierson was a mentor to Glover, encouraging his interest in production and direction. He and McLaren would attend parties at the Griersons', and Glover noted that Grierson himself "never stood on formality—even after hours he was apt to drop in at their homes for a drink and chat."[33] But Glover embodied many of the qualities that Grierson publicly questioned.

Glover's love of theater, ballet, and the arts, and his connections to networks of gay men, were an asset when it came to the "creative treatment of actuality" in *Challenge*. But they also helped to subvert Grierson's moral compass, and to create an ironic subtext to the movie. Perhaps as a consequence of his interest in the arts, Glover helped to introduce into *Challenge* the work of the prominent homosexual artist, Pavel Tchelitchew.[34] Glover himself had been questioned by the RCMP in its investigations of subversion within the NFB, and there was an irony in the fact of a homosexual producer and homosexual artist shaping a work intended for two governments—Canadian and American—that saw homosexuality as a Cold War threat to national security.[35] There was also an irony in a homosexual producer producing a movie in which the character of the scientist—at least the male scientist, even if he embodied some of Grierson's positive characteristics—is portrayed as suburban, married, and (presumably) heterosexual, albeit keeping his love at home while he attended to his other love, his science.

Meetings

Parker's remembrance is of a series of meeting with Glover where they discussed not only who was available within the NFB, but also how the film might be put together.[36] The shooting script had already created a structure for the film, which would help with the planning both he and Glover expected. It also provided some of the key symbolism that would help them structure the creative interpretation of reality—the symbolic patient and scientist, the image of the cell as universe, and other symbols they could use to subordinate naturalistic representation to symbolic expression, and so rise above the mess of details on screen: the creative interpretation of reality as Glover echoes Grierson. But the shooting script was only a start. Glover and Parker would meet regularly during the making of the film, discussing what worked and what did not, changing the script along the way, with Constant's input and that of the animators, cameraman, editors, and special effects people. However, attention had now begun to shift from the paper technologies of the script to the other technologies of the film.

CHAPTER 6

Animating the Movie

O NE OF PARKER'S AND Glover's first tasks was to involve the animation unit in the movie (figure 6.1). To this end they turned for advice to Norman McLaren (1914–87), the head of the unit, and eventually two of his protégés—Evelyn Lambart (1914–99) and Colin Low (1926–2016)— were assigned to the film. Both Lambart and Low had trained at the NFB: Lambart had learned her craft as a student of McLaren; Low had learned his craft from both Lambart and McLaren. It was no small wonder then that they approached the film using animation techniques developed by McLaren in the 1940s, fleshing out the Griersonian and animator's perspectives of the producer and director. The latter perspectives might have guided how Glover and Parker approached their commission, but McLaren's animation techniques were what allowed the filmmakers to conjure up the worlds of the body, cancer, and the cell so central to it. The film was to inspire and challenge young audiences through its portrayal of these worlds, and McLaren's techniques were the foundation on which these depictions were built.

Having close connections with the animation unit, Glover likely advised on the use of these techniques, as did McLaren, but the surprise for all of them was the film also employed animation techniques that were brought to the film from outside. The NFB had appointed a scientific adviser, Vito Faustin (V.F.) Bazilauskas (1915–87), to guide Lambart and Low as they illustrated the cell, the body, and cancer. But Bazilauskas, a physician, medical illustrator and filmmaker, went beyond his remit. Not only did he guide Lambart and Low on the science, but he also provided an animation technique that solved some technical problems with the environmental and biochemical cancer sections of the movie. The paradox is that in so doing he also helped to move the animation away from a strict focus on scientific accuracy. He helped Lambart and Low conjure up symbols such as the cell-as-universe that seemed to some viewers to be more fantastical than factual.

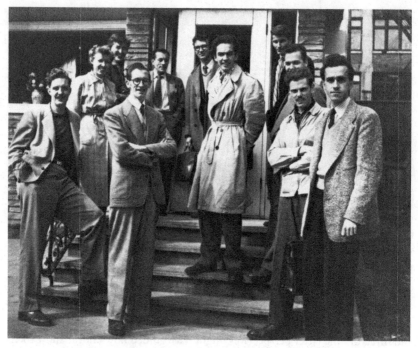

FIGURE 6.1. The NFB animation unit, no date, probably late 1940s or early 1950s. From left to right: Barry Helmer, Janet Young Preston, Evelyn Lambart,* Sidney Goldsmith,** Guy Glover,* Norman McLaren,** Colin Low,* Robert Verrall,** Marcel Racicot, Wolf Koenig, Grant Munro. The asterisks refer to those who contributed to *Challenge*, * = credited, ** = uncredited. Source: National Film Board of Canada, reprinted courtesy of the NFB.

The use of such symbols did not begin with animators. The shooting script had explicitly labeled the world of the cell as a universe or outer space in miniature, and Lambart and Low adapted McLaren's animation techniques to illustrate travel through the cell as if it were outer space with the various parts of the cell like planets or constellations, seemingly at great distance, separated by the darkness of this outer/inner space. In the Griersonian imagination, such symbols were a means to a more abstract or generalizable reality. To the scriptwriters and the animators, the vast scale of outer space was to be symbolic of the enormity of the cancer problem, the darkness encountered there was to be symbolic of scientific ignorance or uncertainty and by extension the opportunities for researchers entering the field, inspired by the majesty and awe of it all. This approach, the animators hoped, would create the symbolic language that would enthuse and challenge young scientists with the wonder of the body and cell and the threat posed by cancer. For scientists viewing the film, however, there were tricky questions about the boundaries between the real and imaginary: they wanted scientific accuracy. To the animators, however, strict adherence to scientific accuracy would make for a very dull film. Symbols such as the cell-as-universe might not be entirely accurate, but they were a key to the animators' efforts.

But the animation was about much more than about cancer, recruitment, and science. For Low—and likely also for Lambart—this was an opportunity to begin dialogues with other artists and film genres. Low, for example, saw himself as commenting on the work of the artist Pavel Tchelitchew, not only borrowing the idea of his so-called x-ray images to portray the inner world of the body and cell, but also engaging with his ideas about the meaning of such images, or more accurately the meanings as interpreted by Tchelitchew's critics. The film thus emerges as a mix of visual references to the arts—not only Tchelichew, but images of the anatomized body produced by Bernard Albinus and Vesalius, and the Apollo Belvedere. Bazilauskas's mysterious, otherworldly environmental imagery helped cement the connections with space travel—intermingled with allusions to scientific illustrations of the cell and time-lapse photography, so that visually it was sometimes very difficult to tell where the arts began and the science ended.

Structure

Of the fourteen sequences in the film, six are animated. The first, normal and abnormal growth, was, as the title suggests, a demonstration of normal and cancerous growth, and of what is wrong with Mr. Davis, the symbolic patient (table 4.3: sequence 2). Most of the rest of the animation (sequences 4, 6, 8, and 10) function as a series of introductions to the live-action sequences on the work of science and the character of the scientist: animated sequences on cell division, on chromosomes and heredity, on cell biochemistry, and on environmental threats to the cell were to be followed respectively by live-action sequences on tissue culture, genetic, biochemical, and epidemiological research on cancer. The final animation sequence (14) is there as a background to the closing credits, and to give visual emphasis to the lecturer's comments in the preceding live action (13) that, in converging on the mysteries of the cell, scientists are grappling with an "enormous problem. . . . the problem of life itself." [1]

Each animation sequence is framed by the live-action sequence that precedes and (except for the last sequence, 14) succeeds it. Visually, each begins with a sequence in which the live action mutates into animation and ends (except for 14)

with one in which the animation mutates back into live action again, often via a
fade or dissolve created on the NFB's optical printer that allowed the live action
and animation to briefly overlap. Aurally, they often begin with a question posed
by the narrator (which the animation sequence then answers) and with the first
musical chord: often an electronic-sounding "Special Effects"[2] (as the composer,
Louis Applebaum, labels it in in the score). Music also marks important transitions within an animation sequence (recall how in sequence 2 the script wanted
the music for cancer to be a demonic perversion of the normal growth theme),
and it also helps to mark the end of the animation. As each animation sequence
concludes, so does the music. Most of the live action is without music.

Although the beginning and the end of each animation sequence is well
marked, the borders between the live action and animation are often porous.
The filmmakers used the NFB's newly acquired optical printer, operated by the
Optical Effects specialists Arnold Schieman and Gordon Petty, to allow the
live action and animation sequences to briefly overlap, the animation intruding
into the live action, and the live action into the animation.[3] It should also be
noted that sometimes the ambient sound of the live action and the music of the
animation bleed into each other. Thus, in some transitions between sequences,
Applebaum's special effects seem to be an extension of the ambient sound in the
preceding live action, as when the sound of a centrifuge becomes the opening
chords of the succeeding animation sequence (transition sequence 9 to 10). At
other times, the ambient sound in a succeeding live action takes up aspects of
the musical theme of the animation, as when the rhythm of the music in the
animation finds an echo in the rhythm of a live-action scientific instrument
(transition sequence 8 to 9).

Maclaren, Lambert, and Low

Parker recalls that the animation began with a series of discussions between
Glover and McLaren, joined later by Lambart and Low as work began on the storyboards, an early step in turning the script into a film.[4] Parker himself did not
take the lead here. While he attended some these meetings and wanted clarity
on how the animation and live action would fit together, he did not have Glover's
experience of animation, and was content to step back. Glover knew Lambert
and Low and, as Low's comments on his creative input in the last chapter suggest, Glover was more comfortable than Parker discussing the technicalities of
how the animated sequences might be approached and the visual symbols they
might employ.

It might be asked why McLaren himself did not animate *Challenge* given its importance to the NFB. In fact, McLaren was abroad in Asia, including China, from August 1949 to April 1950, when the bulk of the animation was undertaken.[5] Moreover, despite their close personal relations, Glover and McLaren rarely collaborated on a film, and McLaren's status as Canada's preeminent animator meant that he could resist projects he was not attracted to.[6] His interests in the late 1940s were elsewhere, in experimental and increasingly abstract animation: often joyous entertainments like *Hoppity Pop* (1946), *Fiddle-De-Dee* (1947), or *Begone Dull Care* (1949) that married music to techniques of animation influenced by a wide range of visual styles, including surrealism and abstract expressionism.[7] *Challenge* was to be a very different type of movie, and he may have been reluctant to get involved.

This is not to say McLaren did not lend a hand. Low recalls that McLaren helped on the movie behind the scenes.[8] However, this must have been at a very early stage, since the real work of animation did not get going until July 1949, and McLaren did not return from China until after the film was released. Nevertheless, McLaren's influence is evident in the movie, and shaped—likely guided by Glover—how the animators approached the task of turning the sponsors' demands into a film, not least because both had been trained in McLaren's unit.

Lambart had joined the NFB in 1942 as a letterer, the same year as Glover, just as McLaren was establishing the Animation Unit.[9] A story goes that one day McLaren asked Lambart to help with some heraldic devices for a film he was working on, which turned out to be the beginning of an enduring collaboration in which Lambart moved from letterer to animator, and from McLaren's film assistant to perhaps his closest film partner.[10] Colin Low had joined the NFB three years after Lambart in 1945.[11] Much as Lambart before him, Low started out as a graphic artist, hand-lettering titles. After a dispiriting start on the *World in Action* series, he came under Lambart's wing, and she, McLaren, and other members of the Animation Unit became important mentors.[12]

By 1948 Low wanted a break.[13] He had recently married, and with his wife he traveled to work and to study film in Europe. The following year, Tom Daly (the executive producer of the NFB's Unit B) suggested he return to Canada.[14] McLaren had left for Asia, or was about to leave, and they needed an animator. As Low recalls, Daly told him "'Come back, there is work for you to do,' and the main work that he was thinking about was this . . . was that film [*Challenge*]."[15] Low accepted the offer and returned to Canada to find the movie already partly storyboarded. He moved into the animation studios on Sparks Street with the graphic artist, Sidney Goldsmith (1922–2005), renewed his association with

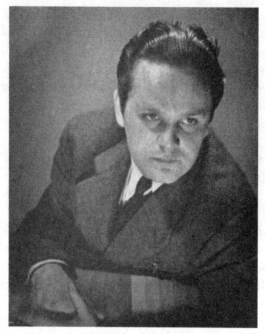

FIGURE 6.2. Vito F. Bazilauskas, c.1942. Source: Archives and Special Collections, The Medical Research Library of Brooklyn, SUNY Downstate Health Sciences University.

Lambart, and started to finish the storyboard. Low also recalls that Goldsmith and the animator Robert Verrall (1928–), neither credited in the film, helped with some of the imagery.

Bazilauskas

The problem for Glover was that neither Lambart nor Low had experience animating scientific subjects, and he began looking for a physician or scientist who might be able to guide them. In June 1949, Ralph Foster wrote to the US Public Health Service's Communicable Disease Center (CDC) in Atlanta asking for Bazilauskas' services for six to eight weeks. He had recently visited the Center as part of a survey for the Association of American Medical Colleges' Medical Film Institute, and had perhaps come across Bazilauskas then, or he may have been pointed in Bazilauskas's direction by David Ruhe, when he was briefly loaned to the MFI.[16] Bazilauskas was apparently unaware of this approach. Foster explained that the NFB film would involve a relatively large amount of important animation in a field to which the NFB's animation department was new. He noted that the animators they had assigned to the job were "excellent technicians and artists but will need the supervision of a scientific authority, preferably a medical illustrator."[17]

Born in Brooklyn, Bazilauskas had attended medical school at the Long Island College Hospital of the City of Brooklyn and held an internship at Kings County Hospital in East Flatbush, Brooklyn.[18] His son describes him as a self-trained illustrator, but he was skilled enough for the biologist Alfred F. Huettner to hire him to produce some of the illustrations for the 1941 edition of his *Fundamentals of Comparative Embryology of the Vertebrates*.[19] After graduating from medical school (1942), Bazilauskas spent the war as a medical officer in Miami, then moved to Georgia to join the CDC. His son recalls that film was Bazilauskas's passion, but that he was generally unable to make a living from it, and family finances were often precarious. They lived in "the projects," as he describes them, in Marietta, outside Atlanta, and his father supplemented his income by working as a physician in a country practice. He became friends in Georgia with the filmmaker George Stoney (who had joined the Southern Educational Film Production Service in 1946) and worked on several films for the CDC.[20] It was probably with this experience in mind that Foster wrote to the CDC.

But Bazilauskas was no longer there. He had held a war-service appointment at the CDC, but had not passed the examinations for permanent status and had left.[21] On hearing of this, Foster picked up the phone and called Bazilauskas at his home in Marietta, and arranged for him to consult on the film for six weeks at $20 a day beginning the last week in July, with the possibility of a longer-term arrangement that might keep him in Ottawa after the cancer work was over.[22] An official invitation followed the phone call, but Bazilauskas did not respond. Concerned by the silence, Foster telegraphed David Ruhe at the Medical Film Institute asking him to pursue the matter. Bazilauskas responded two days later on July 14, with a telegram confirming his acceptance of the offer and that he would be in Ottawa on July 25.[23]

True to his telegram, Bazilauskas arrived in Ottawa and signed a contract with the NFB on July 25. The contract committed him to act as consultant and animation assistant on the film for six weeks from July 25 for a sum of $840 (Can$420 and US$420) plus travel, accommodation, and living expenses.[24] "Hope that Baz is not demoralizing your staff with his peculiar talents,"[25] David Ruhe (perhaps jokingly) asked Ralph Foster in early August shortly after Bazilauskas had moved to Ottawa. If the comment betrayed any worries about his recommendation of Bazilauskas, he need not have been concerned. Bazilauskas' contract was renewed for a further eight weeks in September (US$1,120, plus expenses),[26] and then a further three days after the end of the second contract (US$60).[27] Bazilauskas thus worked at the NFB from July 25 to November 3, 1949, but even when his final contract ended the NFB was reluctant to let him go completely. The animation was progressing slowly, and parts of it would not be ready when the rough cut was shown to the various groups involved in financing the movie in December 1949. (See chapter 8.) Bazilauskas agreed to be available as consultant and animation assistant (at US$25 per day plus expenses) for brief periods after November 3 until the movie was finished.[28] Foster enthused about Bazilauskas' involvement shortly after his last contract expired: "Glover's hunch that we should have someone like Baz here for the animation has paid off in pure gold. Apart from the pleasure of having him here, our animators report that he has been a tremendous source of inspiration and information—with emphasis, by the way, on inspiration."[29]

Animation techniques

Following their appointment to the film, the animators began to explore how they were to approach the themes set out in the shooting script, and one of the key issues was what sort of animation techniques to use, since these would be the foundation on which these themes would be brought to life. With Glover (and at the beginning, McLaren) to advise them, Lambart and Low adopted a range of techniques deployed in the Animation Unit, but Low notes that two were particularly important to this movie: staggered mixes and overlapping zooms, techniques that had earlier been developed by McLaren in the 1940s. Lambart and Low were familiar with these since both had worked with McLaren when he first developed them, and they adapted them to the themes of the new film, the first applied especially to the normal and pathological growth sequence, the latter especially to the cell-as-universe sequences. Thus, the representations of the inside of the body and the cell and the allusions to space travel would all be grounded in these techniques, and when he joined the team, Bazilauskas would add a further technique that allowed the filmmakers to portray the cell as if it was surrounded by threatening gaseous clouds or as a dynamic, living organism: cinemotifs as he called them.

The first of these techniques—staggered mixes—is employed throughout the animated sections. Its use is well illustrated in the first animation sequence—normal and abnormal growth (sequence 2)—animated by Colin Low. In this sequence Low notes that he used a series of single frame drawings that he brought to life using single frame movement (the illusion of movement created when a series of slightly different single frame drawings are shot one after the other, like a flip card) and staggered mixes. The last was a technique he had learned from McLaren, during the making of *Là-Haut sur ces montagnes* (1945), which was being shot when Low arrived at the NFB in 1945.

In *Là-Haut sur ces montagnes,* McLaren sought to capture the changing light on a mountainside by filming a pastel drawing of the mountain. McLaren would film the picture for a few frames, at the end of which he would fade out and stop the camera. He would then make a modification to the picture, with perhaps the addition of a shade or of light. Then the film would be rewound a few frames, and the new shot would be made of the changed picture. The shot would start with a fade in, followed by a fade out. The camera would be stopped, and the procedure undertaken again until the end of the sequence, so that each position had been overlapped several times, but at different levels of exposure. The procedure was risky in that no one knew if it had worked until the shot was finished, and the film removed from the camera and developed. The outcome—if it worked—was a slow transformation in the mountain in which the light changes constantly over the scene. Essentially, as Low puts it, McLaren was animating chiaroscuro

Low recalls watching McLaren make *Là-Haut sur ces montagnes*: one of the first titles he did was for this movie, and McLaren tried him out with drawing some of the pastels.[30] There were other opportunities to learn the technique, for it was used in a number of other films that McLaren made for the NFB—*A Little Phantasy on a 19th-Century Painting* (1946) and *La Poulette grise* (1947), both completed while Low was in the animation department, before he left for Europe. By 1948 Low was proficient enough to employ the technique in the first film he directed alone, *Time and Terrain* (1948), a classroom movie on geology for the NFB, which illustrated the slow geological changes to Canadian terrain over millennia, some sequences of which employed staggered mixes, albeit in color not black-and-white. When he came to animate *Challenge*, he turned once again to staggered mixes.

The opening frames of the first animation sequence of *Challenge* (sequence 2) employ this animation technique. This sequence—a story of the cell and the embryo and its growth and development—consists of a series of staggered mixes, with some single frame shots. An illusion of the cell or embryo growth is achieved using the same method McLaren had earlier used in *Là-Haut sur ces montagnes*: a series of images on black card shot one after the other, the fade-out on one image overlain with the fade-in for the next, so that there is an appearance

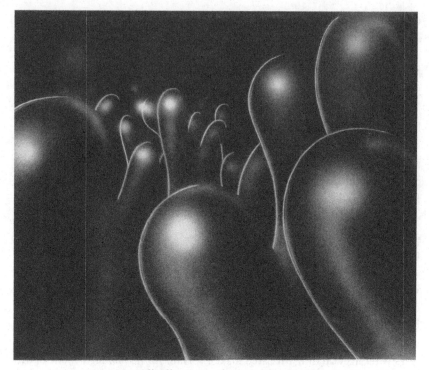

FIGURE 6.3. The Villi, illustrating the use of the airbrush to imitate edge-lighting. But where did the light come from in the darkness of the small intestine? Source: Frame grab from *Challenge*.

of growth and development. As the story reaches the embryo and we see how the cells and body parts begin to specialize we are shown a series of a hand, an eye, and so on. (According to Low, the hand was drawn by Sidney Goldsmith, his colleague in the animation department at Sparks Street.) Each subsequent growth scene—the organs of the body, the delicate network of arteries, the embryo, the villi, heart, muscles—each drawn, exposed to the camera, the film wound back, the fade-outs and-ins. Low recalls spending most of his time on the images of growth, but each image had its own challenges. Figuring out how to pan across the organs and tissues while continuing the staggered mixes; how to give the impression of lighting (the edges of the cell or the villi were drawn with an airbrush to imitate soft luminous edge-lighting); and how to create a sense of depth to the body as when, for example, the camera pans across the delicate network of veins and arteries, the background panning at a slower speed than the foreground, one pan superimposed on another.

The second animation technique—that of overlapping zooms—can be illustrated by the second animated sequence—created by Evelyn Lambart—where the technique generates an impression of traveling through interstellar or intracellular space (sequence 4).[31] The technique had been developed by McLaren in the 1930s, and employed in another movie, *C'est l'aviron* (1944), and the opening and closing shots of *La Poulette grise* (1947).

C'est l'aviron (1944) was part of the *Chants populaires*, a series of films made by McLaren of French-Canadian folk songs. It was a canoeing song about a man who meets a woman but fails to follow up on her interest in him so that she leaves him. As we listen to the song, the movie illustrates themes from the lyrics between shots of a canoe traveling in a straight line down a river. In the canoe scenes, the viewer is in the canoe, looking forward, with the bow of the canoe bobbing in front of him or her. The viewer watches the scenery on either side of the river coming toward the canoe and passing behind, giving the suggestion of the forward movement of the canoe down the river. It was this effect of traveling down the river that the staggered zooms were used to create, employing a motorized zoom acquired by the NFB shortly before production of *C'est l'aviron* began.[32]

The technique worked like this: zooms were made from a twenty-four-inch to a three-inch field, the field being the area of the card viewed through the camera. Each drawing consisted of a large black card with some small details of landscape painted just outside the three-inch field. At the start of each zoom, the landscape details appeared very small, as if they were in the distance. As the zoom progressed the details would enlarge, and just before the end of the zoom they passed out of the edges of the field, leaving only a black card. McLaren would then rewind the film some way back (but not to the start) and begin another zoom with a different picture, creating the sense of forward motion from one landscape to another. The procedure was risky in the same way as the staggered mixes technique was risky: no one knew if it had worked until the sequence was finished and the film removed from the camera and developed.

The sequence of traveling through the cell was achieved in the same way as the sequence of moving down the river in a canoe, using a set of motorized staggered zooms. But instead of landscapes passing on the banks of a river, the viewer now sees parts of the cell passing by, seemingly at great distance, like interstellar constellations as the script wanted. To create this effect, Lambart made white gouache drawings on black cards, which she photographed with overlapping zooms to suggest the forward movement of a space traveler/scientist past constellations of cytostomes and centrosomes, and the Golgi network, each starting

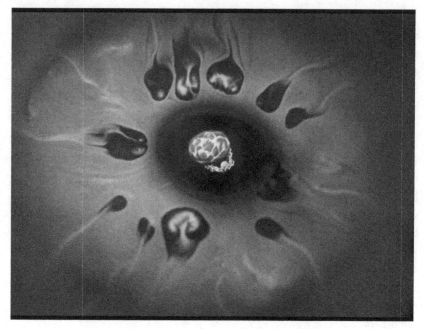

FIGURE 6.4. Cinemotif surrounding drawing of a part of
the cell. Source: Frame grab from *Challenge*.

as a small pinpoint of light before enlarging and passing behind the viewer. This
may have been one of the first sequences to be filmed, since Low recalls McLaren
helping Lambart with the sequence before he left for Asia.[33]

A challenge of this sequence is that instead of traveling in a straight line
(as in, for example, McLaren's *C'est l'aviron*), the shot curves through the cell,
side-slipping toward the end of the sequence. Lambart achieved this effect by
shifting the final position of the camera sideways across the image, a technically
difficult thing to do, since—to retain the appearance of a smooth, even speed of
travel through the cell—it involved precise calculations of how much to slow the
camera as it did its zoom. At the end of the shot the camera passes through some
cloud-like structures before the next live action sequence was appended to the
film using the NFB's optical printer: the cloud-like structures are reminiscent of
the sequences in *C'est l'aviron* where the trip down the river is interrupted by several moments in which we pass through clouds to view scenes illustrating themes
from the song. (Low would later use similar cloud images, and curving shots in
The Universe.) It might also be noted that the end of *C'est l'aviron* includes a
starry sky not dissimilar to the constellations we view in *Challenge*.

The third technique that produced the cinemotifs was developed by Bazilauskas, who later unsuccessfully tried to interest Hollywood studios in it.[34] It will be noted that Bazilauskas' contracts described him as consultant and animation assistant. Much of his work involved ensuring that the animators accurately represented the biological structures and processes they sought to portray as a science illustrator might. But Bazilauskas also helped to solve some of the animation problems. In particular, Low recalls that he provided the solution to a technical problem of the environmental cancer section of showing the cell surrounded by threatening gaseous clouds, and also of the portrayal of the fluid interior of the cell in the biochemistry sequence (9).[35] A drop of some paint-like substance was made to fall onto a flat sheet of liquid, and the camera then recorded the "strange and beautiful diffusion patterns"[36] that resulted, a swirling effect used in several sequences in which the filmmakers combined with the animation using the NFB's optical printer (figure 6.4). According to a publicity leaflet, the technique "was ideal for suggesting the mysterious laws of matter, those forces of nature which govern as well in the sub-microscopic depths of the living cell as in the astronomic furies of the sun's corona."[37] The cinemotifs were a means to create some of the symbolic imagery that the filmmakers hoped would help inspire young viewers with the majesty and beauty of the inner world of the cell and its environment. However, as later chapters will show, viewers found it quite unclear what was real in these sequences and what was imaginary. Bazilauskas had been hired to ensure scientific accuracy; he also, however, contributed to the fantastical imaginary within the film.

Visual symbols

The shooting script asked the filmmkers to portray the inner world of the cell as if it were outer space, the viewer a traveler in this vast emptiness, passing parts of the cell that appeared like planets, moons, or constellations: points of light surrounded by a darkness—Low and Lambart's black cards—symbolic of scientific ignorance and by extension the opportunities that awaited a young scientist entering the field to shed some light. The sheer scale of it all would establish the cell as a place to marvel at, akin to the contemporary excitement about the possibilities of space travel generated by science fiction.

Much of this work would be undertaken by Lambart, the principal animator for the cell-as-universe sequences, but in an interview Low disclosed that he also hoped to anticipate such themes in his own animation (sequence 2), marrying references to the cell-as-universe with the interior images of the body, in ways

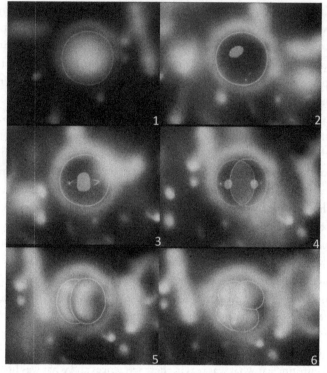

FIGURE 6.5. Cell Division. "Mitosis, the biologist calls
it." Source: Frame grabs from *Challenge.*

that acted as subtle harbingers of themes explored more fully in Lambart's later
cell-as-universe sequences: creating parallels, for example, between the blackness
of outer space and the inside of the body.[38] The point can be illustrated by a close
reading/viewing of the first half of sequence 2: normal and abnormal growth.
As the title suggests, the sequence is divided into two parts, the first, according
to the shooting script, aimed to show by means of a "time-lapse"[39] technique
(Bazilauskas' bailiwick here), "the wonder of the human body as a purposeful,
planned, and smooth-functioning machine, in order to provide maximum contrast for the uncontrolled, disruptive, purposeless activity of the cancer cells."[40]
In the second part, the filmmakers aimed to show how cancer grew, "irresponsi-
ble, indifferent to the laws and life of the body . . . indifferent to the good of the
whole."[41] The narrative thus moves from the wonder of the human body and cell
to the danger of cancer and its harm to the body.

The sequence starts when the figure of Mr. Davis (in the opening live-action
sequence (1) with the physician and two scientists) turns into a ghostly white

figure in the same pose as Davis, set against a black background: the optical printer had done its task, and Low's work with white gouache on black cards had begun.

This ghostly figure shimmers, and a single ill-defined circle of light emerges out of it. It is a mysterious light, and Low does not immediate provide any visual clues as to what it may be, except that it has emerged from the figure of the man. Now the figure of the man fades away, and the circle of light briefly fades, before returning, and gaining a distinct edge or linear outline (figure 6.5, image 1). Low has created an image of a cell that could have come from any school science textbook.[42] He has also indicated that the earlier ill-defined circle of light was in some way the origins of the cell, though it is unclear from his animation whether the origin is in biology or just in the film: it works as visual transition between the ghostly image of the man and the image of the cell, perhaps as a symbol of the beginnings of life, or the light of science in the darkness.

Now Low begins to illustrate the development of the cell and its environment. As backdrop, he painted a series of ill-defined white shapes outside the edge of the cell and moving behind it, all against a black background. A gray oval shape appears in the cell, and two smaller gray shapes (figure 6.5, image 2) one of which merges with the oval, which then shimmers or wobbles, while the other small shape surrounds the merged shape with a ring not unlike that surrounding the planet Saturn (figure 6.5, image 3). Something is going on in the cell, but Low does not immediately indicate what it is. Then the converged shapes split into two oval shapes (figure 6.5, image 4) still surrounded by the ring, at which point the cell in which they are encased splits, each with one of the new ovals, plus a pinpoint of light, seemingly the remains of the ring. Now Low elaborates on the theme: the two cells seem to cloud over so that their insides are no longer visible (figure 6.5, image 5). Instead, we are watching something like two small dark spheres, side-lit from the left, clinging to each other, both of which split into two (figure 6.5, image 6), then the four into eight, and so on, all still clumped together. Low has brought us back to an image of dividing cells that could be found in many textbook illustrations.

So far, the animation has moved between the mysterious and the readily recognizable, disorienting the view momentarily in in its transition from the man to cell division. Now a further disorientation allows Low to introduce subtly the theme of outer space. The dividing cells fade away, to be replaced by a pinpoint of light near the top center of the screen that travels directly down the screen leaving a faint trail behind it (figure 6.6, image 1). The backdrop now is full of dark rounded hillocks and round holes or craters filled with blackness, the

ment
124CHAPTER 6

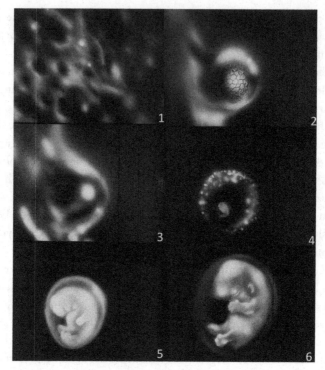

FIGURE 6.6. From Fertilized Egg to Fetus: Source: Frame grabs from *Challenge*.

hillocks seemingly lit from the top, and slightly curved as if part of a sphere. Low has departed visually from common illustrations of the passage of the fertilized egg to the womb, in film or on paper, so that it is not immediately clear what the relationship between this and the earlier images of cell division might be, except that it follows chronologically from the previous sequence.[43] It is almost as if we are suddenly watching from a great distance a comet or spaceship pass over a darkened planet. Low wanted to introduce a visual anticipation of themes that would be developed in sequence (4), the journey through the cell as outer space, though here it is the cell itself traveling through outer space.

Now the animation changes again. Low has painted a dark spherical object, with a surface crisscrossed with plates like cracks in a shell (figure 6.6, image 2). We are not told what this is in the film: a publicity photo identifies it as a blastula, but it is unlike images of blastulas used in many science textbook illustrations, which generally lacked the dark and cracked appearance.[44] It could be a planet or some other body from outer space, surrounded by a semi-transparent cloud, which seems to wrap around it like a gaseous nebula at first, and to give off its own light, since the source of the light comes from no single direction. (And where could this light be coming from in the darkness of the womb?) The gaseous cloud loses transparency, so that the cracked sphere is no longer visible (figure 6.6, image 3). Low has moved from something that 'Baz' could have told them was readily identifiable to a biology student—the cell—to something the filmmakers recognized as mysterious, perhaps tantalizing, to many students, a gesture towards the mysteries of outer space, planets, and nebula.

Now Low creates a new transition: the cloud fades away, to be replaced by a new spherical object with a lighter object inside, shaped like a comma (figure 6.6, image 4). The sphere disappears, and the comma-like object grows into something immediately recognizable as a fetus surrounded by a transparent sac (figure 6.6, images 5 and 6). As Sara Dubow notes, by the late 1940s Americans (and Canadians) were becoming increasingly familiar with what the fetus looked like. Not only were (generally animal) fetuses depicted in school textbooks, but human fetuses were the subject of science exhibits and sex education classes, and were depicted in museum catalogs and magazines such as *Newsweek* (1946), *Time* (1949), and *Life* (1950), the year that the film was released.[45] In the brief embryo sequence in *Challenge*, Low animates these images so that we see the embryo grow from something he regarded as likely unrecognizable to many students into something that is clearly a fetus, though not in utero, as was, for example, the case in the 1947 *Miracle of Growth* exhibit at the Museum of Science and Industry in Chicago, or the classroom film *Human Growth* (1947).[46] Instead, the effect is closer to the "lonesome space traveler" image popularized in the 1960s by Lennart Nilsson's photographs of fetal development in *Life* magazine, albeit perhaps also anticipated in other films such as *Human Reproduction* (1947).[47] *Challenge's* fetus is alone in his/her transparent sac, surrounded by the darkness that in later animation sequences the animators hoped would conjure up the vast empty distances of outer space. Once again, Low has gestured toward the contemporary enthusiasm for space travel and science fiction.

By this stage of the animation, Low has also given a chronological place to the mysterious blastula sequence, sandwiched between sequences on cell division and fetal growth. Its temporal location in the visual thread of the film suggests it is part of the same process, and perhaps the brighter students might have guessed at what they were watching, even if visual references to comets, craters, hillocks, and cracked spheres evoked associations more to do with space travel than embryological development. For Low, however, these associations were part of the larger argument of the film, for they helped prepare the viewer for the parallels, evoked in later animation sequences, between the universe of the cell and

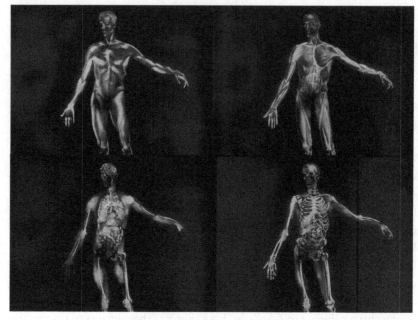

FIGURE 6.7. Dissecting the Apollo Belvedere. Top left: The whole man. Top right: The musculature. Bottom left: Organs. Bottom right: Bones. Source: Frame grabs from *Challenge*.

the universe of planets and starry constellations, much as the fetus as spaceman helped prepare the viewer for later sequences that conjured up the vast distances of outer space. Besides, the spectacle of it all would, he hoped, carry all students, the inquiring and those less curious.[48]

It should be clear by now that Low's allusions to outer space were very subtle and ambiguous—maybe outer space, and maybe not. All he wanted to do was to visually suggest themes that would be developed later in the film and then to move on, leaving the ambiguity of the imagery. So the rest of the sequence on normal growth keeps the black background, without any emphasis on its earlier suggestions of outer space. Instead, Low begins to highlight connections between the fetus and the adult man. The hand of the fetus is illuminated, and an adult hand appears; the fetal eye is illuminated, followed by an adult eye. We next watch something beating behind a rib cage (the fetal heart, followed by the adult heart), after which we return to the fetus, which is then replaced by the adult man (an Apollo Belvedere figure, surrounded by black, maybe outer space or maybe not). This figure is then "dissected" to reveal muscles, organs, and bones (a Bernard Albinus figure, again surrounded by black) before we move to a sequence on the functioning of a healthy body with a panning shot of working heart muscles, images of blinking sugar storing cells in the liver, and blood (a clear liquid, not obviously red) running though semi-transparent veins and arteries.

It should be clear from this that Low's animation leaves much unexplained. It creates a visual thread that moves from events that filmmakers thought would be easily identifiable to a student or his or her teacher (the cell, the dividing cell, the fetus, the hand, the eye, the heart, the adult man, like science illustrations helping to highlight certain features of body and cell, signposts along the way) to others that they thought were likely less easily identifiable, mixed with some elements of the imaginary or fantastical. It is also clear that Low had created a temporal space for the less familiar and the fantastical by situating them between (and sometimes within) the familiar images, and so, he hoped, evoking themes about space travel that would be explored more fully in later cell-as-universe animation sequences but not fully establishing them, since their symbolic meaning remained ambiguous. It would be left to Lambart to explore these themes more fully in her cell-as-universe sequences, built on McLaren's technique of over-lapping zooms, themes—as I shall indicate in the next chapter—meshed with some of the live-action sequences that sought to construct the cancer research scientist as an explorer, akin to a space explorer, dwarfed by the immensity around him.

Pavel Tchelitchew

As the preceding suggests, the visual references and symbols in this film were about much more than the problems of cancer, science, and recruitment. They gestured toward the contemporary enthusiasm for space travel, the body imageries of the Apollo Belvedere, Vesalius, and Bernard Albinus, alongside quasi-scientific imagery of the fetus, cell, and internal organs. Indeed, for Low—and maybe Lambart—the film was also an opportunity to develop a commentary on the work of other artists and about the roles and meanings of visual imagery. The case of Tchelitchew illustrates the point. At first glance, it might seem as if all Low and Lambart did was take some of the imagery of the artist's interior landscapes and apply it to the film using McLaren's techniques. As Low later noted, "Eve [Lambart] and I were doing it [the animation] in the manner of Pavel Tchelitchew, the famous transparent artist. So I began doing chiaroscuro animation, which was Norman's [McLaren's] principle of staggered mixes, and I combined it with linear outline."[49] (Linear outline is the use of white outlines—a contrast to the black cards used for the backdrop—to depict the edges of the illustrations being animated.) However, in an interview it became clear that the reality was more complex. Low not only applied Tchelitchew's approach to the film but also saw himself engaging with issues raised by the artist, or more correctly how they were interpreted by some of the critics who promoted him, sometimes in harmony with them, sometimes diverging.

Low has two stories about his first view of a Tchelitchew painting. In one, it was during a visit to the Museum of Modern Art in New York on his way to Europe in 1948, so he was familiar with Tchelitchew before he started on *Challenge*.[50] In the other story, he learned of Tchelitchew from an art magazine given to him by Guy Glover, who suggested that he use the transparent images as a model for *Challenge*.[51] In both stories Glover's magazine, and Glover himself, play important roles in helping Low to adapt Tchelitchew's style to the cinema screen. Low had lost the magazine by the time I interviewed him in 2007 and could not remember its name, but he recalled it had had an image of a transparent Tchelitchew head on the cover. Tchelitchew's interior landscapes feature in a variety of magazines including *View* and the *Magazine of Art*, and it is possible that Low's recollection is of Tchelitchew's picture of a transparent head, interlaced with a network of veins, arteries, or nerves that had recently been reproduced on the cover of the Spring 1947 edition of *View* magazine (figure 6.8), which also included an article by the art critic Parker Tyler on Tchelitchew's shift toward X-ray images, making man a "spectator of himself as a transparent envelope in the center of which he exists."[52] Ironically, when Low turned to his interior landscapes, Tchelitchew himself was abandoning the approach, moving instead toward representations of weightless, transparent, dematerialized forms. From 1950–51, Tchelitchew created a series of drawings of geometric heads consisting of thin, nearly parallel, sometimes intersecting, circular lines set against dark backgrounds.[53]

In a 1948 article, published the year before production began on *Challenge*, the critic Lincoln Kirstein noted that Tchelitchew's interior landscapes were quite literally *landscapes*, "portraits of places":[54] "Sometimes the place is the antrim [*sic*], the vaults of the sinus, the spiral labyrinth of the inner ear, the corridors of the semicircular canal, the tree of the nervous system, the rivers of lymph or the pools of glands and vessels."[55] He argues that Tchelitchew's interior landscapes "contain nothing of the melodrama of the dissected but resurrected cadaver. Their interiors have not yet been penetrated by the scalpel but by light."[56] Tchelitchew had little interest in pathology or dissection, according to Kirstein. On the contrary, he argued, the artist was interested in portraying dynamic,

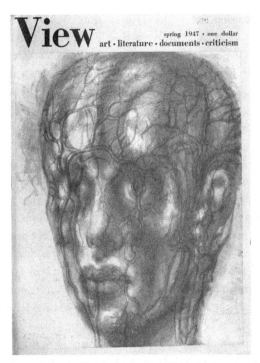

FIGURE 6.8. An interior landscape by Pavel Tchelitchew, on the cover
of the last issue of *View,* Series 6, No.3 (March, Spring 1947).

functioning, living bodies: "The drama in them is that the tubes, sponges, vessels and processes are not drained away but active in full force, motile, dynamic."[57] Echoing a common theme in *View*'s assessment of Tchelitchew, Kirstein came to praise the humanism of his neoromantic art, his humanistic judgement of society: the stance of the figure in Tchelitchew's *The Golden Leaf,* for example, conveys "the humanity in the inclination of its quivering silhouette, the solidity inside its complexity fuse in a sense of living completeness within a transparent, fluent luminosity. The profile flickers steadily like an alcohol flame, but the interior also flows with light."[58]

In an interview, Low noted that he played with many of these themes in his animated sections, but also transformed them for the purposes of the movie.[59] Like Tchelitchew, Low wanted to create a dynamic, functioning, living body, viewed as though by means of x-rays through the flesh, as in Low's panning shot of a beating heart, blinking images of sugar storing cells in the liver, and blood running though veins and arteries, all brought to life using Maclaren's staggered mixes, and perhaps the NFB's newly acquired optical printer to create a sense of depth to the animation, much like cel animation, to allow the different layers of veins and arteries move at different speeds (sequence 2). Much as Kirstein claimed that the *Golden Leaf* was "no stripped corpse but a revealed and burning existence,"[60] so Low wanted to reveal the vitality of the functioning body, echoing the humanism that Kirsten and others detected in Tchelitchew's art.

Yet, in *Challenge* this functioning body is married to the sort of dissection that Kirstein informs us Tchelitchew eschewed in his transparent paintings and drawings. For Kirstein's Tchelitchew, Vesalius was only a starting point. Unlike the anatomist, he was not interested in cataloguing the results of his dissection, he was no scientist. Instead, Kirstein argued, Tchelitchew selected elements from anatomy, choosing the topographies of his paintings as other artists might select trees, rocks, or clouds, which he then arranged into landscapes, such as the vine-like veins that cover a skull or head as in the cover of Spring 1947 issue of *View*. At times Low followed Kirstein's Tchelitchew in arranging the elements that made up his landscapes, but he was also limited in how far he could move away from the anatomy. Thus, while Low wanted to create landscapes within the body—think of the intestinal villi (figure 6.3) waving delicately back and forth, like the tentacles of a sea anemone, populating a place like a dark cavern, partially lit from one side—he also had to create one recognizable to scientists.

Thus, for example, as we end the embryo sequence (sequence 2) of the movie we are shown a pastel drawing of a grown man posed like the Apollo Belvedere, which as discussed above is slowly dissected by means of a series of staggered mixes (figure 6.7).[61] Coming at the end of the embryo sequence, this dissection distanced Low from Tchelitchew. It was a harbinger of death, and an anticipation of the danger of cancer that the animated sequence will later explore.[62] It also distanced the animation from Tchelitchew's landscapes with their compositions of elements at the whim of the artist. Low might have taken inspiration from Tchelitchew's so-called x-ray images, but he could not move too far from the anatomical body to arrange the topography of the body as he liked.

Finally, Low differs from Kirstein's Tchelitchew who had no interest in pathology. For all the symbolism of the skull, with its echoes of death and decay, for Kirstein, Tchelitchew is interested in functioning living bodies, not ones in decay. The skulls wrapped in nerves and other vessels might hint at eventual decay and death, but they are alive, kept alive by the network of vessels around them. And if these networks give a sense of luxuriant, profusion, it is not the uncontrolled growth of cancer. They are, to Kirstein, dynamic, living, complete, in harmony with the body. Low echoes such themes in the sequence on normal growth, but only as a prelude to the following sequence on pathological growth where he sought to show how such dynamic harmony could turn against the functioning body when growth became uncontrolled. The delicate networks and organs keeping the body alive would be overwhelmed and could lead to death. Thus, where Kirstein's Tchelitchew sought to portray life and wholeness, Low also sought to show how life and wholeness could be destroyed.

Thus, while Low sees Tchelitchew as a model for the images of the body in *Challenge*, he mixes this with other imagery that presented a different agenda to that of Tchelitchew as presented by critics. As noted above, in the article that accompanied the Spring 1947 issue of *View*, the critic Parker Tyler (another enthusiast for the humanism of Tchelitchew) interpreted the artist as making the viewer a "spectator of himself." [63] Tchelichew, according to Tyler, sought to clothe a naked skull with a skin of sorts, countering a tendency within modern art "to alienate man from this very sense of his own death,"[64] an almost pathological situation involving the problematic separation of a person from his future demise. Low shared with Tyler's Tchelitchew a desire to transform this pathology into something healthy by confronting the viewer with the possibility of death. But where Tchelitchew was content, according to Tyler, to reveal a center "overflowing with unnamable sweetness,"[65] Low introduced a darker theme of mortality and disease so as to set up the possibility of a cure and the need for research. If Low distanced the animation from Kirstein's Tchelitchew by introducing a dissected view of the body and at times a scientifically organized body landscape, so he also distanced himself from Tyler's Tchelitchew in introducing science as the solution to man's alienation from his own sense of death.

It should be clear by now that while Low might have seen himself as commentating on Tchelitchew or his critics and enthusiasts, he also needed to differentiate his work from that of the artist in a film that served a more utilitarian function. In *Challenge*, the humanism of Tchelitchew's art would become the humanism of science; his celebration of dynamic harmony would become the prelude to cancer and science's attack on the disease. Thus, Low wanted—or needed for this commission—to create a series of visual symbols that would be different from Tchelitchew's visual symbols, at least as interpreted by Kirstein and Tyler. Where scientists often saw Tchelitchew as invoking technologies such as the X-ray, Kirstein and Tyler saw him creating a symbolic world that might have distant roots in science but was trying to do something quite different. Low's appropriation of Tchelitchew transformed this symbolic world into something opposed to the artist's intention. Low's Tchelitchew-esque imagery brought the artist's work back into the realm of science, even as Low himself sometimes strayed into the fantastical with its hints of outer space.

The sponsors had wanted a film that educated students in the biology of the body, the cell, and cancer, and that also inspired them to think about cancer research as a career, to understand the mystery of cancer. The scriptwriters had taken these ideas and combined them with visual metaphors of the cell as universe, which the animators brought to life with McLaren's and Bazilauskas' techniques. The animators added other visual references that allowed them to comment on artists such as Tchelitchew and to mix images, some of which were based on science illustrations, others in which the image is imaginary or even fantastical, and others where there may be gestures toward other themes, or where it is unclear what an object might be. Such a seamless mix might have helped the film to inspire and challenge, but later viewers would see this as a problem. This was film about science sponsored by leading biomedical and health agencies. How could they support a film where it was sometime unclear what was based on fact and what was illusory?

CHAPTER 7

Live Action

WITH THE ANIMATION SECTION of the movie underway, in July 1949 Glover and Parker turned their attention to the live-action sequences. The live action was to be directed by Parker himself, with the sound recordist Clarke Daprato (1923–82) and the cameraman Grant McLean (1921–2002). The three men had all joined the NFB in the early 1940s—McLean in 1941, Daprato in 1942, and Parker in 1943—and all had recently collaborated on *Family Circles* (1949), directed by Parker. In *Challenge*, all three traveled to the live-action locations, Parker directing, McLean operating the camera, and Daprato recording the synchronized sound. Other sound effects would have been added later at the editing stage, probably by the editor Douglas Tunstell.[1]

As was the case with the animation, the filmmakers' approach to the live action was shaped in part by the culture and practices of the NFB. Following Grierson's belief that filmmaking meant that naturalistic representation had to be subordinated to symbolic expression, Parker and his colleagues sought to present the themes of the film through two key symbolic figures—the patient and the scientist. These symbols had been there in the scripts, refined and modified, likely in discussion with the sponsors. Now the filmmakers had to bring them to life in dramatic recreations by means of the actors, their props, the ambient sound, and (as we will see in the next chapter) the music, editing, and narration. The dramatic recreations also sought to illustrate the character of scientific work: its ceaseless activity. In these ways, the filmmakers attempted to transform the sponsors' demands for a film that encouraged young people to think of science as a possible career. If the animation was intended to inspire them with amazing views of the inner worlds of the body and cell, the live action set out the character of the scientists who undertook this work and the patients for whom this work would ultimately be undertaken, and gestured toward the nature of scientific work.

In many ways, these symbols would have been congenial to the sponsors. The patient was obedient and respectful of physicians and scientists, calmed by their reassurance, an object of medical and humanitarian need that science could—both in the long- and the near-term—help. At the same time, the scientist was heroic, an explorer (of the outer/inner space of the cell), and completely absorbed in his or her dedication to their work; an ordinary person, but exceptional all the same; driven by the science, the product of years of training and research, but also someone whose work would in the end serve a humanitarian need. The two symbols thus helped to shape each other—the needs of the patient an inspiration for science, the knowledge and skill of the scientists a reason for the respect of the patient, his or her confidence in medicine. Both, the filmmakers hoped, would help to tempt viewers into seeing cancer as a problem for science, and to think of cancer research as a potential career.

However, the filmmakers struggled at times to get a consistent message across. Some of this was because there were tensions within the symbols (for example between the images of the scientist as both extraordinary hero and ordinary man or woman), but also because of the limited acting range of some of the actors and the limited visual palette of some of the filming locations. The film might have been shaped by the culture and practices of the NFB, but it was also shaped by the exigencies of filmmaking. Problems of this sort were not unique to this film, but they introduced uncertainties to the movie that meant that the symbolic figures central to establishing the broader themes of the film were not entirely stable and did not do the work the director hoped. The features of the character of the scientist and patient outlined in the script were dependent on the acting, the locations, the props, and sound as much as they were dependent on the script.

The structure

Of the fourteen sequences in the film, eight are live action. They begin with the introduction of cancer as the latest challenge to science with the dramatic arrival of a symbolic cancer patient (Mr. Davis) in the hospital (table 4.3: sequence 1), which sets the stage for the animated sequence (2) illustrating normal and abnormal growth. There follows a live-action sequence (3) where after meeting with his physician and some scientists, Mr. Davis is reassured that he has a curable form of cancer, after which his physician contemplates a magnified slide of Davis's tissue and walks into it so that we begin to travel (sequence 4) through an animated representation of the cell as if it were interstellar space.

Then comes a live-action sequence (5) on tissue culture research.[2] According to the shooting script, this sequence had two goals: to illustrate how such research was contributing to knowledge about cancer and biology; and to marvel at the idea that cells could live longer in tissue culture than the animals from which they were derived. Thus the opening few shots are of a Carrel flask, a caged mouse next to it, and a dripping tap. "Through a careful, almost Dali-esque handling of three elements," the shooting script notes,[3] "(the Carrel flask, the animal from which the tissue was taken, and a dripping faucet) we create a receptive mood for the novel and somewhat philosophical idea presented in the commentary, where the limited life of the individual is contrasted with the immortality of the isolated tissue taken from it." Whether the Dali-esque effect was truly created on celluloid is open to question, and immortality is never mentioned in the final cut. However, the point about tissues living longer in tissue culture than the lifespan of the animal they came from remains as part of this sequence, which also includes an account of how (in order to study, for example, the effect of chemicals and diet on the disease) cancer cells might be introduced into animals and eggs and grown in culture. There is also mention of the enormous effort and time it takes to do this work, a theme taken up again in later sequences.

The following sequences (6 to 11) follow a similar pattern to that of 4 and 5, in which an animation sequence is followed by a live-action sequence on scientific or medical efforts to understand the aspect of the cell in the previous animation, or to intervene against cancer. Thus, the animated sequence (6) that illustrates cell division and chromosome separation is followed by a live-action sequence (7) on the genetics of cancer; an animated sequence (8) on the cell as a complex industrial organism is followed by a live-action sequence (9) on the biochemistry of cancer; and an animated sequence (10) on external threats to the cell is followed by a live-action sequence (11) on environmental and occupational cancers and cancer prevention.

As in sequence 5, the live-action sequences (7, 9, 11) seek to do more than provide an account of the work of science. Thus sequence 7 on the genetics of cancer not only explores the work of genetics (the different animals used in genetics research, why each is chosen, and the role of radiation in creating hereditary changes), but also introduces first, the idea of the mouse—"looking terribly curious and cute"[4] according to the shooting script—as the hero of cancer research; second, the curiosity of the young boy depicted in the sequence, his fascination with animals, as a future driver of research; and third, the parallel between animal and human heredity. "There is an obvious resemblance,"[5] the script tells us, between the boy and the two adults (not so obvious in film itself), and the male scientist informs the boy in the script that "Our friend here isn't just an ordinary mouse. He's quite special. And he, and many others like him, can help us find out a lot of things . . . for example, why you got to be so much like your mother."[6] The woman bats her eyelids in response in the film itself. Sequence 9, in the shooting script, tells us as much about the character of the scientist (his or her complete absorption in science) as about the work of biochemistry (see discussion below). And sequence 11 is as much about the various causes and risk factors of cancer (sunlight, occupation, sex, chemicals, radiation) as it is about research into them—interviews in the field and the clinic, the collection of statistics, the mechanization of their analysis, and the study of chemicals for carcinogenic properties.

After this last sequence, the pattern changes. The live-action sequence on environmental cancer (11) is followed by another live-action (12) sequence on the therapeutics of cancer and the search for a test for the disease (also highlighting the humanitarian and medical impulses behind cancer research), and by a further live-action sequence (13) as the shooting script tells us on the character of the scientist, his or her long period of training and preparation, dedication to work, and the vast international effort against cancer (again see discussion below). The final sequence—the closing credits (14)—is an animation that returns us to the cell-as-universe theme of sequence 4.

Where to go?

As with the animation, Glover and Parker began with conversations and meetings. They had the shooting script that set out the structure of the film and the substance of the live-action sequences, and the characteristics of the symbolic patient and scientist and the work of science. However, things did not end there. Parker's version of the shooting script is full of scribbled notes and pieces cut, pasted, and rearranged, and dialogue added suggesting some ways the early planning had to be adapted to the practicalities of filming. Some of these changes were likely undertaken in the meetings with Glover and other members of the team as the filmmakers sought to address the exigencies of filming. The soundman, Clarke Daprato, for example, had to work with the NFB's antiquated, often unreliable sound-recording equipment, make up for its deficiencies, and address the difficulties of synchronizing sound with the 35-mm equipment used in *Challenge*.[7] Grant McLean—the cameraman, and son of the NFB's controller and nephew of Ross McLean, the government film commissioner[8]—had to figure out which cameras, lenses, filters, zooms, and other equipment would be needed for the shots, and likely was responsible for cleaning, testing, and transporting it to the film locations. He also evaluated potential challenges (other than cancer) during filming, helping with setup, distance, angles, and lighting. All these practical efforts facilitated the transition from script to film.

Preparations for the live-action scenes began in earnest in August 1949 when the NFB started to scout for locations, looking at the possibility of filming at Chalk River, the Canadian nuclear research facility (for experiments on induced gene mutation), the University of Rochester, Roswell Park, Memorial Hospital, Queen's College Kingston, the IBM Company (for statistical machines), and the NCI in Bethesda, Maryland.[9] Concerns about the cost of travel, however, prompted Ruhe to urge the NFB to cut back on the number of locations. In his view, most of the necessary footage could be obtained in Canada.[10] Thus by September 1949 the number of locations had been reduced to two cities: Toronto (Toronto General Hospital, the University of Toronto—the Wallberg Memorial Building and the Connaught Laboratories, and some outside locations) and Rochester (the Strong Memorial Hospital and University of Rochester) just over the Canadian/US border in New York State. The plan was to do the location shots in Toronto and Rochester back-to-back, and on September 30 they planned to hire a car for eight weeks for CAN$400 for shooting in Toronto and Rochester, and also for transporting a few members of the crew from Toronto to Rochester.[11]

It is here that one begins to understand some of the reasons for the annotations and changes in Parker's version of the shooting script. The live-action sequences, hamstrung by a 35-mm technology that made it tricky to synchronize sound (Daprato's province), required extensive scripting and rehearsal, which Glover would have endorsed from his animator's perspective. Yet ideas that worked on paper did not always work on location, and Constant traveled with the crew to advise on how the script might be modified, while Parker and McLean figured out the camerawork, layout, and lighting and Daprato worked out how to synchronize the sound. The risk was that the constant writing and rewriting and the many rehearsals and changes to the script might result in a loss of spontaneity, especially among the amateur actors hired for the film. In October 1949, the first contracts were signed with actors. (See table 7.1) In October and November, permissions to use their images were also signed by physicians, nurses, and others who appeared in the film.

The Toronto shoot took place in October and early November.[12] Those were busy days, filming at a variety of locations in the Toronto area, with time allocated for moving and setting up and removing equipment, as well as the actual filming itself. The filming started with the crew at Toronto General Hospital (October 3–9), where they shot some of the opening sequences of the movie—the waiting room scenes where Mr. Davis first appears (sequence 1); the stairs and corridor where Davis is led by a nurse (sequence 1); a conference room scene (perhaps where Davis meets the the physician and scientists, sequence 1) and some general hospital scenes. The crew then moved to the Wallberg Memorial (October 10–15) where they shot the night laboratory scene, the college corridor, and a lecture theatre scene (all sequence 13). "This has been a furious week, the past one,"[13] Parker informed Glover, the day after shooting started at the Wallberg Memorial. "We have tackled some our major set-ups and have them in the can now—I fervently hope."

Now that he was on location, Parker began to understand some of the practicalities of filming in working hospitals, laboratories, and classrooms. The point was brought out by the realization that the allowance for overtime (15 percent) had been grossly underestimated; it was more likely to be 70 percent. "The hard fact is that from here on in it will not very often be possible to begin the working day at 9:00 a.m.,"[14] he informed Glover, not only because they were shooting night scenes. The filmmakers had to fit in with the routine of the places where they were filming. "Not only is it very difficult, or almost impossible to interrupt lab or classroom routine, but in some major cases it may require our breaking down the set-up each night to leave the rooms clear for the regular work taking place there during the daytime." [15]

So the filming went on. From October 17 to October 20, they shot the scientist's office (location unknown, possibly the Wallberg Memorial), the factory and exterior scenes (Mr. Davis) (sequences 11 and 12 respectively), before moving to the Connaught Laboratories (October 21–29) for the tissue culture (sequence 5), biochemistry (sequence 9), and micromanipulator scenes (cut from film). On October 30 and 31 they were either in a hotel or in the university shooting the international conference scene (still in the film at this point, likely transformed into the educational scene at the end of the movie), and filming concluded (November 1–2) with some general exterior shots and some other exterior shots involving Mr. Davis.[16] The next day—November 3—Foster informed Dallas Johnson that the first batch of stills was ready.[17]

At the time Foster wrote to Johnson, the film crew was on its way to Rochester. On November 3 they crossed the border in a passenger car and an NFB truck.[18] Morten Parker reported "that, almost invariably, the Americans seemed to be more sympathetic and anxious to help than our own compatriots."[19] But such cooperation tended to come more from the scientists than the US border authorities. In the month or so before the trip, the Canadians had spent long, anxious times, and prepared much paperwork clearing the bureaucratic path for the film

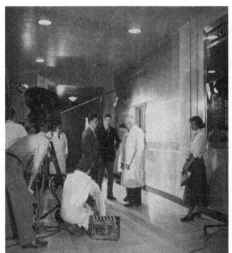 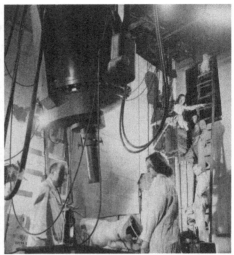

FIGURE 7.1. Left: Shooting in the Wallberg Memorial building, University of Toronto, Scene 172, Take 5. From left: Grant McLean, Morten Parker, unknown (possibly Clarke Daprato or Maurice Constant), various unknown actors. Photo by Christian Lund, October 1949. Source: NCI archives, AR-4900-010785. Right: Shooting at the University of Rochester Atomic Energy Project. On ladder from top: Grant McLean, Morten Parker, two unknown members of the crew. On the ground, various unknown actors. Photo by Christian Lund. (The NFB dates this as October 1949, though the visit to Rochester was in November 1949). Source: National Film Board of Canada, reprinted courtesy of the NFB.

crew—including some uncredited individuals—and its equipment to visit New York and return to Canada.[20] The shoot, however, seems to have passed uneventfully, and the car and truck escaped safely back across the border into Canada afterward. There might have been some relief among the crew that all went smoothly. Maurice Constant and Grant McLean believed themselves to be regarded as unwelcome by the US authorities: Constant had been a Communist, and McLean had recently filmed *The People Between* (1947), which had been banned by the Canadian government, largely under pressure from the United States. The film showed the Chinese Communists in a positive light and portrayed the Chinese as pawns exploited by nationalist ideologies, both Eastern and Western. *Challenge* provided a retreat from the controversy, an opportunity for McLean to rehabilitate himself, and to work on a collaborative venture with the Americans.[21]

In Rochester, the filming took place at several locations at Strong Memorial Hospital and the University of Rochester. We do not have as detailed a shooting schedule as for Toronto, but the impending arrival of the camera team generated some excitement among the medical faculty. Austin Deibert noted that Dr. John Morton—a member of the NCI's NACC, and professor of surgery at the University of Rochester, "facetiously told me that I should not be surprised, when the film is finally produced, to see his visage in many scenes, multiply occurring, as peering into a microscope, wielding a knife, watching bubbling retorts, and even scrubbing floors. He really is a grand guy!"[22]

Challenging actors

The shoots in both Toronto and Rochester raised several problems for the film-makers. One related to the actors. The cast included a mix of professional and amateur actors with a range of acting ability. Many of the scientists, physicians, and students in the film were scientists, physicians, and students who worked at the locations in their life outside the film; others were local actors, and other members of the production team (figure 3.2)—and not all were endowed with great acting ability. (For a list of actors and their professions, where known, see table 7.1.) Parker had to struggle (not always successfully) to coax more than a wooden performance from his amateur cast members. For example, Mr. Davis (the main symbolic patient) was played by an amateur actor, Emerson Houghton (1889–1965), the owner of Houghton's Silverware and Plating, then on Church St. in Toronto, which specialized in ecclesiastical pieces in sterling, silver plate, and brass: a nice man, recalls Parker, but of limited acting ability.[23] These ama-teurs were leavened with a selection of professional actors and speakers, includ-ing the writer and raconteur W. O. Mitchell (1914–98), who plays Dr. McVicor;[24] Larry McCance (1928–70), a local Toronto actor, who plays one of the scientists sitting behind a desk holding a test tube over a Bunsen burner (Parker used him in a number of other films);[25] and the actor Murray Westgate (1918–2018), who plays a male scientist in the tea scene, in the center of the group that discusses a scientific paper during their break (figure 7.2).

This is not to say that professionals always succeeded in the acting or that amateurs were always stilted. In the tea scene, for example, Parker recalls that he struggled unsuccessfully to make the scene come alive: the actors were unable or unwilling to inject life into their lines. This happened despite the presence of the professional actor Murray Westgate, who engages the other mainly amateur actors in a conversation about research.[26] Cinematic results were as much the product of the ensemble as of the individual actors. And it was also the case that some amateurs could give strong performances. Thus, the scientist in the night scene (which begins with him talking on the phone to his wife before leaving

TABLE 7.1. The Cast of *Challenge*

Name	Address	Profession	Pay (dates of appointment)	Role (if known)
Bamford, J				
Belling, Babs				
Buckham, Rosemary				
Chevrier, Helen				
Dawe, Olive				
Dearden, Ruth				
Doyle, Dr.				
Duffy, Owen				
Dussault, Jacques				
Field, Barbara				
Fisher, Dr. A. M.				
Gillespie, Mrs. G. N.				
Graham, George Wm.	Strong Memorial Hospital, Rochester, NY	Assistant director, Strong Memorial Hospital		
Graham, Miss J.				
Hammond, Shirley M.	216 University Road, Rochester, NY			
Hillman, Elleen				
Houghton, Mr. E. (1889–1965)	313 Church St., Toronto	Shop owner	$125 October 12– November 18, 1949	Mr. Davis, the symbolic patient

(Cont.)

Name	Address	Profession	Pay (dates of appointment)	Role (if known)
Hundal, Jerry (Mr. J. S.)	Y.M.C.A., 40 College St., Toronto	Unknown, sometime clerk	$40 October 15–17, 1949	Dr. Ramm
Kaiser, Martha/ Campbell, Margaret	Strong Memorial Hospital, Rochester, NY			
Kerr M. D., John W.	Strong Memorial Hospital, Rochester, NY			
Kibsey, Rose				
Kirkwood, Mrs. M.	149 Augusta, (Toronto?).			
Lacey, Erucata R	601 University Park, Rochester, NY			
Lake, Dorothea W.				
Ljunch, Esse				
Linton, E. H.	55 Belmont St., (Toronto?)			
Martin, Doris				
Mason, Sopie				
McCance, Larry (1928–1970)	372 Glen Manor Drive, Toronto	Actor	$29 October 18, 1949	Biochemist.
McNaughton, Grace				
Millard, Ross		Actor		
Miller, Dr.		Radiologist: Toronto General Hospital Dunlap Clinic		
Mitchell, C				

Name	Address	Role	Amount	Dates	Notes
Mitchell, Mr. W. O. (1914–1998)	140 Springdale Blvd., Toronto	Actor, writer, and raconteur	$40	October 15–17, 1949	Dr. McVicor
Parker, Dr. Raymond (1903–74)	193 Carlton St., Toronto	Scientist: Tissue Culture research, Polio			
Praff(sp.), E. P.					
Rapkin, Maurice (?–1964)	34 Wineva Avenue, Toronto	Actor (producer of singing commercials for radio stations)	$105	October 20–31, 1949	
Raz, Ben					Scientist working late at night
Rae, James J.		Chemist			
Reardon, Dave					
Robertson, George H. (1922–2003)	48 Summerhill Gardens, Toronto	Radio announcer/ actor/ narrator	$19	October 18, 1949	Scientist(?)
Scott, Dr.					
Telford, Joan					
Trout, Elizabeth					
Walker, Miss T.					
Ward, Mrs. L.					
Westgate, Murray (1918–2018)	26 Northumberland St., Toronto	Actor	$89	October 23–31, 1949	
Williams, Katherine C.	64 Avondale Park, Rochester 20, NY				
Williams, Miss S.					
Woolford, Miss B.					

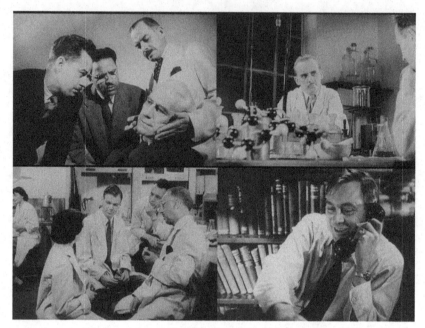

FIGURE 7.2. *Challenge's* actors. Top left: W. O. Mitchell (left), Jerry (J. S.) Hundal
(second left), and Ross Millard examine Emerson Houghton. Top right: Larry
McCance in an environmental cancer sequence. Bottom left: Murray Westgate
(third from left) in the tea break scene. Bottom right: James J. Rae, professor
of chemistry and amateur actor. Source: Frame grabs from *Challenge*.

for home) is played by the Toronto University chemist James J. Rae.[27] Rae was
not a professional actor, but Parker recalls that he played the role of the scientist
fluently and naturally. In sum, the director was never able to fully control the
scene, dependent as he was on unpredictable acting skills of his cast.

A dull palette and the interference of scientists

A second problem had to do with location and subject. The film aimed to represent both the work of science and the character of the scientist, which meant
lots of laboratory scenes and of shots of men and women in white coats, lab animals, and equipment. As Bert Hansen has shown, such images had long been a
regular feature of still photographic representations of scientists, and they were
also common in entertainment films.[28] Nevertheless, they also made it difficult to maintain visual interest. For example, in the laboratory scenes there was
the problem of avoiding repetition of shots of men and women in white coats,

glassware and equipment. So Parker and McLean enlivened the action by varying the lighting (sometimes shots were taken at night; sometimes they used high
contrast and shadows), using a range of camera angles (high shots, low shots,
near shots, distance shots, shots through the equipment, shots over it, inside
scenes, outside scenes), a variety of different people (some absent a white coat),
and shots of different pieces of equipment, sometimes moving, sometimes still,
sometimes with ambient sound, sometimes silent. So it was that the filmmakers
sought to maintain visual and aural interest. The danger was that it might all fall
flat even in the skilled hands of Parker and McLean.

There were also some problems in ensuring that the concerns of scientists
in the sponsoring agencies were addressed. Dallas Johnson had tried to involve
NCI scientists in the filmmaking, and Gilchrist had NCIC scientists as advisers,
as well as people in the DNHW. Many of their concerns were fielded by Johnson, Gilchrist, and Foster behind the scenes before filmmaking even started,
but the live-action sequences themselves raised some unforeseen problems. For
example, in one sequence a "girl"[29] picks up two mantels and places them in the
centrifuge. This sequence was made in Dr. A.M. Fisher's laboratory in Toronto,
and Fisher (as the laboratory chief) had been the adviser on these scenes. The
problem—one that Parker was entirely ignorant of beforehand—was that this
technique was not used in every lab. Not only did this raise the question about
what constituted a representative portrayal, but it was also a revelation to scientists in the sponsoring agencies who were not aware of the variety of different
techniques applied in different laboratories until they viewed the film.[30]

Scientists were also anxious about what to show what not to show. Dr. George
B. Mider (professor of cancer research at the University of Rochester) commented that the activities of the American Society for the Prevention of Cruelty
to Animals and the anti-vivisectionists were so alarming that he felt that "we
should be extremely cautious in demonstrating diseased animals . . . [and] that
if, by one device or another, normal animals could be shown, that this would be
very advantageous and would prevent a full scale assault on everyone involved
in the film production."[31] Susan Lederer has shown how both research scientists and anti-vivisectionists had lobbied the Hollywood studios in the 1930s
to reflect their opposing ideological views.[32] Mider's comments suggest that
anti-vivisectionist activities also had an impact on a film intended to recruit
people into scientific research, including laboratory research. Thus, the NFB
filmmakers restricted themselves to showing unharmed mice, portraying them
as heroes (as one character states in the genetics sequence) and the nearest we
get to harmed animals are the circulating rats and leapers, and damaged flies.

Nevertheless, Morten Parker recalls having to leave the room at one point when the scientists showed how a rat was killed.[33] It might not have been politic to show this on film, but apparently it was politic to show it to the filmmakers.

Mr. Davis: The main symbolic patient

For Glover and Parker, the representation of the patient was crucial to their efforts to portray science as a humanitarian calling, to indicate the hope that it offered, and to organize their efforts to evoke empathy/sympathy for the plight of those with cancer. It also served to portray patient confidence in modern medicine and science. The sponsors believed that an appeal to humanitarian sentiments might encourage young, idealistic high school and college students to enter the field. The filmmakers' task was to find a way to encourage such humanitarian impulses, and also to ensure a portrayal that addressed concerns about the tendency of patients to seek care too late when the cancer had so advanced that a "cure" was impossible. The patient's trust in science and medicine was to be a key here.

Part of the reason for this focus on trust in science was continuing medical concerns about the willingness of patients to follow the recommendations of the Canadian and American cancer organizations.[34] Such concerns can be traced back to the beginnings of anti-cancer campaigns in both countries, where cancer organizations sought to persuade patients to seek early detection and treatment at the first sign of what might be cancer. The problem then—and in the 1940s—was that many did not. Cancer organizations in both countries argued that people with cancer, fearful of a stigmatizing disease and of its treatments (surgery and radiation), often failed to go to the doctor, preferring dubious home remedies or quackery, delaying until the disease had progressed too far to be curable. In both countries, then, cancer organizations urged people to place their trust and hope in medicine. One of the goals of *Challenge* was to establish such trust and to anchor it in the work of science. Just as scientists were to enter research out of humanitarian impulses, patients were to trust in science because of this research.

The main focus of their efforts was Mr. Davis, the key symbolic patient, who is introduced in the opening scene (sequence 1) making a dramatic entrance that disturbs the calm of a hospital waiting room (Toronto General Hospital), and the recitation by the narrator of past "triumphs" of medicine over diabetes, tetanus, and other conditions.[35] Before his arrival, there had been an atmosphere of calm assurance in the waiting room. The room was bright, nurses moved unhurriedly

across the floor, a man lit another's cigarette, and the seated patients were uncon-
cerned, perhaps even bored. Then Davis enters, an elderly white-haired man with
a tumor on his cheek, setting up the new challenge that science itself faced in
cancer. The lighting and camera angles change so that we view Davis from below,
and his entrance is accompanied by a clichéd Hollywood musical alarm chord
added in later by the composer Louis Applebaum. The title of the movie—*Challenge: Science Against Cancer* or *Alerte: Science Contre Cancer*—appears on the
screen in gothic script, and there is a suggestion of gothic horror indicated by
shadowy lighting and slightly skewed camera angles as a nurse takes Mr. Davis
up a flight of stairs, their shadows thrown against the wall.[36] The camera watches
the two from below and slightly at an angle, so that they climb up and across
the screen. The shadows and the dark, gloomy appearance threaten to engulf the
light, which Parker hoped would create an atmosphere of unease.[37]

In the following part of the sequence, the live action returns us to a calm
assurance associated with medicine. Mr. Davis and his nurse walk toward us
along a corridor, the camera angles return to horizontal, the shadows are less defined, and there is little that is visually disorienting. The corridor is dark, though,
perhaps symbolizing the remnants of the uncertainty that Parker had hoped to
capture: darkness would later symbolize ignorance of the cell and cancer in the
animation sequences. Then we meet a man in a white coat, and two others in
suits. Their conversation reveals them as Ross (the physician formerly known
as Doug), and two men he introduces as research scientists, Drs. McVicor and
Ramm (elsewhere identified as the pathologist and his assistant[38]). There is an
atmosphere of calm deliberation. The lighting is brighter than the preceding
sequence in the corridor (symbolic of the hope offered by science and medicine?).
These three men are wreathed in cigarette smoke. They are viewing a photograph of magnified tissue projected from a lantern slide. Mr. Davis enters and is
greeted by the men. He is revealed as formally dressed in a dark double-breasted
suit, polite, respectful. He is asked to wait, and while he does, he transforms
into an outline, the beginning of sequence 2, the animated sequence on normal
and abnormal growth. We return to Davis in sequence 3, which begins with the
animated tumor turning into Davis's tumor, which is being examined by Ross,
McVicor, and Ramm, who then inform him that his type of cancer is one of the
more curable types: ninety chances out of a hundred he will be cured.[39]

Then Davis disappears from the film before briefly reappearing in the environmental cancer sequence 11 when we glimpse him at home in an armchair,
smoking his pipe, his cancer clearly present on his cheek. The narrator asks: "Are
certain cancers more common to men than to women . . ."[40] Only after this are

we returned to the calm assurance of Davis's treatment. (Clinic: sequence 12). We view a brief shot of him walking in the rain, lighting his pipe, and throwing away the match. (The shooting script had two football players tossing a ball in the background, whom Davis briefly watches as he lights his pipe, before moving on.) Davis's understated trust in science and medicine is echoed in the narration. The narrator tells us that patients can approach treatment (as Mr. Davis is about to do) with confidence. There follows a sequence on research on radiation treatments, which as the narrator notes, sets the background for the treatment of the patient with cancer. Mr. Davis now enters a hospital or clinic from the rain, and we see him begin his treatment, under a large, multimillion voltage piece of X-ray equipment. The narrator then briefly notes medicine's inability to cure many patients not as fortunate as Davis (accompanied by a brief shot of a patient being wheeled into an operating room), before moving on to highlight the hope offered by scientists' research, and the search for a test to identify cancers early, when according to the narrator they could be most effectively treated: a zoom in on an elderly female patient in bed, mixed with a montage of research scenes that fade away as the woman turns to face us—she symbolizes vulnerability, medical and humanitarian need, and perhaps the fear or concern of those with cancer.

The problem for the filmmakers in constructing this story of reassurance and submission to science was the actor. It will be recalled that Emerson Houghton, who plays Mr. Davis, did not have the acting range that the director, Morten Parker, had hoped for. In Parker's view (and that of some reviewers, see following chapters), he gave a wooden performance, and failed to express adequately the emotional journey of cancer—from fear to reassurance and relief—which would be essential to the portrayal of science as a humanitarian activity and the confidence that patients should have in it. Thus, while in sequence 3, for example, the filmmakers tried to get Houghton to express relief at being informed that his character had a cancer that was likely curable, they were unable to do this. While he smiles after receiving the news, the filmmakers and some critics felt that Davis's inner feelings—unlike his Tchelitchew-esque inner biology—were never fully transparent.

So the filmmakers had to figure out other ways of getting the emotional cost of cancer across. Some of this was done through the camerawork and lighting (recall the use of gothic horror-like lighting and camera angles to highlight the threat of cancer in the open sequence [1]) and the darkness that the filmmakers saw as symbolizing uncertainty); through the action and dialogue of the other actors (Ross reassuringly pats Davis on the shoulder when he gives him the good diagnostic news); through the editing (which structured the path of Mr. Davis from diagnosis to treatment, and its pacing); through the narration (which stressed the point about reassurance); and through the props—his smart suit, his pipe, and the X-ray equipment to which he submits. Houghton's Mr. Davis thus gained some of his character through components of the movie other than his acting, which also served to establish his role as symbolic patient, and the themes the filmmakers wanted him to symbolize: human vulnerability to disease, the emotional costs of cancer, and hope and assurance in medicine and science.

The rain sequence (part of sequence 12) illustrates some of these themes, since the filmmakers wanted it to portray Davis's calm confidence in medicine. Thus, the June 1949 shooting script informs us that Davis stops and lights his pipe in the rain, a tranquil moment before he enters the clinic for radiotherapy. Such a moment was a godsend for Parker given Houghton's limited acting range. His unexpressive features might have had difficulty in projecting an emotional journey from fear to relief, but the pacing of the moment where he stops to light and smoke his pipe on a rainy day countered such difficulties: calmness and confidence was there in the slow, deliberate timing of the sequence, the care with which he stops to light his pipe, and his peaceful puffing away as he walks slowly to his appointment. He was one of many symbols in the film—the symbolic scientist and nurse, the symbolic lighting, and indeed the rain—and their conjunction helped to construct Davis's character and narrative

The rain itself had an important if changing symbolic role in the film that helped to indicate the environmental threats faced by Davis, the treatments he undergoes, and his confidence in medicine. In the June 1949 shooting script, the rain was part of a visual thread that can be traced back to the preceding sequence (11, in the final version) on chemicals and environmental cancer. The thread began with a chemist pouring a clear liquid into a glass container (test tube, in the shooting script): the instruction is "MIX to Cell-as-universe, to give momentarily the effect of contents of test tube pouring into the cell."[41] There follows, in the script, a short cell-as-universe animation sequence, which then transitions to the live action, so that the liquid poured into the glass becomes the threat to the cell and eventually the puddle into which Mr. Davis steps. "Transition: In the last shot of cell-as-universe, an effect of rain obscuring all detail."[42] "Mix to MCS [medium close shot] of puddle of water in rain. Foot enters frame and steps into puddle."[43] Thus there is a complex connection between environmental cancers and the rain which affects Mr. Davis, so that when he eventually leaves the rain to enter the hospital, he is actually also stepping out of the environmental threats symbolized by the liquid rain and into the hope of the hospital and that radiation therapy offers: Davis is to have radium therapy.

TABLE 7.2. Comparison of the Structure of the Rain Sequence in the June 1949 Script and the 1950 Film

Script	Environment	Cell-as-Universe (animation)	Davis in rain. Lights pipe.	X-ray therapy	Davis enters clinic	Davis has radium therapy
Film	Environment	Davis in rain. Lights pipe	Radiation treatment and research: including radium.	Davis enters clinic	Davis has X-ray therapy	

This diagram represents only the sequence of events, not the time allotted to each sequence.

(Elsewhere in the shooting script, the mist was also intended to suggest "possible menace in the environment."[44])

At some point the short cell-as-universe animation (sandwiched between the environmental and the therapeutic sequences) was cut out of the film, and the symbolic role of the rain changes. Thus, in the final version of the movie, we move directly from the live-action pouring of the liquid into the glass container to the foot entering the puddle, without the intervening animation. The liquid link is still there but the emphasis on the environmental threat posed by chemicals to the cell is diminished, and with it the connection between the environmental threat and Mr. Davis's encounter with the rain.

In the revised version of the film, the first of the two rain segments (where Davis lights his pipe and does not glance at the now nonexistent footballers) is less about the threat of environmental cancer than an introduction to the sequences that follow on the role of radiation in combating cancer. This first rain sequence always had this introductory role, but in the revised version of the film the visual link with environmental cancer is lessened, and a greater emphasis is given to radiation research. Thus, Davis's lighting of his pipe in the rain, and the calm assurance this scene suggests is followed by a more extended (compared to the shooting script) look at the role of radiation in tackling cancer, before we view his exit from the rain. In the shooting script, Mr. Davis's exit from the rain was also an exit from the environment threat symbolized by the rain. In the final cut, his reassurance has more to do with the hope offered by radiation therapy.

In the shooting script, after Davis enters the hospital or clinic from the rain, we are treated to a sequence on radium therapy. We see a doctor hovering over and obscuring a seated patient. "Enter nurse with tray. As doctor reaches for the needles on tray he reveals Mr. Davis as the patient."[45] But while the radium sequence is retained in the final version of the movie, this patient is not Mr. Davis. Instead, Grant McLean shot an anonymous person, his or her eyes and nose framed by a cloth which drapes the patient's hair and two bandages that are taped above and below the mouth, in between which the physician fixes the radium needles over the patient's mouth. (Davis's cancer is on his cheek, but the cancer of the lip from earlier treatments seems to have returned.) Later, when the developed film was back in Ottawa, the editor reordered the segments of the clinic sequence. In the final version of the film, the radium therapy sequence becomes a prelude to Davis's entry into the hospital/clinic out of the rain (the place previously held by the X-ray sequence in the shooting script). By the same token, the X-ray sequence, with its adjustments of the super-voltage apparatus, becomes the sequence in which we witness Davis's treatment. Davis is to be treated by X-rays, not radium. The hope embodied by Mr. Davis, his trust in medicine, is a construct of these other sequences, the rearrangement designed to emphasize the importance of radiation in combating cancer, to compensate for the limitations of Houghton's acting range, and to set up the symbolic role of the scientist.

Not every viewer would be satisfied with Houghton's portrayal (chapter 11) but his presentation as an obedient patient, following his doctor's instructions, and his calm assurance in science and medicine, aided by the doctors and more important, the nurses who care for him, would have been agreeable to the sponsors concerned about patient delay in seeking appropriate help. But he was a malleable figure. He had started life as a woman in Constant's first script anxious about her diagnosis, whining like a dog, and was now transformed into a man, whose tumor had migrated around his body in the different iterations of the script; someone calm, even stoic, in his response to the diagnosis, and placid in the face of his upcoming treatment. This construction of the patient was also a product of the other major symbolic figure in the film, the scientist, whose steady work to understand and intervene against the disease had already led to triumphs that meant that Davis's cancer was treatable, and whose continuing work would lead eventually to many more cancers being caught early and treated successfully—at least that was what the film suggested.

The scientist and the work of science

The problem the filmmakers faced in constructing the image of the scientist and his or her work was similar to that of the patient—the varied acting abilities of the mix of amateur and professional actors used in the film. As with the patient,

the character of the scientist and his or her work was not only constructed by
what the actor did in front of the camera, but also through the other components and symbols of the movie: the narration, music, staging and ambient
sound, in addition to the other actors with whom an actor shared the screen.
Together, these allowed the filmmakers to generate a complex—and sometimes
contradictory—character that would serve the broader argument of the film
and (they hoped) persuade audiences. This character was sometimes heroic (and
sometimes not), sometimes explorer, sometimes ordinary family man, and sometimes completely absorbed in his or her dedication to his work: a special sort of
man or women, but also a small cog in a worldwide effort against the disease.

The construction of the scientist as medical hero was not new to this film. As
Bert Hansen shows, this construction can be traced back at least to the late nineteenth century and the co-emergence of both a new form of laboratory-based,
scientific medicine and new business models and technologies that helped the
development of mass-circulation newspapers and national magazines. In particular, Hansen argues that media reports of Louis Pasteur's 1885 announcement
of a vaccine for rabies helped create a long-standing transformation in public
portrayals of medical science that nurtured both popular anticipation of medical discoveries and media confidence that medical breakthroughs would be
news: a fascination with medical breakthroughs that lasted until the 1950s, the
highpoint of popular admiration and optimism, also propagated by media such
as radio and film. *Challenge* thus built on a long tradition of portrayals of the
laboratory science as a key to medical progress, and it used nineteenth-and early-twentieth-century figures—Pasteur, Koch, and Ehrlich are briefly mentioned
as we scan the calm, waiting patients in the opening sequence (1)—to set up
cancer as the next challenge for science, encouraging audience anticipation of
future medical discoveries.

The construction of the scientist as hero had been present in the shooting
script, long before the NFB hired its actors. It will be recalled that the June
1949 script had closed with a shot of a scientist in heroic composition—in deep
concentration, at a micro-manipulator, delicately making adjustments—and
that this sequence seems to have been discarded sometime later. Morten Parker's shooting script seems to suggest that the scene was in fact shot, but I have
found no footage of it, so we know little about how this composition might have
looked. One might have expected that a film aimed at recruiting scientists into
cancer research would portray the scientist as hero. However, without the heroic
compositions, the final version of film makes less of it than might be expected,
in part because it also wanted to portray the scientist as an ordinary figure (of

which more below), perhaps playing on the idea of the ordinary man as hero propagated during the Second World War. Indeed, the film at times seems somewhat ambivalent about the heroic status of scientists. It is true that the narrator invokes the heroic image of the scientist at the beginning of the movie: the list of great names provides models for future cancer researchers as well as explaining the reassurance and calm hope of the hospital waiting room (sequence 1). However, when the narration came to be written it had the narrator portraying the work of science as "The steady, unheroic search for shaft of light."[46] The only hero in the film, named as such, is a mouse in the genetics sequence.[47]

The one area where the scientist seems unequivocally a hero is in the film's portrayal of the scientist as an explorer. This character was created with a mix of camera angles, lighting, special effects, animation, and narration. It begins in sequence 3 after Mr. Davis and the two research scientists, McVicor and Ramm, have left the room, and Ross is left alone with the slide of Davis's tumor on the screen. He replaces the slide with another and sits on the table on which the projector stands and contemplates the slide. At this moment, the camera is behind Ross and the projector and at a distance so that we also see what Ross is watching projected on the screen. Then the camera position changes. It has moved into a low angle in front of Ross, so that we look up at him, while he looks over and above us to the unseen screen behind the camera. The narrator asks why the answer to the cancer problem is so difficult, the composer provides a percussion special effect, we (the viewers) see a closeup of the image on the screen, which transforms before our eyes (accompanied by another special effect created on a different musical instrument), before the camera returns to face Ross. Ross stands up and walks slowly towards us so that we are looking up towards his chest and head. If there is a heroic composition of the scientist in this film it is this, for the low angle shot of that emphasizes the stature of a hero had been employed in American cinema since at least the 1910s.[48] But it is also a composition that hints at the questions that the narrator (and Ross) are asking about the difficulty of the cancer question, the attraction of the question (to Ross), and the beginnings of the view of the scientist as explorer of the strange unknown universe of the cell, someone with the cachet of the then contemporary space explorer (fictional or otherwise), able—as discussed in Chapters 3 and 4 on his portrayal in the script—to promote cancer research just as portrayals of spacemen promoted the budding space program.

At this point the camera angle changes. We are now once again behind Ross, looking at his back and the image on the screen in front of him. We are at the transition from sequence 3 to sequence 4, where Ross walks into the universe of the cell, shrinking as he does, like an explorer entering a strange new world. His diminishing stature is in marked contrast to the heroic composition we viewed a few moments before. Now Ross serves not only to visually represent the scientist as explorer (a point highlighted by the narrator), but also to evoke visually the vast size of the cancer problem: Ross's shrinking figure means that parts of the cell come to tower over him, as he eventually vanishes into the darkness, leaving us to journey on through the cell without him. This image of the scientist as explorer is thus created not only by the actor, but also by the animators (who conjured up the images of the internal world of the cell); the special effects cameramen (who melded the live action and animation); Grant McLean, (who filmed the actor from various angles); the lighting (which leaves Ross surrounded by the darkness, which eventually comes to symbolize the vast reaches of outer/inner space as well as the mystery of the cell and cancer, and scientific ignorance), the narrator who describes the cell as "a universe to be explored"; [49] and the composer who conjures up the cell-as-universe with special effects that sometimes sound like electronic music, albeit created with a conventional orchestra.

If the filmmakers represented the scientist as a hero (albeit sometimes) and explorer, he or she was also, paradoxically, an ordinary person. This is "a man like other men," [50] the narrator informs us at one point. As I have already noted, Steven Shapin maintains that the idea that scientists were ordinary people was increasingly asserted during the twentieth century, especially after World War Two.[51] Following the explosion of the atomic bombs in Japan, scientific knowledge received greater public respect, but of a different type than that achieved by earlier icons of science such as those mentioned at the start of *Challenge*. In the United States, scientists were increasingly represented in popular culture as emotionally cold, sometimes scary experts, and by the government as too sophisticated, too independent-minded, or too ethically sensitive to be entirely trusted. Under these conditions, Shapin argues, the idea that "scientists are human, too" was invoked as a reassuring, counter-stigmatizing self-defense. The narrator's invocation of the scientist as a man like other men may reflect such counternarratives. But there were additional motivations for this portrayal. One was that it allowed an appeal to humanitarian instincts, which scientists shared with other individuals concerned about the suffering of patients such as Mr. Davis. Another, as I've mentioned, was that it allowed a play on the language of ordinary heroes deployed to represent servicemen during the war. And yet another was that it allowed the sponsors to reassure potential recruits to science that they could have the lifestyle of their peers, despite not having the income of an industrial researcher.

The filmmakers used this last image of the scientist most clearly in sequence 13, which portrays the scientist as both a dedicated researcher and also as a family man as imagined in the 1950s. In this scene, the scientist, played by the Toronto University chemist James J. Rae, is on the phone discussing day-to-day issues of family life with his wife. He is in his office or lab late at night. As he chats with her, the camera pans over his bookcases stuffed with medical publications, over liquids bubbling in glassware, over a photo of his wife, while the narrator tells us about the many years he trained to become a scientist, and how this training prepares him to identify the clues to the disease (should they come his way). As noted before (chapter 4), the shooting script informed us that the visuals were to reveal the nature of the office and character of the scientist.[52] This character involves both dedication and complete absorption in his work, and also marriage, children, and a middle-class lifestyle. The sponsoring agencies—the NCI and the Department of National Health and Welfare—had worried that many men were put off a career in biology and cancer because its uncertainties and poor pay made it difficult to start a family, purchase a house or car, or live a normal middle-class life. One of the functions of *Challenge* was to reassure would-be scientists that this was not the case.

The filmmakers thus had to juggle potentially conflicting images of the scientist, as someone who did not go into science for material reward but who nevertheless was able to share in the lifestyle of his or her middle-class peers. One of the ways in which they sought to resolve this potential conflict was to appeal to an older idea of the scientist as uniquely virtuous, given to stoic fortitude and self-denial in the service of truth. Thus, after informing us that the scientist is a man like other men, the narrator also states that this is a special sort of man, "whose intelligence has been alerted, his imagination given special edge. He has stored within him a vast fund of knowledge drawn from the scientific harvest of the world. And in him is the agitation of a problem. The search . . . The question mark . . ."[53] He is a man who has accepted what the narrator calls a challenge: Someone who cannot leave the laboratory or office till late at night: The darkness here coming to symbolize not so much uncertainty or ignorance as in earlier sequences, but dedication, and likely his sacrifice in separating from his wife and family. The sequence ends with Rae leaving work, walking down an empty corridor alone, his back to the camera (an echo of the earlier explorer scientist, Ross, who had walked into the world of the cell), leaving the machines in the laboratories to carry on in semi-darkness. The machinery of science continues even after the scientists have gone, and its sounds—echoed in the music—emphasized the mechanical, automated nature of this work.

A final tension in the portrayal of the scientist in this sequence is between dedication to work and desire for a life like other people, a family, fun, and economic security. In the scene with Rae, it seems to be resolved by posing a gendered division of labor, with male scientists working late at night in the laboratory and their wives caring for the children at home. But many—perhaps most—of the white-coated scientists in the film were women, and they too were represented as completely absorbed in their work. The film never raises the question of what this dedication meant for their home life, and no women scientists are portrayed working late into the night or calling their husbands from the office.

It is unclear to what extent the large numbers of women in the laboratory scenes reflected the desire of the sponsors to recruit women to cancer research, or the contingencies of filmmaking: the choice of laboratory locations that employed lots of women. Whatever the case, the filmmakers seem to have struggled with the issue of what dedication meant for women scientists. Take, for example, sequence 9: Biochemistry. This is the sequence set in a laboratory at lunchtime. An older male scientist brews some tea in the laboratory glassware, and then calls everyone to join him. Most do except Barbara, who continues with her experiment, unwilling to break for lunch, while the others gather around the older scientist, surrounded by laboratory equipment, discussing a recent scientific publication, the progress of their own research, and the problems of grants. "The purpose of this lunch scene," the shooting script notes,[54] "is to capture a little of the character of the scientist and his co-workers . . . their complete absorption in their work."

The shooting script had portrayed a gendered vision of absorption that is not present in the final cut. In the June 1949 script, the male scientists talk seriously about the latest research, while the female scientists mix discussion of work with plans for a dance in the evening, one "ruefully regarding her fingernails"[55] and commenting: "Look at my hands. I'm supposed to be going to a dance tonight."[56] The work of science, it seems, could be a handicap to a woman seeking to make an impression in the dance hall. In the final cut, the comments about dancing and fingernails disappeared, as did a scene in which a male scientist fills his pipe from a laboratory desiccator which is being used as a humidor.[57] Instead, while the older male figure is clearly the senior scientist, there is little in the way of a gendered division of absorption in the laboratory. The men might talk about the results and publications more than the women, and there is a distinction between the English-and French-speaking scientists, the latter including one male and one female who join in the lunchtime discussion, and struggle with the English word "progress."[58] However, the scientific chatter of the scientists at tea (added during the filming, as annotations in Morten Parker's shooting script suggest),[59] highlights not only their interest in research, but Barbara's as well. She never joins them, and the noise of the laboratory instruments around her and to which she is attending almost drown out the chatter of the scientists. The rhythmic ambient sound of the instruments symbolically highlights the constant work of science, and the dedication of the scientists, male and female.

In such ways the filmmakers sought to appeal to young scientists, men and women. Those who entered this field might never have the income of someone who worked in industry, but the film reassured them that they could have a middle-class lifestyle, and that at least the men would continue their chosen path after marriage. These men and women were engaged in something as exotic and thrilling as work in atomic physics, but also something that would eventually benefit the many millions facing cancer. The women are never portrayed as explorers like Ross, nor are they visually portrayed as heroes. But both men and women join teams of dedicated researchers, completely absorbed in their work, forming part of a select international group of men and women. "There are men like this," the narrator informs his listeners, omitting women, "in places like this . . . in Montreal and Washington, New York and Paris, London, Rome, Geneva, Stockholm".[60] Their search might result in international recognition, but the path to such recognition (if it came about) was not glorious. "What is man, that thou art mindful of him"[61] the narrator asks, quoting Psalm 8:4, invoking an image of God's care for humans, and associating the scientist with it in the "steady unheroic search for shaft of light," mentioned above.

It was here that the film focused on the work of science. Machinery provided a visual and aural symbol of science as an incessant, even mechanical activity, as when the machines continue their work in the dark of night, with no human intervention, just the musical imitation of their rhythms. But here was no message about the subordination of man to machine, but rather the opposite. Such scientific work does not survive long without scientists. In this film world, they are needed to give meaning to the routine work of the machines, the arrays of glassware represented in many sequences, the liquids and chemicals, and the living animals, eggs, tissue cultures, and microscopic slides.

Moreover, the incessant nature of cancer research may in some ways be a counterpoint to the incessant spread of cancer in the body. It is orderly, controlled, disciplined, and subject to the scientists who run it, unlike the undisciplined nature of cancer, its disorder, uncontrolled growth, not subject to the laws of the body. The script also emphasized the insatiable nature of research perhaps a counter to the ravenous nature of cancer. Nature was controlled within the laboratory, no matter how ravenous. Thus, in the tissue culture scene described in the shooting script an assistant brings a diet of media for the tissue culture to feed off, prompting one scientist to comment, "More food for the hungry little mouths, eh?"[62] The phrase is cut from the final version, and while we get a closeup in which the frame is filled with the mouths of flasks and test tubes containing tissue cultures, perhaps even "lined up with openings gaping into the camera,"[63] it is doubtful they achieved the image required in the shooting script, "to give effect of numerous hungry squabs with their beaks open."[64] Perhaps they avoided it because the greediness of nature in the laboratory presented here could also blur into a portrayal of science as itself ravenous, greedy for the sorts of recognition – financial, professional – written out of earlier treatments of the film (chapter 4).

So the filmmakers strove to marshal all these elements to show how scientists were making cancer and the cell objects of science, and their hope was that this—the animation with its depictions of the inner world of the cell, the live-action representations of the patient, the work of science and the character and training of scientists—would help enroll young scientists in the endeavor. But before it could be presented to audiences, the footage had to be edited together, the music and narration composed and performed.

CHAPTER 8

Pulling Together

WITH THE ANIMATION AND live-action sequences nearing completion the filmmakers began to think about the final aspects of the movie—the music, editing, and narration. In different ways, these parts were about pulling the film together to make the film's "argument" for the overlapping projects of making the body and cancer objects of science, and of attracting would-be scientists and the public. Following Grierson, the animation and live action had sought to promote this argument through a range of visual symbols and metaphors. In the animation, the metaphor of the cell-as-universe and the darkness of outer/inner space served to symbolize the vast scale of the cancer problem, the wonder of the human body and cell, and the opportunities that opened for someone who would venture into this world. In the live action, there were the symbolic figures of the patient and scientist, and the ceaseless work of science, all mobilized to conjure up the sorts of people who might be attracted to science, and to invoke the humanitarian and medical need for their calling. The editing, music, and the narration were about imposing order on this mix of symbols.

The filmmakers had begun to create the argument of the film in the scripts and treatments discussed in chapters 3 and 4. Likely it began in meetings between Constant, Foster, and perhaps others in the NFB before Constant put pen to paper and sketched out his first script, establishing a structure for the film. After that began an iterative process that continued with the many later revisions of the scripts and treatments and into the filming. The structure helped to frame the argument, which was then to be fleshed out by details of the script, given visual form in the animation and live action, and then taken up by the editors who would string the whole thing together and match sounds with visuals. Just as the live action and animation sought to mobilize visual symbols to advance the themes of this film, so too the sound introduced aural symbols, sometimes reinforcing those of the visuals and sometimes not. The narration would often abandon literal description in favor of metaphorical allusions. The composer would use a variety of aural symbols: allusions to science fiction, leitmotivs, and imitations of events on screen or counterpoints to them. Even the ambient sound could have a symbolic role, as when, for example, it sought to evoke the mechanical nature of some scientific work. Thus, the symbols so central to the argument of the film were not only products of the live action and animation, they were also created through the music, the sound, and the narration.

The narration holds a key place in this film, which, like many NFB educational films, used a voice-of-god narrator to explain the events on screen, set out the argument, and highlight the distinctive roles of the key individuals and subjects of the film—the cell, the scientist, the patient, and the work of science. Yet the narrator was not the only one to help audiences interpret the film. The composer, Louis Applebaum (1918–2000), would use the music to interpret the film though tone paintings of cell division, rhythmic evocations of the growth of the body, musical suggestions of the work of science, the wonder of nature, the danger of cancer, and the harmony of the body. The ambient sound, too, could be used to help viewers interpret the film: listeners might detect allusions in the ambient sound to the Cold War fascination with science and mechanism, the character of the scientist, and the calm hope of a hospital waiting room with its unhurried footsteps and silent patient patients. Finally, when the editors opened the film canisters and began to figure out how to piece it all together they also helped to interpret the movie. The pace of the editing helped to set mood as did the mixing of sound, while the transitions between animation and live action helped to mark the structure of the film and create the narrative. All would help with symbolic expression—symbols of science (and assurance in it), the patient, the scientist, the cell-as-universe and more.

The challenge of composing

By the time Louis Applebaum was appointed composer, the film was almost finished. The live-action sequences were complete, and the animation was almost done. At some point, the composer met with Parker and Glover in an editing room or small theater and reviewed the movie. Douglas Tunstell—the editor—may also have participated, since he (and perhaps Clarke Daprato, the soundman) would be responsible for editing the sound, and making the final edits to the film when the last of the animation sequences came in. During this and other meetings, Parker recalls, they talked about what parts of the movie needed music, what its function should be, and perhaps something about the styles of music appropriate to these sections.[1] Together this group decided to focus on the

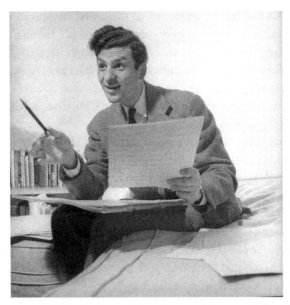

FIGURE 8.1. Louis Applebaum, December 1945, photograph by John F. Mailer. Source: Library and Archives Canada, accession number 1971-271 NPC, item number 11975, reproduction number PA-193042.

animated sections of the movie; all the animated sections are accompanied by music, but only three of the live-action sequences are: the opening title sequence where Mr. Davis appears in the hospital waiting room, and two sequences later in the film illustrating therapeutics and the ceaseless activity of research. Then it was up to the composer to produce a score.

Born in Toronto and trained at the Toronto Conservatory of Music, Applebaum had worked for a brief time with Grierson at the NFB in the early 1940s, before moving to Hollywood, where his film work culminated in his nomination for an Oscar (jointly with Ann Ronell (1905–93)) for the score of *The Story of G.I. Joe* (1945), Robert Mitchum's first major movie.[2] But by the late 1940s he had become concerned that his association with Grierson would lead some to label him a Communist or Communist sympathizer, a situation perhaps not helped when he composed the score for McLean's film on China, *The People Between* (1947). (He continued to compose for the NFB while in the US.) Consequently, he moved back to Canada in 1949, fearful that he would not be employable in the United States, and started to work under a series of contracts for the NFB.

On December 22, 1949, Applebaum signed a contract with the NFB for CAN$500 plus living and travel expenses to provide the score, orchestration, the preparation and cutting of the music track, and the special music effects work for *Challenge*. He also agreed to conduct the score.[3] The contract specified that the score was to be ready for recording by January 25, 1950, and Applebaum seems to have produced it before time: his copy of the score is dated January 20, 1950.[4] The recording session took place on the afternoon of January 28, 1950, at St. Barnabas Hall, the parish hall of the Anglican Church of St. Barnabas, Apostle and Martyr, in central Ottawa.[5] It lasted 5½ hours, beginning at 1:30 p.m.

Applebaum's score called for a small orchestra.[6] Most of the musicians are unknown, but an invoice notes the names of three out-of-town musicians who were given travel expenses and living expenses for the recording:[7] the cellist, Jean Belland (1895–1965),[8] clarinetist, Joseph M. P. Delcellier (1876–1957),[9] and flutist Marcel Baillargeon (1928–2019).[10] Only Applebaum's copy of the score seems to have survived, and it is likely that some aspects of the score and how it should be played would have been worked out in conversation between Applebaum and the musicians. Likely these were dealt with in the rehearsals at St. Barnabas Hall, or perhaps by phone or in person beforehand.

Interpreting *Challenge*

Applebaum had a singular position within the film. Since his score was produced almost at the end of the production process, he was able to create a personal musical interpretation of the film. Such freedom was likely constrained by his position as a contractor, by his conversations with Parker, Glover, and Tunstell (and the possibility of a Parker or Glover veto), by directions within the script that compelled him to use certain themes, styles, or quotations, by directorial prescriptions for placement of music, by the sound editor's final mix, or by last-minute alterations made by others. Nevertheless, Applebaum seems to have had considerable scope to develop the musical materials as he wanted.

One of the early discussions with Parker, Glover, and Tunstell resulted in an agreement that the music would provide a narrative frame for the film and the sequences within it. Thus, Applebaum bookends the film with musical arrangements, which accompany the main title and end credit sequences. Music also serves as a frame that separates the animated sequences from the surrounding live-action sequences. It generally begins at the start of an animated sequence and ends at the beginning of a live-action sequence. Elsewhere, it helps to structure the narrative within a sequence, for example, in the few times it is used in the live-action sequences: in the opening sequence (1) it announces the arrival of Mr. Davis and the subject of cancer, and accompanies Davis and a nurse until they reach the scene where Davis is introduced to the the physician and two scientists; in the therapy sequence (12) it marks transitions between the incessant work of science and the hope it offers, and in the night laboratory sequence (13) it both marks the unending work of science, and serves as a frame between the exit of the last scientist late at night and the entry of others the following morning.

Applebaum used the music as much more than a framing device. He also uses it to interpret the visuals or the spoken text, sometimes by creating a mood (as in the opening scene, where it helps to create a mood of tranquility and trust in science in a hospital waiting room), sometimes by imitating an idea (like cell division, cancer, or the mechanical movement of scientific equipment), sometimes by building on a concept (as when he tried to invoke musically the otherworldliness of the cell-as-universe), and sometimes by intensifying a dramatic event (like the sudden change from the tranquility of the opening scene to the dread of cancer signaled by a clichéd Hollywood alarm chord). Within the score there are subtle references to the work of other Hollywood composers such as Korngold and Bernard Hermann, for example in the solo clarinet and its melodic fragments, or what Applebaum labels "special effects" that accompany the cell-as-universe animation sequences.

Much of this was in the background. The source of the music is never represented in the film: no musical instruments are shown in the movie, or sound collecting instruments such as microphones, though sometimes the music imitates what we see, so that it might appear that the music comes from a scientific instrument. But in general the music is just there, accompanying the visuals, with no indication of the work that has gone into its composition and performance. Its source is hidden, "inaudible" to use Claudia Gorbman's phrase, subordinated to the narration and visuals, the primary vehicles of the narrative.[11] As I shall show in chapter 11, the music was in fact not "inaudible" to all viewers/listeners, but there is evidence that Applebaum and the filmmakers wanted it in the background, as was the musical convention or "grammatical rules" for film music that had emerged in Hollywood in the 1930s and '40s when Applebaum had worked there.[12]

Compare, for example, the music with other sounds in the film. While the source of the music is invisible, this is not true of all sounds in the film such as the rhythmic moving of certain scientific instruments, the splash of liquids, the falling rain, or the dialogue of the actors. This contrast between the music and other sound effects is one way in which the filmmakers tried to keep the music in the background. A sound—such as the splash of liquids, a dripping tap, the sound of a machine, or an actor's voice—that originates from a source within the film (a diagetic sound) is part of the world created in the film in a way that the non-diagetic music is not. In addition, while the music might help move the narrative forward, it does not push the narrative forward in the same way as the (also non-diagetic) narration. It tends to be subordinate to both diagetic sounds and narration.

Having obscured the source of the music, and subordinated it to the narration and diagetic sounds, Applebaum is free to use the music in the various ways he wants. Likely some of these themes were discussed with Glover and Parker in their meeting(s) before the composer began work on the score, and several approaches are apparent from the score and the soundtrack. Thus, when he wants to show humanity, organic harmony, completeness, normality, or hope in medicine, Applebaum tends to use a tonal structure, and often uplifting or reassuring harmonic, sometimes melodic, fragments. When he wants to evoke the unknown or alien, the uncontrolled, deadly growth of cancer, and sometimes the work of science, he extends tonality, and employs dissonant musical textures (tonal clusters), and orchestration that produces something akin to electronic sounds and music.

There is a comparison to the music of science fiction films here.[13] Beginning in the 1940s, composers began to use discordant and/or unusual instrumentation or orchestration to convey otherworldly or futuristic themes. Typical of the new instrumentation was the use of the theremin to signify otherworldliness, the unknown, the future and/or alien threat; themes that were also invoked using conventional instruments (sometimes with electronic instrumentation) but using unconventional orchestral arrangements to produce sounds derived from the repertoire of modern avant-garde music. In these scores, the future, otherworldliness, or the unknown were often invoked using chromaticism, dissonance, tone clusters, and unconventional instrumentation. Applebaum makes no use of the theremin, but his score—especially the special effects sounds of the cell-as-universe sequences—employ many of these orchestral techniques, and sometimes mimics the glissandi or portamento of the theremin, to draw a parallel between the unknown, the otherworldly, the future, and alien environments of outer space, and the unknown, the otherworldly, the future, and alien environments of the universe of the cell. The theremin had earlier been used within film to signify mental instability, but Applebaum does not invoke that theme in this movie.

If the cell-as-universe musical arrangments evoke the sound world of science fiction films, the music that accompanies the first animation sequence (2) on normal and abnormal growth imitates some of the action on the screen. For example, when cell division is explained, Applebaum utilizes a technique called "tone painting." The composer begins with a tiny melodic fragment, played mainly by the clarinet: the single cell. As the film's narrator explains that the cell divides, and we see it happening in the animation, additional layers of music are added to the first fragment, creating an aural image or imitation of cell division and growth. Then again, when the sequence comes to a discussion of the body as an organic living whole, Applebaum uses a throbbing beat to imitate the expansion and contraction of muscles including the heart depicted in the film. The layers culminate in a serene, harmonic musical fragment that accompanies the image of the fully formed biological man. So as the cells multiply into the unified vibrant creature, the musical layering culminates in a unified consonant harmony. Applebaum has "painted" cell division and life.

When we come to cancer in the same sequence, Applebaum again imitates cancerous growth. As we watch the first cancer cell emerge, Applebaum starts with one instrument, perhaps signifying the small, localized beginnings of cancer, and then adds other instruments as the cancer grows and proliferates. But whereas Applebaum resolved the normal growth sequence with the harmony that accompanies the complete man, the cancer growth sequence is discordant, fails to find a resolution, and does not complete. Applebaum maintains a holding pattern, for example, when the clarinet and bass play two and three notes repeatedly—an ostinato, a short melodic, rhythmic, or harmonic pattern that is repeated throughout the section, never resolving, never moving forward. Thus, while the visuals and narrative depict uncontrolled growth and metastasis, the music tends to hold back as more and more instruments are added to the painting, until, with metastases, the timpani rolls us forward, an echo of an earlier use of the timpani to evoke alarm in the opening scene (sequence 1) when Mr. Davis appears with a cancer on his cheek. All this alarm in the animation, however, is resolved not musically, but in Mr. Davis's consultation (sequence 3), where the fear of cancer is followed by the reassurance message of Ross when he informs Mr. Davis that his type of cancer is curable.

The last point also highlights how Applebaum—and Parker, Glover, Tunstell, and likely Daprato—sought to create a dialogue between the music and the other sounds in the film: the ambient sound and the narration. One example of this is the opening sequence where a brief series of melodic arpeggios played on the harp dissolve into the subdued chatter and noise of the hospital waiting room depicted in the live action. Applebaum and Daprato have sought to evoke a mood of calm assurance, the muted sounds of the waiting room being a resolution Applebaum's short melodic opening. Later in the same sequence,

Applebaum seeks to heighten the emotion of Davis's first appearance: the narrator talks of a new challenge facing science, while Applebaum employs the horror chord and timpani roll mentioned above to heighten the urgency of the new challenge and the danger of cancer. This continues with the following secondary chords, which fail to resolve, and eventually return as aftershocks of the initial alarming chord: tremolos that might denote uncertainty (when the nurse and Mr. Davis climb the staircase with its lighting evoking gothic films). The mood in the sound world is one of alarm, unease, and urgency, until the music fades away, and is replaced with the scientists' calm conversation about Mr. Davis's tumor and their greeting to him when he arrives. We have moved from the calm chatter of patients to the narration to the horror chord and back to calm conversation, the various aural elements working together to transform mood.

In such ways, then, the music sought to create aural symbols to accompany the visuals, often in conversation with them, and with the ambient, diagetic sounds and narration. Listeners could hear evocations of science fiction films in the sequences on the cell-as-universe in miniature, alarm and calmness in the opening sequence, and musical imitations of what is going on screen—normal cell division and cancerous growth, and elsewhere the unending work of science as Applebaum's music imitates the rhythm of the machines running late in the night scene. The film was not only a visual experience but also an aural one, and Applebaum sought to conjure a sound-world that described and played with the themes of the film, helped to structure it, and drew comparisons with other types of film.

Editing together

With the animation, live action and music coming together, attention focused on the editing and narration. Douglas Tunstell, a veteran NFB editor, began the process, helped by Arnold Schieman and Gordon Petty who operated the optical printer that mixed the visuals of the live-action and animation sequences, and used a photomicrography camera stand adapted from a drill press to film live-action sequences showing the growth and spread of (cancer) cells.[14] Tunstell probably also acted as sound editor, mixing in the music, and the ambient (diagetic) background sound to help set the mood and sometimes to interpret the narration. As with the music, the use of ambient sound would have been decided by Glover and Parker, with perhaps the help of Applebaum and the sound recordist, Clarke Daprato (himself a trumpet player) and Tunstell.[15] Some may have been recorded by Daprato during the filming of the live-action sequences.

However, it is also possible that other diagetic sounds were added later as special effects sound—footsteps, dripping water, the sounds of machinery.

Little documentary evidence remains of the editing process but given the Griersonian interest in the interpretative potential of editing, it had an important place in the making of the film. For Grierson, editing was a key to the creative treatment of actuality, a means of using the symbolic to depict the real through the phenomenal that the camera recorded. The script—the revised one printed after or during the live-action shooting—laid out the general structure the editor had to follow, and some of the goals of the editing, as for example animation blended into live action. But there was much more to do in the editing room, much revision, figuring out how best to piece together the strands of film to get at the essence of the subject: what should be cut, the order and pace of the sequences, how the transitions between sequences should be handled, where sounds and music needed to be added or removed, and what functions they might have. It was in these decisions that the symbolic patient and scientist, the work of science, and the visual metaphors would be honed from the raw material coming in from the live action and animation. In short, these symbols and metaphors would be revealed through the manipulation of footage by creative editing techniques, and so the broader themes of the film about making the body and cancer objects of science.

Although there may have been some editing before October, Tunstell probably began the first serious editing around the time that the first live-action shots came back from Toronto in October/November 1949 and would also have been affected by the delays in finishing the animation sections. The bulk of the editing probably happened between mid-November 1949 and January 1950, with a rush of final editing before the interlock—when the visuals and the sound were locked together—which happened sometime in February 1950.

Most of the discussions about editing were carried out internally within the NFB, primarily between Parker, Glover, and Tunstell with input from the American consultants. Parker recalls dropping into the editing room several times, sometimes by himself and sometimes with others.[16] But it was clear that the sponsoring agencies would also want a say, and this happened on Monday afternoon, December 19, 1949, when the NFB screened the rough cut—the first-draft attempt to stitch the film together—to an audience of NCI scientists and administrators along with representatives of the NFB, the AAMC scientific advisers, and the Canadian Department of National Health and Welfare.[17]

Many portions of the film were still missing at the time of this screening, particularly sections of the animation. A Department of National Health and

Welfare memo on this screening noted that there were no major criticisms of movie—just a few minor comments.[18] Physicians thought that Davis's cancer was very convincing, and they believed it real until the sequence where the doctor in the film massaged the cheek revealed otherwise. They also thought that there should be more emphasis on early diagnosis in the film and that Davis should be "cured" by its end, and there were various concerns about the meaning of certain shots and, as mentioned in chapter 7, about laboratory practices shown in the film. The NCI virologist Howard B. Andervont (1898–1981) thought the film was slightly out of balance in favor of the scientist, but others did not agree.[19] It was also suggested that the phrase "early cancer is curable" should be qualified: "early cancer is often curable".

The filmmakers likely breathed more easily after this. Scientists were something of a wild card in the production process, and no one knew what would happen if they objected to major parts of the movie and wanted parts of it reshot or new scenes added (probably at considerable expense), and Glover and Parker feared they might dilute the cinematic quality of the movie. The NCI scientists' participation had reflected, in part, Johnson's desire for their involvement, but even she recognized they could be trouble, and she tried to ensure that those invited to the meeting were sympathetic to the project. Nevertheless, it was still a worrying experience for the filmmakers, and even more for those who had promoted the film at the NCI, and who stood to lose credibility if scientists were unhappy with the film. It was here that the MFI had an important role to play. Men like David Ruhe (and perhaps Dryer and Bazilauskas) acted as mediators between the filmmakers and their scientific sponsors, and one of their roles was to forestall any major proposals for change at this late stage.

There remained the problem of the title. Dallas Johnson had pressed for the title to be changed to *Challenge: The Scientist Against Cancer* back in August to coordinate publicity for the film and for Lester Grant's book. By the time of the December meeting this was still a tentative title, and a small subcommittee was formed to look into this issue.[20] Subsequently, the title seems to have gone through a number of permutations including *Cancer—The Challenge to Science*, and *Cancer—Challenge to Science*[21] before agreement was reached on a final title—*Challenge: Science Against Cancer*.

So it was that by December 19 a considerable portion of the editing was complete. The screening seems to have resulted in some minor reediting to take account of a few criticisms raised, and Tunstell also had to include the animation sections that had not been ready on 19th, along with the soundtrack, and any ambient sounds not recorded on location. Thus the editing continued up to the fine cut in January, shortly before the commentary was recorded in early February 1950. The narrative was to be recorded using the fine cut, and (given concerns about fitting the commentary to the script) it is unlikely that major changes would be made after that. But a synopsis of the movie prepared for the Canadian premiere of the movie on March 19 suggests that the first animation sequence—normal and abnormal growth—may at one point have been slightly earlier in the movie than in the final cut.[22]

The challenge of narration

With the animation, live action, and music coming into the editing room, attention focused on the commentary. By late January the NFB was optimistic that they could get the actor Raymond Massey to read the narration, and a tentative agreement was reached with his agent that his fee would be small ($150), which he would hand over to a cancer fund.[23] Massey offered the possibility of reaching a broader audience than might otherwise have been reached, but there was an increasing urgency to tie him down to a date if the movie was to be ready for the US premiere, now scheduled for March 13. Dryer wrote to Massey's agent urging that he record in the first week of February.[24]

The impending premiere and the difficulties of getting Massey to commit to a date gave added urgency to efforts to complete the text of the commentary. During December and January, Constant, Parker, and Dryer had written and rewritten the narrative, trying to fit it to the evolving film. "Enormous effort has gone into literally every word of it," Foster and Dryer explained, "every phrase has been precisely timed with a stop watch to fit the film."[25] There are several versions of the narration in the NFB production files: some which are heavily annotated and edited, while another is the final script read by Massey, and the changes to the text seem to confirm Foster's and Dryer's account of the stopwatch.[26] They may also have sought to adapt the commentary to Massey's reading style as they imagined it. Massey was to deliver the narration in a slow, authoritative pace, poetic but spare, and many changes to the narrative seem to have been made so as not to interrupt this style of delivery.

Fitting the commentary to Massey's delivery style and to the pace of the film was a tricky task. It was exhausting work, under pressure, and there was always the risk that someone might object, that the revision would continue, that the whole thing would unravel in the rewrite, and that deadlines would be missed. Given the concerns of its scientific advisers and sponsors that the movie reflect the current state of scientific knowledge, Foster and Dryer were particularly worried that scientists might call for more revisions. During the rewrite, scientific accuracy had sometimes been sacrificed to the flow of the commentary: details had been cut, vague metaphorical allusions introduced, and dull, plodding facts removed, despite their technical accuracy as when a metric (1/2000 of an inch) became a metaphor (pinpoint fragment of life), or a technical term (centrosome) became a philosophical or mystical one (astral body).[27] Foster and Dryer pleaded against any further changes: "There are one or two key points in the script where, it can be argued, we have over-simplified our information almost to the borderline of inaccuracy.... we must ask that you grant us sufficient poetic license in these few instances."[28]

Fortunately for Foster and Dryer no one seems to have called for change. The writing was over, and Massey came into the studio on February 6, 1950, and recorded the commentary.[29] Massey wrote to the Canadian Minister for National Health and Welfare, Paul Martin, that the movie was a "superb achievement:" "I found it very difficult to do my commentary because of the absorbing interest of the film itself."[30] Morten Parker had a different memory of his visit to the NFB, remembering him as a snob who looked down his nose as he read the narration.[31] He recalls that Massey refused to take any advice on how to read it. His stentorian delivery, to Parker, overdramatized the commentary.

But Massey's narration was not the end of the story. Complicating all their efforts to complete the film on time was the fact that the sponsors had contracted for two films, one in English and the other in French. The two films were essentially the same, except that the titling and the narration were in French, as were the subtitles used to translate the English dialogue of the actors. Thus, as Parker, Glover, and Constant sought to finish the English narration, Alberte Sénécal (Department of National Health and Welfare) and Jacques Bobet (1919–96), one of the few French Canadians in the NFB, were frantically translating and adapting it for a French audience.[32] It was not an easy task, and the problems of the English writers in completing their narration had a knock-on effect on the French version and threatened to derail its schedule. Thus some of the poetic phrases and metaphorical allusions introduced into the English version were abandoned and replaced in the French version, which opens, for example, not with the phrase "Look beneath the roof-tops of the world, through all the lands, into the houses of healing,"[33] but with a longer version of a line from Ecclesiastes 4:10 that had been cut from the English version: "Si un homme tombe, dit l'Écriture, un autre le soutient; mais malheur à l'homme seul; car lorsqu'il sera tombé, il n'y aura personne pour le relever"[34] ("For if they fall the one will lift up his fellow; but woe to him that is alone when he falleth").[35]

Sénécal and Bobet wrote and rewrote and cut and changed the text to fit the pace of the movie, much as Glover, Constant, and Parker had done with the English version, and there is evidence of the changes they made in different versions of the narration that have survived in the NFB archives. They also had to find a new narrator, since Massey could not do the French version. After a quick search, the NFB recruited the French theater and film actor Claude Dauphin (1903–78), who had recently narrated the film *Van Gogh* (1948), which would be awarded an Oscar for best short subject in 1950. Dauphin came into the studio to record his narration on February 7, the day after Massey had recorded the English version.

There is little documentary evidence on the filmmakers' response to Dauphin's narration, but with it and Massey's work complete the filmmakers now had to ready the film for its premiere in less than a month. Cards had to be ordered for some subtitling in the French version (these were to be ready by March 10).[36] And the titling had to be completed for both the English and French versions of the film.

The titling might not seem a major issue, but it posed some tricky political problems given the sensitivities of the various organizations involved: font sizes came to symbolize both hierarchies and relations of equivalence.[37] Thus the titler was instructed that the text for the National Cancer Institute had to be the same size as that of Public Health Service (though one was to be in script and the other in roman type), and both were to be smaller than the font for the Federal Security Agency (FSA), of which they were both a part: the FSA's font was to be twice the size of the other two. Also, given the international collaborative nature of this film, the text for USA had to balance in size with Canada, two equal partners symbolized in the size of the text. In the end, someone—a subaltern titler?—subverted these goals. In the film itself the FSA had the same size font as the NCI and the PHS (both in the same typeface); Canada got a larger font than the USA, and the DNHW had the largest font of all the sponsors.

As the filmmakers strove to show how scientists were making cancer and the cell objects of science, the sponsors had their doubts. In their view, the film could not achieve the goal of attracting young scientists alone. Audiences had to be prepared to accept their arguments, and the curious had to be provided with much more information about cancer, biology and research than the film alone could provide. Even before filmmaking began the sponsors started planning ways of marketing the film to ensure that its case would reach an audience already prepared and open to the message. It is to the efforts at marketing that we now turn.

PART 3

PACKAGING

CHAPTER 9

Between Production and Promotion

T HE MARKETING OF THE movie began shortly after the contract between the Americans and Canadians was signed. Dallas Johnson, on the American side, and Lt. Col. C. W. Gilchrist, on the Canadian side, began to correspond regularly on how to attract media interest in the film, and on how to coordinate the publicity for the elements of the broader educational package. This packaging would come to include a booklet to accompany the film, a teaching guide (to help with its use in the classroom), a filmstrip (for situations where a movie event was not possible or desirable), and a number of different versions of the film to target different audiences. This was to be huge effort for Johnson and Gilchrist and their small teams at the NCI and the Department of National Health and Welfare, and would take up much of their time in 1949 and 1950.

As Johnson and Gilchrist began their promotional work, it soon became clear that promotion could not easily be separated from production. If they were to successfully market the movie, and the broader package of which it was a part, they wanted some say over what was in the film. The film was as much a promotion as it was a production. Thus, both Johnson and Gilchrist found themselves corresponding with the filmmakers on production issues, asking to review storyboards and scripts. At the same time, those on the production side also began to get involved in promotion, including David Ruhe, at the MFI. The boundary between promoting the film and determining what should be in it and how it should present its message was increasingly unclear.

Johnson's and Gilchrist's involvement in questions of production resulted in part from their common desire to get media organizations involved early on, but they also had two other reasons for taking an interest in questions of production. The first was Johnson's desire to coordinate the booklet—to be produced by an award-winning science writer, Lester Grant—with the film, a desire that Gilchrist likely shared. The second reason concerned the vulnerable position of Johnson's Cancer Reports Section within the NCI. She wanted to strengthen the place of her newly created section within the agency, and this meant keeping NCI scientists on board with this project. Gilchrist may also have had similar reasons for wanting to keep Canadian scientists on board given the need to consolidate the position of information services within the recent reorganization of the Department of National Health and Welfare. But Johnson faced particular problems with the research side of the NCI. She wanted her very new section to be at the center of public outreach for the NCI, which meant that she had to have the cooperation of the research side. If such a high-profile project as this went wrong, it could damage her section's credibility and undermine any future educational or publicity projects it might wish to develop. For all these reasons she felt compelled to stray into questions of production, correcting technical errors, passing on the comments of NCI scientists, suggesting themes, urging the NFB to coordinate the booklet and film. Promotion bled into production, and the filmmakers at the NFB found themselves "swamped" (as Ralph Foster put it) with letters from Johnson.

Beginning promotion

Promotional efforts began between April and July 1949, when Johnson and Gilchrist started to put out feelers to the press, radio, and television, sounding out their interest in the film. At first there was little response, perhaps just an occasional glimmer of curiosity from the media. Johnson and Gilchrist were probably unsurprised. The major promotional push would not happen for some time after the contracts were signed and there was not much that they could give the media in the early days. Constant's original script was undergoing revision, the NFB's new treatment would not be ready till May 1949, and a new script was not expected till June. Still, any interest from the media at this stage could be valuable and might help to guide the NFB as it developed its plans for the film. If Johnson and Gilchrist got any response to their inquiries before the scripts were ready, however, no records of them have survived.

All this changed when the writing of the new script was complete, and work began on the storyboards. By July 1949, David Ruhe had become convinced that there was a real possibility that *Life* magazine would do a big spread. A *Life* researcher, Geraldine Lux, had visited him and requested a copy of the storyboard. Ruhe had originally been brought in as mediator between the NCI and the NFB on the production side, and he was also supposed to be involved in distributing the movie, but the interest from *Life* magazine brought him into efforts to promote the film. It is not known whether he had a copy of the storyboard to give to Lux, but even if he had one, he could not give it out without informing the other organizations involved in the film. He wrote to Ralph Foster at the NFB recommending that they supply the storyboard "after suitable delay,"[1] and use it "to bend Life into becoming one of our publicity channels."[2]

A *Life* magazine spread would have been a real publicity coup. As Bert Hansen has shown, the magazine was one of the most widely read US periodicals, often saved and reread over months, years, and even decades.[3] Copies could be found all over the country, strewn across people's houses, piled up in garages, and perused while waiting for a haircut, attorney, or physician. It was a magazine that people leafed through time and time again, Hansen notes, as much for the excellence of the photographs as anything, imaginatively framed and produced on high quality special-coated paper. Before the rise of broadcast television, Hansen argues, *Life* was the United States' most reliable supplier of visual impressions, including portrayals of the medical world, not only facilitating public awareness of medicine and medical discovery but also helping to sustain public interest in and support for medical research and researchers.

Medical stories appeared frequently in the magazine. They averaged two or more a month, depicting new kinds of medical care, recent breakthroughs, and ongoing medical research. The magazine printed numerous striking photographs of medical figures, making some into household names. It not only provided images of scientists and science but also sought to explain the science, both in the text and through the magazine's pictures and diagrams. *Life* magazine was a vehicle by which Americans could visit specialized medical settings such as cancer clinics and operating rooms, normally off-limits to them, Hansen claims, and so helped to normalize those settings, perhaps reducing anxiety for patients and their families. Most important for *Challenge*, *Life* magazine promoted biomedical research: it presented it in imaginative and interesting ways, explained the need for research funding, celebrated the use of animal and human experiments in biomedicine, and promoted science as a glamorous activity that a young scientist might wish to pursue. No small wonder that Ruhe was enthused.

The early signs seemed to be promising. In August, Ruhe had a follow-up visit from Lux, this time accompanied by a reporter, Kenneth MacLeish (son of Archibald MacLeish, the American poet, writer, and Librarian of Congress). According to Ruhe they "gobbled up the story boards ... and apparently intend to do the thing up as a good story of some 6–8–10 pages, in short a super-colossal spread,"[4] and he pleaded for more information on locations, scripts, and other aspects of film production that *Life* could use in the article. For Ruhe, this seemed like a turning point. The early days of planning seemed to be coming to an end.

The film was going into production, and promotional efforts were gearing up: "We're spoiling for the real push, after the skirmishes of ideas and treatments . . . thank God with real people!"[5]

Ruhe was not alone in his enthusiasm. Dallas Johnson expanded on Ruhe's points a few days later to Gilchrist. She noted her surprise at how little persuasion *Life* magazine needed. The publication had made its mind up to do the story. "McLeish [*sic*] said with some glee that the only person who had some misgivings at first was Joe Thorndike, the Managing Editor, but that he had quit Life the week before and now they wouldn't have to worry about him."[6] She also noted that *Life* magazine was thinking of devoting nine to eleven pages to the film, and that they desperately needed the script and schedule so that they could assign photographers to accompany the film crew that would shoot the live-action sequences. Gilchrist had been working behind the scenes to get *Life* interested, and Johnson seemed certain that he had much to do with the magazine's enthusiasm. "As a promotion man, Colonel Gilchrist, you deserve a gold star!"[7]

By October, the early hopes that *Life* magazine might do a major piece on the film had begun to fade. Instead of assigning their own photographer to the production, *Life* now indicated that it would rather depend on the NFB's own coverage. Ralph Foster seems to have had doubts that the NFB could produce images of a quality that would work for *Life* magazine and saw the unwillingness to send a photographer as a sign that the magazine was losing interest. "I have no real confidence that the story will make Life, but we should in any case try to produce something that would be reasonable for them."[8] The crew was by then on location, filming the live-action sequences. It was a week later—November 3, 1949—that Foster informed Dallas Johnson that the first batch of stills from the Toronto shoot was ready.[9]

Foster's concerns about the quality of images produced by the NFB was likely not shared by all. Since its creation in 1941, the NFB's Still Photography Division had become the country's official photographer, ironically sometimes likened by its photographers to working for *Life* magazine.[10] Like the Farm Security Administration and other agencies in the US, the NFB had used photographs and still images to serve the nation. Division photographers shot everything from official state functions to the routine events of daily life, producing some of the most dynamic photographs of the time, seen by millions of Canadians—and international audiences—in newspapers, magazines, exhibitions, and filmstrips. But despite this pedigree, the NFB struggled to produce images that appealed to *Life* magazine. It was becoming increasingly clear that Foster's doubts had proved prescient, and that nothing would come of the early enthusiasm. And so it turned out: *Life* did not produce a major piece on the film. The reasons for its declining interest are unknown. However, Johnson and Gilchrist would find this a common pattern. Media organizations would express interest in the film, but it would come to nothing, with no explanation.

Life magazine was only one of several outlets that Johnson and Gilchrist approached. By August 1949, the two information officers had stepped up their efforts to attract media interest. In that month, Johnson reported that she had talked to CBS television, which wanted to cover the preview. All they needed was a location. Ruhe and she favored New York, unless it turned out to be impossible to get "the Washington hierarchy at that distance,"[11] by which she meant the leadership of the National Cancer Institute, the National Institutes of Health, the Public Health Service, and Federal Security Agency.

Also, in August/September, Johnson talked to Albert J. Rosenberg, the manager of the Text-Film Department at the McGraw Hill Book Company, who was keen to distribute the film. McGraw Hill had launched its first Text-Films in October 1947, and by 1950 had already distributed several NFB movies. Rosenberg saw *Challenge* as a chance to expand its text-film activities further by distributing other movies produced under the sponsorship of the US Public Health Service for school and adult audiences—general adult audiences as well as those in the medical profession. The market in text-films was beginning to expand rapidly, and other book publishers were entering a field which they had previously largely ignored.[12]

Johnson also began to talk to Robert Rendueles, WHO's information chief, and the United Nations Film Board (founded 1947), which aimed to coordinate the film activities of the UN and specialized agencies and to stimulate the production, distribution, and use of films. In October 1949, the film board voted preliminary endorsement and sponsorship for the film. "This is the first time this had been done for a health film, and it will mean a lot in our promotion and distribution,"[13] Johnson told Foster. But the meaning of this "provisional approval for sponsorship" is unclear.[14] At its next meeting the UN Film Board dissolved itself, and its functions were brought within a technical subcommittee of the UN's Consultative Committee on Public Information (CCPI). This group retained the name UN Film Board, but it worked under the rules of the CCPI and consisted of members of the CCPI. There is no further mention of *Challenge* in the records of this committee, and it does not seem to have gained final approval.[15]

The Package

With the beginning of efforts to interest the media in the film, Johnson began to work on other parts of the package to be associated with the film—a booklet on the challenge of cancer, a teacher's guide, and the filmstrip. The booklet was to be targeted at a broad general audience, the teaching guide and the filmstrip directly at schools. Her hope was that these would be ready for the premiere of the film sometime in early 1950, when they would benefit from the publicity around the film and would help to promote the film itself. The package was important to Johnson for while each part could be marketed individually, the impact was likely to be much greater if everything was ready at the same time. Johnson also hoped that different versions of the movie would be available as part of this package—a twenty-minute theatrical version of the film, and shorter ten-minute versions of the film, all tailored to different audiences than *Challenge.*

Planning for the booklet began in early 1949, about the time that the NCI began to foresee a future collaboration with the Canadians on the film. Johnson recalled that it initially proved a more difficult project than the film.[16] She tested several writers, assigning them single chapters to write, but none proved satisfactory. Then, by chance, the science writer Lester Grant came to Bethesda to talk to NCI scientists for a series of articles on cancer research commissioned by the *New York Herald Tribune*—a series that won the 1949 Westinghouse Science Writing award, administered by the AAAS.

Born in Taft, Kern County, California, Grant had had a long career as a journalist.[17] He had worked as a copy boy at the *Oakland Post-Enquirer,* where he eventually became a sportswriter. Grant took his sports writing talents on the road, working for the *Sporting News,* the *Washington Times-Herald,* the *Evening Star* and, by the middle of World War II, the *New York Herald Tribune.* He was excused from wartime service for health reasons, and after the war won a Nieman Fellowship in journalism at Harvard for the 1947–48 academic year. Soon after he started the series for the *New York Herald Tribune* that gained Johnson's attention. Grant seemed to her to be a perfect solution to the problem of the book.

In April 1949, shortly after the memorandum of agreement between the Canadian and American film sponsors had been signed, John Heller, the NCI chief, wrote to the publisher of the *New York Herald Tribune* asking if a version of Grant's articles, with some additional material, could be republished to coincide with the release of the movie. Heller noted that the NCI was undertaking a program to explain cancer research to the public, and the need for long-time, continuous research in the cancer field, as opposed to "any speed-up attemp [sic] to 'buy a cure' as we 'bought the bomb.'"[18] The institute also wanted to develop this project in such a way as to recruit promising students, both at the high school and college level, into the cancer research field. Grant's articles, Heller explained, could be made into a book to accompany the film. The *Herald Tribune* agreed, and Johnson arranged with the paper to reprint the complete series as a book—for which Grant was to write three additional chapters.[19]

With Grant's book underway, Johnson also began planning the teaching guide. She got the backing of the US Office of Education and the National Education Association, and approached the school superintendent of Prince George's County, Maryland, near Washington DC, who provided eleven science teachers (the chair, and two members each from biology, chemistry, physics, botany, and general science), all given time off to help prepare the guide that would make it easier for schoolteachers to utilize both the movie and book. The hope was that the subject of cancer could be worked into existing courses of study, to motivate a lesson, indicate a practical application of a scientific principle, illustrate a research method, or dramatize the progress of a science. Presented in this way, the NCI hoped, cancer education could enhance regular teaching and enrich rather than overload the syllabus.[20] The plan was to have the teaching guide, booklet, and filmstrip ready for the premiere in 1950, along with different versions of the film targeted at different audiences, including theatrical audiences.

Titles

The commissioning of the booklet in April 1949 marked the beginning of Johnson's efforts to coordinate the promotion of the book and the film. It continued with efforts to coordinate the title of the film and the book. She told Ralph Foster in August 1949 that she wanted to steal the title from the Lester Grant series. "The Challenge of Cancer" was an excellent movie title, she noted, that would have the added advantage of matching the title of the book, which would help promotion and simplify distribution. Grant was happy to let them use the title of the book for the film.[21]

A week or so after writing to Foster about the title, Johnson sought the advice of Morris Meister (1895–1975) on promotion and distribution: Meister was a recent president of the National Science Teachers Association (1946–8), the principal and founder of the Bronx High School of Science in New York City, and an influential figure in school science education.[22] According to Johnson,

Meister liked the title "The Challenge of Cancer," which he thought a very good one for school audiences. He also argued that the idea of cancer research as a challenge should be stressed throughout the film, particularly in the cell animation sequences. A pioneer of science clubs, fairs, and congresses, Meister had devoted a career to figuring out ways of stimulating youth interest in science. He was the founder of a highly selective specialized school, who lamented that the most scientifically promising students tended to languish in comprehensive high schools. He wanted programs that revealed high school students' special aptitudes, and this meant not only challenging but also tantalizing them. "If you can illustrate for the youngsters what we know about the cell and tell them what we don't know—leaving them with a feeling that here is a great riddle to be solved—you will be taking the approach that we have found a most successful recruiting device," Johnson quoted Meister. [23] "They must be made to feel that it is a great challenge—that they may be the ones to solve the problem." In Meister's view, it was crucial that the film do more than explain how the challenge to science emerged; it also had to offer up a vision of the future: "Technical people may want to leave the animation at the point where the challenge begins; that isn't enough if you want to interest youngsters. Tell them what we know, then where we want to go."[24]

Meister's comments show how easily questions of promotion turned into questions of production. In order to promote the movie, the filmmakers had to do what its sponsors wanted, and that meant structuring the movie and its message to fit the broader effort to persuade children and young adults that cancer could be a career. Meister was particularly critical of the genetics section of the movie, which he described as awfully spotty, hinting at all kinds of complicated things without explaining what the problem was, much less what must be done to solve it.[25]

At first, Johnson confined herself to the issue of the title. She began writing regularly to Foster, prompting the latter to respond cautiously: "You are a tireless campaigner, Dallas. I am led to suspect from a few subtle references in your last four or five letters that you would be pleased to have THE CHALLENGE OF CANCER as the title of the film. Well, maybe we will . . . maybe we will. . . ."[26] There are hints in this August 1949 letter that Foster would welcome a respite from the epistolary flood from Bethesda, but Johnson was not to be put off. "My enthusiasm springs from a knowledge of the 'cancer public' rather than the 'movie-going public,'" she explained to Foster, perhaps hinting that the NFB did not understand this "public." [27] "The general public thinks of our subject-matter area as something that is awful, dreadful, and fearful. The shock value of the word 'challenge,' I think, would not only produce audiences for you, but would also put them in an inquiring, receptive frame of mind." She incorporated the new title *The Challenge of Cancer* into some of the draft publicity.[28] The title *Challenge: Science Against Cancer* was officially adopted sometime between late December 1949 and early February 1950.

If Johnson's efforts to ensure the movie reached "youngsters" and the "cancer public" prompted her to suggest how the movie might be modified, so too did her talks with various NCI scientists. It will be recalled that the NACC had had some reservations about the capacity of a movie to recruit people into the field, and such reservations may also have been common on the NIH's Bethesda campus. So once Johnson received a copy of the storyboard from the NFB she began showing it around campus to drum up interest in the movie and to maintain good relations between her section and the NCI scientists. Whatever hesitations they might have had about the value of movies as a form of public education, few scientists, physicians, or administrators could resist the opportunity to tell the filmmakers how the movie could be improved. Most of their comments aimed to correct what they saw as factual errors in the storyboard. Others seem to have been motivated in part by professional rivalries (as when environmental cancer experts worried that too much attention was being given to tissue culture technique), and others suggested ways in which visual metaphors might be extended.

Johnson passed all this on to the NFB, as part of her broader effort to ensure that the package—the film, the booklet, the teaching guide and the filmstrip— helped those on the promotional side reach out to the intended audience, but also in an effort to maintain good relations with the research side of NCI. She explained to Ralph Foster, "I have a problem at the NCI that I don't believe any of the rest of you have to face. Our scientists are not only extremely interested in this film but they feel strongly that it must reflect the so-called 'scientific accuracy and integrity of NCI.'"[29] She further noted that if she didn't work closely with them on this, and they didn't like the film, "it would be almost impossible for my [Cancer Reports] Section to work closely with the research people again."[30] "That's the story, and I hope you understand it. After all Ralph, when you finish the film you can forget the scientists you deal with for quite a long time—until the next film in fact. But really, we can't."[31]

Foster would not have been surprised that the scientists and others within the NCI would want a say in the making of the film. It will be recalled that he had commissioned the first script written by Maurice Constant in part to rope in cosponsors for the film, and to kick-start the broader NFB international coproduction program. He did not expect that the original June 1948 script would go into production unchanged. It would be adapted to the needs and concerns of its new sponsors, and as discussed in chapter 4 the subsequent May 1949 treatments and June 1949 scripts were very different than the original Constant script, some of the changes reflecting the fact that this was no longer a simple Canadian production but an international coproduction with the Americans. Nationalistic themes that worked for the original Canadian production did not work for a production that involved another country, and internationalist themes came to trump nationalist ones. Some of these changes were probably made internally among the scriptwriters. But scientists, physicians, and administrators at the various sponsoring agencies also felt free to suggest changes, and indeed were encouraged to do so to allow the writers to ensure that their treatments and scripts addressed the concerns of the sponsors.

The backdrop to Johnson's comments was an effort to reshape the relations between her Cancer Reports Section and the Research Branch and Research Grants Branch of the NCI. In developing *Challenge* she had wandered into the territory of the research side. At first, she sought to involve the research side on an ad hoc basis by creating a committee of NCI scientists to evaluate the film and provide advice. But this was to be only the first step in her broader effort to harmonize relations, and in May 1949 she produced a memorandum setting out how she envisaged the future relations of her section and the research side of NCI.[32] There are hints in this document that there were problems in the relationship between the Cancer Reports Section and the research side. Despite Johnson's efforts to involve NCI scientists in its evaluation, the cancer film had emerged as a focus of tension. Its precise cause is not documented in the files, and no one I interviewed for this book remembered it. However, there had been tensions over an earlier public education booklet written by William Hueper on environmental cancer, which had been cleared by the Cancer Control Branch of NCI but apparently not by the research side. The Cancer Reports Section had published the Hueper book.[33]

In her May 1949 memorandum Johnson set out her hopes for the Cancer Reports Section. In her view, it should do much more than simply report on the work of the NCI. It should provide public information on the field of cancer more generally, and this meant that it should also be the choke point through which all public communications should pass. To this end, she proposed that all press contacts by the research side of the NCI be cleared by her section (apparently something that had not happened consistently before) and that conversely her section should clear all their scientific reports with the research side. She also proposed ways in which her section could help with the production of the *Journal of National Cancer Institute* (the NCI's major scientific journal), inquiries from the public, visitors to the NCI's Bethesda buildings, and how the Cancer Reports Section might be better integrated with the work and aims of the research side of NCI. Given these broad ambitions, Johnson was particularly concerned that the film that would become *Challenge* should be approved by the research side. Her ambitions for the Cancer Reports Section would be endangered if the film did not reflect the research side's views or if the Cancer Reports Section was perceived to be acting unilaterally.

Johnson's efforts to bolster the position of the Cancer Reports Section—and public information specialists more generally—within the NCI had thus led her to trespass more and more into questions of production. In part this had come about because the NFB agreed that scientific input was needed at the storyboard stage of the project, and Johnson was best placed to get the NCI's perspective on this. But, as Johnson herself noted, it had also come about because of her efforts to promote the role of public information specialists and in particular her Cancer Reports Section within the NCI. However, if Johnson felt that the status of her Cancer Reports Section was vulnerable to the whims of NCI scientists, it also turned out, ironically, that she and the filmmakers were placed in the position of adjudicating on the science. The problem was that NCI scientists not only sought to correct the science, but also to ensure that their specialist field of research did not lose out to others. Johnson and the filmmakers had a difficult political task in figuring how to respond to such suggestions. A wrong move could alienate support for the Cancer Reports Section not because the film got the science wrong, but because it seemed to promote one field of science over another.

Is it technical advice?

The point about the filmmakers unexpectedly and sometimes unknowingly adjudicating on the science has been mentioned before. In chapter 7 it was shown that scientists were concerned that the film presented scientific practices untaken at one laboratory as representative of practices at all laboratories, and that they were also concerned about the possibility of anti-vivisectionist reactions to scenes depicting animal experimentation. In both instances scientific concerns about accuracy blurred into concerns about science politics, both internal to science and the politics of its broader relations with the public.

The ways in which technical advice on science could turn seamlessly into more professional concerns is also evident in the environmental cancer sections of the movie. Johnson had been asked to check the environmental cancer section of the storyboard, and she spoke to several scientists about this, including William Hueper (director of the NCI's Environmental Cancer Section, 1938–64), Isaac Berenblum (biochemist, special research fellow at the National Institutes of Health, Bethesda, Maryland, 1948 to 1950) and Ummie (Booth). The identity of Ummie Booth is unclear, but it may have been Florence H. Booth, member of Johnson's Cancer Reports Section and later an administrator in the Scientific Reports Branch, the NIH's equivalent of Johnson's section, headed by Judson Hardy.

Hueper and Berenblum thought the section was handled very adequately, though they suggested some changes to the character of the cancer patient, Mr. Davis. At that point in the production, Davis had a carcinoma of the lip (not the cheek we see in the final version), and Hueper and Berenblum wanted a backstory that would allow the filmmakers to explain more about the origins of the cancer. They thought Davis should be identified as a farmer, and a scene included of this "past middle-aged"[34] man working in the hot sun. Also, they wanted the point made in the beginning about the connection between long hours of working in the sun and skin cancer. In other words, they asked for a cancer for which there was both a cure and a known cause.[35]

A week or so later Johnson had a further talk with them. Now they suggested that in addition to being past middle age, the man with the skin cancer should be a Nordic type, and that instead of having a cancer on the lip he should have it on the back on the neck or the hand—two areas where this type of cancer developed because of long exposure to the sun. In the view of the environmental cancer scientists, the hand was probably better than the neck since it had the added advantage of being a part that could be shown in its entirety and of being a part of the body that people are used to having things happen to. Children in the audience would shudder, they claimed, if something happened to a lip, but they would not respond that way to a cancer of the hand. (An echo, perhaps, of the concern behind Constant's June 1948 instruction that the filmmakers gauge the horribleness of the cancer they intended to use.) The hand was also suitable for the cell growth scene, the introductory animation sequence (2) where normal cells grow to complete organs, the eye, the heart, and the hand. They also proposed a modification to their suggested opening scene: the farmer working in the hot sun should have his hands exposed to the sun—perhaps in closeup showing bright sun on hands on a plow.[36] Dallas Johnson endorsed such views, and her early drafts of publicity for the film describe the patient as a farmer with a cancer of the hand.[37] Indeed, one version of the shooting script included a shot of farmer's head in the sunlight, "His face is weatherbeaten and heavily wrinkled. With the odd wart it is suggestive of a precancerous state."[38] The environmental scientists also had some other corrections to make. For example, the shooting script suggested that the animal used in the tissue culture sequence (5) might be a rabbit, but Berenblum and Hueper disagreed. In their view, it was illogical to use rabbits in tissue culture, since they were used less than any other experimental animal in such a field, and they suggested a young chick or a rat.[39] The environmental cancer scientists also worried that some of the beakers and glassware drawn by the storyboard artist were not actually used in scientists' laboratories. Johnson indicated that this would be taken care of automatically since the film was to be photographed in laboratories.[40]

NCI scientists were not only concerned about correcting what they saw as errors in the science. They were also keen to ensure that their fields were adequately represented in the film vis-à-vis other fields of science. Thus, in the view of the environmental scientists, the film treatment gave "a little too much emphasis"[41] to tissue culture, while the biochemist Jesse P. Greenstein (1902–59) suggested the film was thin on the biochemistry—as Johnson noted, about all that was shown once the cell animation was out of the way was a lot of glassware with somebody making tea in a container of boiling water (sequence 9).[42] Such suggestions were difficult for the filmmakers or for Johnson to resolve. While it was relatively easy to swap a rat for a rabbit, or one piece of glassware for another, it was much less easy to determine the balance between different fields or specialties because the scientists themselves did not necessarily agree on the balance. The filmmakers were caught between the disciplinary and professional rivalries of NCI scientists, as were Johnson's efforts to secure recognition for her Cancer Reports Section from the research side of NCI. There would be no easy way of solving this issue, for what was "too much emphasis" to one scientist was too little emphasis to another.

Nor was it clear how the filmmakers and Johnson were to deal with the scientists' enthusiasm for suggesting scenes or images for the filmmakers to include. The environmental scientists provided perhaps the most detailed suggestions, but they were not alone. Greenstein strongly advocated for a "factory" analogy to describe the biochemistry of the cell, which he thought was much better than "industry." Normal cells, he claimed, had one "factory plan," cancer cells had another, where the "central control" had "gone haywire:" "It's as if the administrator has gone nuts. We know one thing—that the converters (the enzymes) don't convert the same way. This screws up the works and the result is that the factory turns out the wrong stuff."[43] In his view, "What we have to do is to find a way to bring the administrator under control; get those converters working properly; convert the cancer cell to a normal cell."[44] Johnson also talked to the NCI tissue culture expert, Wilton R. Earle,[45] about the tissue culture sections, and he had some suggestions regarding the location and made some technical corrections: microns were not thousands of an inch as the filmmakers had it. He agreed with the environmental scientists that a rat or mouse would be better than a rabbit, and had some ideas for demonstrating tissue growth.[46] He also added his own bizarre ending: "He [Earle] made merry with what he termed a real 'Hollywood' ending, suggesting that the picture close with an autopsy on our cancer patient. I protested that our patient wasn't supposed to die. 'But you've got to kill him if you are going to pull out his intestines,' Earle said, 'and you'll need several yards of intestines to spell out "The End" as the picture closes.'"[47]

In the end the NFB filmmakers seem to have been quite selective about the suggestions they included in the film. Earle's fantasy ending did not make the cut, nor did Greenstein's metaphor of the cell as factory (replaced with "complex industrial organism"[48]), nor the analogy with foremen, and the idea of converters gone wrong. Despite Johnson's concerns, they did not do away with the tea-making sequence. Mr. Davis's cancer migrated from his lip not to his hand or neck but to his cheek;[49] and the rabbit in the tissue culture sequence became a mouse. Other suggestions were adopted, or changed, or ignored. Mr. Davis is not identified as a farmer; he is not shown plowing, and he is not exposed to the sun. In addition, the sequence depicting the farmer's head, the sunlight and warts suggestive of precancers disappeared in the finished film—though the link between outdoor work/living and cancer is mentioned in the scenes on environmental and occupational cancer.

Such choices meant that Johnson had her work cut out keeping the scientists on board with the project. She constantly informed them about what was going on, repeatedly sought their advice, and notified them of the filmmakers' responses and the reasons they accepted or rejected proposals. No doubt it was not always a comfortable time for Johnson, with the tricky question of how to deal with the balance within the film between different scientific specialties and fields, the detailed suggestions that some NCI scientists made regarding what should be included in the film, and so many suggestions rejected. Johnson herself seems to have been able to calm much of the disquiet with her constant efforts to keep NCI scientists involved and informed, and she seems to have had a gift for cultivating support from the scientists. But there were limits to her persuasive powers. As mentioned above, the film itself became a source of tension between her Cancer Reports Section and the research side of the NCI. While,

as mentioned above, the reasons for this are unclear, the continued efforts of
scientists to shape the content of the film may be suggestive of disquiet, and the
continued tension over the balance of attention given to some areas of science
cannot have helped. In addition, Johnson's broader efforts to create a central
place for the Cancer Reports Section did not fare well: she failed in making it
the choke point for all NCI public communications, and did she not gain full
support for her other suggestions. The tensions over the film likely contributed
to some of her frustrations.

Johnson had the important backing of David Ruhe and other members of
the Medical Film Institute, and they stepped in to try to ease tensions between
the filmmakers and their scientific paymasters, as occasionally did Gilchrist,
explaining why certain scientific suggestions did not work cinematically, and
pressing the scientists' points to the filmmakers where necessary. Advice went
back and forth between the NCI, the DNHW/NCIC, and the NFB in an iterative process, and that many scientists continue to support the project despite the
rejection of so many of their ideas is a tribute to Johnson's, Gilchrist's, and the
MFI's skill in fielding their suggestions. But Johnson was becoming frustrated
with the NCI, since her broader ambitions for the Cancer Reports Section were
stymied. The scientists might have given way to her on the film, but many remained doubtful about its value, and unwilling to let Johnson or her section gain
control of all public outreach. Johnson's efforts to promote the film may have
bled into questions of production, but this did not mean that she had achieved
her broader goals for the Cancer Reports Section.

CHAPTER 10

Planning Premieres

I N DECEMBER 1949, JOHNSON dropped a bombshell: she was leaving the
NCI. She had long complained about civil service status and the constraints
it imposed but claimed her move had nothing to do with these concerns, or
her more recent frustrations in establishing the Cancer Reports Section within
the NCI. She had had a "beautiful new job offer in New York City,"[1] handling
the education program of the Public Affairs Committee. She had published
some of her earlier work on consumer issues in their pamphlet series. She reassured Ralph Foster at the NFB that she would continue on as a consultant to
Austin Deibert, the head of Cancer Control at the NCI, on the NCI's film program, which meant that she would work half-time for NCI until the premiere
of the movie. Her replacement as chief of the Cancer Reports Section was to be
Hugh Jackson, who transferred from the Department of the Navy to take up his
new appointment on December 16, 1949.[2]

The consequence of Johnson's leaving was that the center of promotional activities moved from Washington to New York, where Johnson—as a self-styled
"film consultant"[3] to the NCI—was to exploit her networks of contacts to get
the promotional campaign going. Much of this was done quite independently of
the Cancer Reports Section of NCI. She would send periodic reports to Hugh
Jackson on progress, in part because she needed Jackson to see to the printing of
the booklet and teaching guide, and in part to keep others at NCI on board—
but otherwise Jackson had little involvement, at least to begin with. *Challenge*
had been Johnson's special project, and Jackson seems to have been content to let
her see it through while he familiarized himself with his new duties as director.
The promotional campaign for *Challenge* was to be an enormous undertaking,
and Johnson seemed to have all energy and contacts needed to see it through.

Johnson's key contact was Leonard A. Scheele, her former boss at the NCI
(director: 1947–8), and now surgeon general of the United States (1948–56), with
whom she had developed a close working relationship. With Scheele's backing
she began to work feverishly from late 1949 to early 1950 to get the premiere

off the ground, juggling her involvement with *Challenge* with her new respon-
sibilities at the Public Affairs Committee. But despite her periodic reports to
Jackson, disquiet about her working methods and the protection she seemed to
enjoy from Scheele began to be voiced by information officers in Washington
and Bethesda. If in 1949 Johnson had worried that discontent among scientists
might derail the film; in 1950 discontent among her former information officer
colleagues not only threatened the smooth completion of the film, but also the
work that she was doing to promote the movie and the premieres that would
launch it.

While Johnson's working arrangements at the NCI were unique to this film,
the work of promotion would have been familiar to any information officer. It
involved determining which media outlets were important, how to approach
them, what would appeal to them about the film, and ensuring they projected
the message approved by the sponsors, not always a certainty even if media outlets were tempted to report on the movie. This work involved exploiting existing
contacts and connections and making new ones, building on their accumulated
the knowledge of existing media, learning how to approach the new medium of
television, and countless meetings, letters to write, and phone calls. Johnson's
work thus provides a snapshot of the roles of media in educational programs as
imagined by communications experts in the late 1940s and 1950s. It was contingent, uncertain work, and an enormous amount of it. No wonder that Johnson
was often exhausted and overwhelmed, and why the threat from her former information officer colleagues was such a problem, as they likely knew.

Planning the premieres

Johnson wanted the premiere to be a major event, something that would garner
significant media attention, and that would alert medical, scientific, and educational organizations to the existence of the film, in addition to the general public
increasingly regarded as an audience. To this end, she and Scheele began planning for a series of launches: a United States premiere (eventually held on March
13, 1950, at Hunter College in New York, likely the final preview mentioned in
table 10.2), a Canadian premiere (held a few days later at the Elgin Theater in
Ottawa, March 19: the first showing for the French version; the second national
premiere for the English language version), and a series of regional premieres in
the United States and Canada. Most of Johnson's efforts focused on the Hunter
College event. The Canadian event was to be organized by the Canadian health
authorities, notably Lt. Col. Gilchrist, while the regional premieres were largely

organized by local individuals and organizations. Johnson was a keen advocate for regional premieres, which had the potential to bring the film to the notice of groups and individuals that the New York and Ottawa events could not reach. But there were limits to her energy, and the NCI did not provide adequate institutional support so that the US regional premieres were held only when she was able to tempt locals into undertaking the work. A similar arrangement seems to have happened with the local premieres in Canada, with Gilchrist taking a back seat to local organizers, the Canadian Cancer Society, and perhaps the NFB.

Planning for the New York premiere and for other promotion efforts would take up most of Johnson's time from January 1950. She joined the New York Cancer Committee of the American Cancer Society and used this and her contacts in the publishing and media world of New York to get promotional efforts going. Johnson would make the connections, get the recommendations, research the outlets necessary for the promotional campaign, and write the invitation letters that Scheele would sign: Scheele's name promised to bring in some of the big names necessary for the premiere to make a splash, and Johnson had a personal connection with Scheele that would help ensure his continued involvement. Besides, he had little to do except suggest contacts, sign letters, and approve Johnson's activities, and perhaps not even that. G. Bryant Putney, Scheele's assistant in charge of information, was closely involved the organization of the promotional activities, and took much of the burden off the Surgeon General, at least until March 1950 when he left to join the Department of the Interior as assistant director of information.[4] A former Milwaukie newspaperman, he had worked before the war as a reporter for *Editorial Research Reports* and the *Capital Times* (Madison) and, during the war, as an information officer in the Office of Defense Transportation. Besides taking on some of the Scheele's work, he also had media contacts and advice that would be useful for Johnson in organizing the premiere.

Toward the end of January 1950, Johnson circulated a plan for production, promotion, and distribution.[5] The plan portrayed the various premieres as the linchpins of the campaign: the period from January to March building up to the public launch of promotional efforts, and the start of film distribution. It will be recalled that this period was fraught for the filmmakers. Although scientists had had an opportunity to comment on the film at the rough-cut stage back in December, there were still fears that they might demand changes to the film. The final cut was scheduled to be cleared on January 23, 1950 and shown without the narration to media outlets on 23rd and 24th. Any changes after then would be expensive and might complicate the promotional efforts if the film was

significantly different to the version seen by media outlets. They—scientists—
also threatened to complicate completing the narration, still being written at
the time of the showing of the final cut. There may have been some minor edits
to the film before Massey recorded his narration in early February 1950, but the
focus was beginning to shift from production to promotion.

The problem facing Johnson was how to turn a recruitment film into something newsworthy. Scientific recruitment to biology and cancer was not a topic
that would appeal to many news reporters or editors. Most had little background
in science, and little interest in science recruitment, unless perhaps problems of
recruitment threatened a campaign against a deadly disease. That theme could
have given urgency to appeals for young scientists to think of cancer research
as a career, but Johnson did not opt for this approach. Instead, press handouts
tended to portray the film as something that would quench a thirst for more
information about progress against the disease. This focus reflected a growing
tendency within the promotional campaign to see the primary audience for the
film as the general public.

This new focus was relatively recent. The original rationale for the film had
been to target high school and college science students, with the general public
as a secondary audience at least until the theatrical version was available. But
the prospect of a major public premiere prompted a subtle shift in the portrayal
of the film's target audience, perhaps in part because of a growing realization
that the theatrical version of the film might not be ready in time, and a desire
to ensure that *Challenge* might be used to target the theatrical audience at least
until the other version was ready. Thus press briefings increasingly suggested that
Challenge would portray the complexities of the problem to a lay audience. To
this end they provided synopses of the motion picture, mentioned some of the
innovative film techniques that were used, and made constant reference to the
sponsoring organizations, the NFB, and some of the stars, notably Raymond
Massey (known to all Americans, the background information claimed, for his
role as Abraham Lincoln), and Louis Applebaum (who had composed the music
for the feature films *The Story GI Joe* [1945] and *Lost Boundaries* [1949]).

All of these were intended to capture the attention of the new audience, the
general public, and to make the premiere newsworthy. But press briefings were
only a beginning. For Johnson, press briefings by themselves were unlikely to
make the sort of splash she hoped the premiere would make. In her view, it was
crucial that they personally approach media owners, editors, and writers to persuade them to take an interest. Her approach was to identify what was likely
to appeal to each media outlet, and the constraints on each, and then to use

her contacts and the promise of a sensational premiere to encourage a media owner, editor, or writer to report on the event. In some cases, Johnson invited leaders of various media organizations to the event in the hope that they would open the door to publicity. In others, she thought the best strategy was to target the editors, reporters, or other writers. She paid particular attention to science writers, some of whom she invited to the premiere, though she contacted many more.[6] It was to be an enormous effort, much of it behind closed doors, on the telephone, at lunch, dinner, and by letter; all to ensure that each media outlet had the information it needed in a format that worked for it, and that the people who made editorial decisions were encouraged to include a report on *Challenge*.

As a start she began to compile a tentative program of speakers for the New York premiere to include George N. Shuster (US National Commission for UNESCO, and a former president of Hunter College),[7] Brock Chisholm (the Canadian director-general of the World Health Organization),[8] Eleanor Roosevelt (representing the UN), Paul Martin (Canadian minister of National Health and Welfare), Leonard Scheele (US Surgeon General), and James B. Conant (Harvard University, previously on the NACC).[9] She also began assembling lists of people who might be invited to the New York premiere and who might be expected to attract media attention, apparently relying on Scheele or more likely Putney to send out the invitation letters. Particular attention was paid to the *sponsors*; institutions and individuals who lent their names to the event to give it credibility and visibility. These were to include various diplomats and representatives of international organizations (UN, UNESCO, and WHO), government (the White House, Congress, and Canadian government representatives in the US), and various US and Canadian medical and cancer organizations, along with some New York State and City officials. Also included were assorted representatives of the media, and some celebrity individuals—the philanthropist Mary Lasker, the screen actresses Mary Pickford and Irene Dunne, the gossip writer Walter Winchell (1897–1972), the writer and editor Fleur Cowles, and John Gunther, the journalist and author of *Death Be Not Proud* (1949) about his son, Johnny, who died of a brain tumor. Johnson also included a list of lesser invitees, people and institutions who might give the event credibility and visibility but did not lend their names as sponsors of the event. They included representatives of many organizations in the same categories as the sponsors: international organizations, Canadian and US government agencies, medical scientific and professional organizations, public health groups, educational groups, cancer organizations, media organizations, along with prospective buyers and users of film prints.[10] These individuals and institutions were not expected to generate

TABLE 10.1. Dallas Johnson's Proposed List of Sponsors for the US Premiere of *Challenge*

Organization	Name	Position
United Nations	Benjamin A. Cohen	UN, Assistant Secretary General in charge of public information
United Nations	Alva Myrdal	UN, Director of Department of Social Affairs
UNESCO	Milton S. Eisenhower	Chairman, US National Commission, UNESCO
WHO	Martha M. Eliot	Assistant Director General
WHO	William P. Forrest	Assistant Director General
Canadian Government	Humphrey Hume Wrong	Canadian Ambassador to the US
Canadian Government	Kenneth Green	Canadian Consul General
US Congress	-	
NIH	R. O. Dyer	Director, NIH
NCI	John R. Heller	Director, NCI
New York State Government	Herman E. Hilleboe	New York State Commissioner of Health
New York City Government	William O'Dwyer	Mayor
New York City Health Department		
New York City Cancer Committee	Gen. John Reed Kilpatrick	President (sometimes also described as Chairman)
American Cancer Society	James F. Adams	
Sloan-Kettering Institute	Charles F. Kettering or Alfred P. Sloan	

Memorial Hospital	C. P. Rhoads	Director of Memorial and Director of the Sloan-Kettering Institute
Columbia-Presbyterian Medical Center	F. C. Wood	NACC and Director Emeritus, Institute of Cancer Research, College of Physicians and Surgeons, Columbia University
Rockefeller Institute	James B. Murphy	NACC and director, cancer research, Rockefeller Institute
Association of American Medical Colleges,	Walter Bloedorn	Chairman of the Committee on Audio-Visual Education
New York Academy of Medicine	Howard Craig	Director
New York City Medical Society or A.M.A.	-	
Rochester University	J. J. Morton	NACC and Professor of Surgery University of Rochester
American Association for Cancer Research	-	
Canadian Cancer Society	J. C. Meakins	President, CCS
Canadian Cancer Institute	William Boyd	President, NCIC
American Association for the Advancement of Science	-	
Bronx High School of Science	Morris Meister	
US Office of Education	-	
National Science Teachers Association	Ralph J. Lefler	President (elect)
American Public Health Association	-	
Motion Picture Association of America	Eric Johnston	President
Radio Corporation of America	David Sarnoff	
Motion Picture Industry	Spyros Skouras	President, 20th Century Fox

(Cont.)

Organization	Name	Position
Motion Picture Distributors of America	Gael Sullivan	Executive Director, Theater Owners of America
New York Film Council	Irving Jacoby	Chairman, 1949–50
New York Herald Tribune	Helen Ogden Reid	President
Committee on Growth of the National Research Council	-	
National Health Council	Thomas Dublin	Executive Director
White House	Alben Barkley	US Vice President
Others	Mary Pickford	Actor
	Walter Winchell	Newspaper columnist and radio news commentator
	Fleur Cowles	Writer, editor, and artist
	John Gunther	Journalist and author
	Irene Dunne	Actor
	F. E. Adair	NACC
	Mary Lasker	Philanthropist

SOURCE: Adapted from Dallas Johnson, "Production, Promotion and Distribution Schedule for CHALLENGE – SCIENCE AGAINST CANCER," January 23, 1950, NCI archives, AR-4900-01078s, p. 2. Misspellings and misattributions in the original have been silently corrected. A hyphen indicates that Johnson did not propose a person to represent the body listed in the organization column. For a revised list see Dallas Johnson, "List of Invitees," February 17, 1950, NCI archives, AR-4900-01078s.

the same excitement as the sponsors, but they could help to spread the message about the film.

As she began to figure out who to invite, Johnson also began to consider how to attract various media outlets—television, radio, newspapers, and magazines—all of which, she noted, had to be approached in different ways. In the case of network television, she went to the top. Her plan was to personally contact both David Sarnoff (president of RCA[11]) and Frank Fulsom (president of NBC), with a simultaneous approach to the Advertising Council of America to get commercial sponsorship. In her view, NBC was the key to television coverage, and should be approached before others (apparently her earlier contacts with CBS in August 1949 [chapter 9] had not convinced her of the importance of CBS as a news outlet). Once NBC was on board, the plan was to go for the three other New York network channels (CBS, DuMont, and ABC) and the nine local television stations. She drafted a letter from John Heller, the director of NCI, to the nine local stations, asking them to cover the premiere, and mentioning "celebs" as she called them—mostly speakers or sponsors of the event. A key issue was whether the premiere would fit with television schedules. Johnson estimated that the thirty, forty-five, or sixty minutes requested for the opening preview might be too long for television stations, and she speculated about alternatives: "might combine fancy guest introduction with 10–20 minute theatrical version of film on air. Or might follow showing with round table discussion by celebs on value of film. Also possibility of follow up local programs broadcasting film over air."[12] Note that she was still hoping at this stage that the theatrical version of the film might be available by the time of the premiere, despite the lack of lack of progress on the film and the fears that it would not be ready in time.

Johnson's approach was different in the case of radio. Her advice was to spread the load: "Arrange to give information on preview [the NY premiere], not only to key radio personalities, such as Winchell," she recommended (Walter Winchell, the gossip columnist, was one of the invitees),[13] "but also to news commentators, and the little program people all down the line." She was also keen to exploit the connections of other information officers. It will be recalled that she had sought UN endorsement of the movie in late 1949, and she also tried to involve the UN's Information Division in publicizing the movie. She noted that Matthew Gordon could be of help with regard to radio (Gordon was a former news editor at CBS who established the press operations of the United Nations in 1946 and ran its Office of Public Information).[14] She also had another unexpected contact at the UN: Ralph Foster, with whom she had worked closely on the film. He had announced that he was leaving the NFB shortly after she announced she was leaving the NCI. The precipitating event in this case was that Ross McLean's appointment as government film commissioner was not renewed in 1950, and Foster resigned from the NFB in sympathy. Foster's resignation letter became public on December 21, 1949, and he left the NFB on January 3, 1950.[15] Foster subsequently became chief of the Films and Visual Information Division of the United Nations Department of Public Information, shortly after the board had provisionally approved *Challenge* for sponsorship.[16]

In addition to television and radio, Johnson wanted what she labeled "press handling" to include *Time*, *Newsweek*, *U.S. News*, and *Pathfinder Magazine*. She wanted the press to include the event not only in their regular news coverage, but also as Sunday feature stories (the premiere was to happen on a Monday), preferably through the Associated Press and Science Service, with the News Enterprise Association a further choice. She also wanted Sunday "spreads" and mentioned editors and writers who might produce a spread in *Parade* (Rod Motley, executive editor), *This Week* (Bill Nichol, and a tie-in with the *Herald Tribune*), the *New York Times* (Emma Little, Sunday magazine), and *American Weekly* (the Pulitzer Prize-winning science writer, Gobind Behari Lal). In addition to science and medical writers, Johnson also thought that there were story possibilities for film reviewers such as Bosley Crowther and A. H. Weiler of the *New York Times* and John Crosby of the *Tribune*. Nor was she solely concerned with the film. In order to stress the educational value of the film she wanted to promote a tie-in between the movie, the book, the teacher's guide and the film strip: Lester Grant's book, she noted, should go out to book reviewers, including those at the *Saturday Review of Literature*. She urged: "Tie press handling in with preview by good speeches beforehand and good cocktails afterwards."[17] The quality of the cocktails is unknown, but I'll refer to the speeches later.

Johnson noted that each publication required "special handling."[18] In January 1950 she still had hopes of a spread in *Life* magazine. But, she noted "If this looks shaky, we should start early with LOOK and QUICK and the Cowles organization, if possible."[19] It will be recalled that Fleur Cowles had been invited to the Hunter College premiere, and her husband, Gardner Cowles Jr., was an heir to the Cowles organization, which owned a number of newspapers and magazines including *Look*, a biweekly competitor of *Life*, and *Quick*, a pocket-size general magazine.[20] Johnson suggested they should approach Fleur, and other contacts such as Merle Armitage (the modernist book designer hired by the Cowles Publishing Company in the late 1940s to create a new appearance for their flagship magazine, *Look*), and Woodrow Wirsig (editor of *Quick* and executive editor of *Look,* and an alumnus of Occidental College, where Johnson had been educated).[21]

Other magazines, she noted, required different approaches, each requiring the promotional people to exploit whatever contacts they had. For example, in the case of *Collier's* "or that type of magazine"[22] (that mixed fiction, [investigative] journalism, and other entertainment features) she recommended that the best approach was to work with a writer doing an article and make any still photographs they might have available to him [*sic*]. She also recommended talking to several writers who had done work on medical and scientific issues: Lois Mattox Miller (the medical reporter and an editor of the *Reader's Digest* who had worked with the ACS), and Albert Q. Maisel and Albert Deutsch (both of whom had published exposés of America's psychiatric hospitals in the 1940s).[23] She also recommended talking to Walter B. Mahoney, the editor at *Reader's Digest* who had recently called on the NFB with Charles Wall of Ithaca, asking for a story.

It was to be a major effort talking to all these people, and much of it was unlikely to turn into anything. But it should be clear from the above that Johnson employed a mix of her own social and professional contacts as well as those of her colleagues to attract media interest. In her view, a personal touch was the best way of cultivating coverage of a newsworthy event, even for the "little people" down the line. Yet there were limits to her networks, and there were many magazines that either she did not think of as significant, or where she had fewer contacts. She recommended approaching various other categories of magazines: science magazines, medical and health publications, educational film magazines, education magazines with audiovisual departments, and various other education magazines, farm magazines, and church magazines. However, she seems to have had less knowledge of these more specialized publications, and provided no specific advice on who to approach besides listing the editors where she knew their names, and if the magazine had an interest in film (*Country Gentleman,* for example, had a Farm Film Council, she noted.[24])

The lack of information on these categories of magazines should not be taken to mean that the work of raising their interest was any less. Someone had to write or make a phone call; perhaps a blind call, since Johnson or her team may not have had a personal contact. To add to these problems, Johnson was working with little NCI support in New York, and there were limits to her energy. Letters went out and calls were made, but somewhat isolated in New York, and with a new job to familiarize herself with, she could not follow up with every magazine, or all the organizations to which direct mail promotions and material should be sent—mainly buyers of the film, users of the film, and various publicity outlets.[25]

There are indications that her successor at the Cancer Reports Section, Hugh Jackson, may have taken on some of this work, but the bulk of it was undertaken by Johnson in New York.

Anxieties

As the date for the premiere drew closer the NCI and NIH began to get nervous. Information specialists felt sidelined by Johnson and concerned about their lack of control of the arrangements for the premiere, which was being organized in the name of the agencies that employed them. There seemed, however, little that they could do but send missives to Johnson or get senior administrators at NIH or NCI involved. It was humiliating for these officials to be held hostage to a former Cancer Reports Section director, and Johnson, never a lover of government bureaucracy and swamped with the pressure of the upcoming premiere and her new job, sometimes seemed to be riding roughshod over them.

For a while, the administrators did little more than mutter behind closed doors. But that changed when it turned out that Oscar Ewing, the administrator of the Federal Security Agency (FSA), was not included in the ceremonies, and it was not certain that at that late stage he could be added to the program. For the NIH and NCI this was a major problem. The NIH and NCI were both part of the Public Health Service, itself a part of the FSA, and the FSA's name was on the credits and the publicity for the film. It was a huge embarrassment to both the NIH and the NCI. "Putney and Dr. Scheele took active part in developing this scheme, working directly with Dallas Johnson over the past 6 months," Judson Hardy, the chief of the recently created (1948) Scientific Reports Branch of NIH complained,[26] "This is the sort of by-passing of NIH which has contributed to our past troubles—But which will not happen any more if we are to be held responsible."

Hardy's concern was prompted by the reaction of the FSA. The absence of Ewing had aroused the ire of Zilpha C. Franklin, the director of publications and reports at the FSA. A few weeks before the New York premiere, she had written to NCI to demand an earlier screening of the film in Washington.[27] Franklin was dimly aware of the planning for the premiere, but apparently no one in her department had seen the film, and like the NIH and NCI information specialists she felt sidelined. Hardy apparently saw this as the most recent of a long list of instances where the NIH public information officers had been caught unawares, and he and Franklin were not about to let it happen again.

TABLE 10.2. From the Rough Cut to Film Distribution

Date	Status	Place	Who should be present
12/19	Rough Cut	Ottawa	Austin V. Deibert (NCI), C. W. Gilchrist (DNHW), Ralph Foster (NFB), David Ruhe (MFI), O. H. Warwick, (NCIC), William Boyd (NCIC), H. B. Andervont (NCI), H. W. Chalkley (NCI), Guy Glover (NFB), Morten Parker (NFB), Bernard V. Dryer (MFI), Dallas Johnson (NCI).
1/23	Fine Cut (for Clearance)	New York	Deibert, Foster, Ruhe, Warwick, Morris Meister, Parker, Dryer, Johnson
1/24	Fine Cut (for Promotion)	New York	UN Film Board, magazines, movie studios, radio, press
–	Interlock	New York and Washington	Gilchrist, Glover, Parker, Deibert, or Dryer
–	Sponsors' preview	New York	Sponsors plus certain people important to promotion
3/13	Final preview	New York	
3/1-3/30	Prints ready for distribution	From New York	

SOURCE: Adapted from Dallas Johnson, "Production, Promotion and Distribution Schedule for CHALLENGE – SCIENCE AGAINST CANCER," January 23, 1950, NCI archives, AR-4900-010785, p.2.

With Franklin's memo on his desk, Hugh Jackson had the unenviable task of telling Johnson to arrange the screening. He was already aware that Johnson and the filmmakers were opposed to the idea of another showing, and perhaps to avoid the possibility that Johnson would claim that the film was not ready, he had already checked with David Ruhe at the MFI as to when prints would be available. Johnson's concerns are not recorded, but it is likely that she and the others were worried that changes might have to be made, and the whole schedule set back, with the loss of weeks and months of work that would have to be done all over again. She had already ensured that NCI scientists could comment on storyboards before filming began, and they had attended the screening of the rough cut on December 19, 1949; Ruhe and others had been at the screening of the fine cut for clearance. The filmmakers had constantly worried about further interference from the scientists. Now the public information specialists seemed to be making trouble. Jackson made it clear that there was no option but for Johnson to bend to Franklin's will.

> Although, I know that you and others will have strong objections to any preview of this sort, I believe that for various and important reasons that it would almost be fatal if it didn't come off. I want to impress you with the importance of seeing to it that such a preview is made possible. I have a memorandum from Mrs. Franklin which indicates that such a preview is definitely expected.[28]

Shortly after the screening, Ewing was added to the speakers' list for the Hunter College premiere. The FSA's and NCI's information specialists had flexed a muscle, and Johnson had responded. Johnson for her part was discomfited by the prospect of further interference. She was dependent on Jackson and others for the package of educational materials associated with the film and could not afford to alienate them more.

Hunter College and the Elgin Theatre

The organizational issues continued almost up to the day of the Hunter College premiere, March 13. The list of speakers remained unsettled, with Johnson frantically trying to finalize the lineup. Eleanor Roosevelt dropped out, as did Charles Huggins (the Chicago-based cancer researcher, a late addition to the list of speakers), Paul Martin (replaced by G. W. C. Cameron, his deputy), and George Shuster.[29] There were likely other changes or threats of change that are not recorded, and at some point the list had to be finalized. There were agendas to print (Hugh Jackson's bailiwick), speeches to be written (not all by the speakers themselves, but perhaps by their information officers), and announcements to be made.

In the end the lineup was Brock Chisholm (the Canadian director-general of the World Health Organization), who talked about cancer as a world problem;[30] C. P. Rhoads (the director of the Memorial Cancer Center in New York, perhaps replacing Huggins), who talked on the transformations in cancer research;[31] Paul Martin (the Canadian minister of National Health and Welfare, now back on the program instead of his deputy), who discussed Canada's crusade against cancer;[32] Oscar Ewing (the administrator of the US Federal Security Agency), who talked about teamwork in cancer research (perhaps a sly dig at Johnson by his FSA speech writers, for her apparent lack of teamwork in launching the film);[33] George Stoddard, the chair (chairman, US Commission for UNESCO, replacing Shuster), who discussed science and UNESCO;[34] and Leonard Scheele (the US surgeon general). Scheele's talk focused on the "by-products of cancer research." These included research on the role of sex hormones in breast cancer, which had led to the discovery of a mechanism of eclampsia. He also noted the development of a simple method to produce large qualities of optically pure amino acids in a form that the body could safely assimilate through intravenous injection, which could prove valuable when normal intake of food through the digestive tract was not feasible. And he mentioned new tissue culture techniques that allowed the growth of rat pituitary glands outside the body to produce the hormone ACTH (potentially valuable for the treatment of rheumatoid arthritis.)[35]

Johnson had hoped that the other elements of the package—the booklet, the teaching aid, and the filmstrip—would be available by the time of the Hunter College show, but they were not, nor, except for the French version of *Challenge*, were the other versions of the film. Indeed, production of the other versions of the film had not even started. The press releases given out at Hunter College indicated that the booklet, the teaching aid, and the filmstrip were in production, but said nothing about the other versions of the film. A reception followed at the Waldorf-Astoria Hotel, also on March 13.

We know less about the preparations for the Canadian premiere on March 19, though Gilchrist probably had his share of organizational hurdles to jump. Under the patronage of the governor general of Canada, the film was shown at the Elgin Theatre in Ottawa, the English version in the main theater and the French version in Little Elgin (Petit Elgin). Martin and Scheele reprised their roles at Hunter College, joined by the Leslie Bell singers (a popular all-female Canadian choir in the late 1940s and early 1950s), who sang songs from another NFB film in which they had appeared *It's Fun to Sing* (1948), and the Toronto symphony orchestra conducted by Sir Ernest Macmillan. Press releases highlighted Canadian contributions to the film—the fact that it was made by National Film Board of Canada, and that most of the live action was shot in Toronto. They also claimed that this was a Canadian Department of National Health and Welfare initiative which the Americans joined (partly true). The film script might have abandoned a nationalist portrayal of cancer research in favor of one that promoted it as an international endeavor, but the picture was still sometimes packaged in nationalist colors.

Regional premieres

With the Hunter College and Elgin Theatre premieres out of the way, attention shifted to the regional premieres. Johnson explained that the sponsorship pattern here was very varied. She had no help for this part of the operation, for the US Public Health Service did not sponsor these events. All she could do was to let local groups know that the film was available and ask them whether there was a possibility of local sponsorship of a premiere. Plans for all these premieres were left in the hands of local sponsoring groups.

The first showing after Hunter College was held in Cleveland (March 14), sponsored by Bruno Gebhard, director of the Cleveland Health Museum, and included introductory remarks by David Dietz, a Pulitzer Prize-winning science writer and the author of two books on the cancer research published locally.[36] Gebhard telegrammed that the show had been a "great success." "Acclaimed by film critic of Cleveland Plain Dealer."[37] The review by the paper's film critic, W. Ward Marsh—titled "Health Museum Acquires a New, Excellent, 'Hopeful' Film on Subject of Cancer"—warmly recommended the movie as "a film of assurance and cheer."[38] Gebhard later noted that the museum had purchased a copy of the film.[39]

There followed three showings in Boston (at the Harvard Medical School,[40] Tufts Medical School, and Boston Medical School), and premieres in Chicago,[41] Minneapolis, and San Francisco. There were plans for premieres in Houston (Texas), Atlanta (Georgia), Washington, DC, St. Louis (Missouri), and Gary (Indiana). The last was not planned originally, but the Gary Film Council president became interested in the film and asked for permission to have a preview there. A librarian at the Gary Public Library sent sample comments from papers written by high school students after seeing the film—all responding positively to a question about the film's effect on them, with the exception of one E. Sayles who commented, "The picture didn't have a great effect on me."[42]

The Gary screening illustrates the contingent ways the regional premieres came about. Each screening was dependent on an enthusiastic individual such as Bruno Gebhard, Lester Breslow, or Odum Fanning in Cleveland, San Francisco and Atlanta respectively, or was tied to a local event: in Houston it was linked to a groundbreaking ceremony for a new cancer research facility at the M. D. Anderson Hospital for Cancer Research; in Minneapolis it was sponsored by the Minneapolis Division of the Cancer Society, and was linked with the opening rally of the American Cancer Society drive there. Minneapolis also highlights the ways in which local media networks were important to the program. The

TABLE 10.3. Regional Premieres of *Challenge*

Date	City	Location	Sponsors (Attendees)
		United States	
March 14	Cleveland	Cleveland Health Museum	Bruno Gebhard
March 15	Boston	Harvard Medical School	Dr. L. S. Snegeriff, Harvard School of Public Health
	Boston	Tufts Medical School	Dr. L. S. Snegeriff, Harvard School of Public Health
	Boston	Boston Medical School	Dr. L. S. Snegeriff, Harvard School of Public Health
March 21	Chicago		Chicago Film Council (Attended by officers of: Chicago Welfare Council Association of American Medical Colleges. American Medical Association. Illinois Division of the American Cancer Society UNESCO representatives in Chicago Public health officials, including representatives from the FSA regional office)
March	Minneapolis		Minneapolis Division of the American Cancer Society
	San Francisco	Fairmount Hotel	Lester Breslow (California State Health Department) with the FSA regional office, the University of California School of Public Health, the California Cancer Society, the San Francisco Film Council and other groups
	Houston (Planned)		M. D. Anderson Hospital for Cancer Research and the Cancer Bulletin

(Cont.)

Date	City	Location	Sponsors (Attendees)
	Atlanta (planned)		Odom Fanning, Information Director, Atlanta Communicable Disease Center, perhaps with the American Cancer Society
	St. Louis, Missouri (Planned)		
March 31	Gary, Indiana (Planned)		
May 4	Washington. DC (Planned)		
		Canada	
March 26	Halifax, Nova Scotia		
Last week March	St John's, Newfoundland		
Last week of March/ first week of April	Montreal, Quebec		
Last week of March/ first week of April	Moncton, New Brunswick		
Last week of March/ first week of April	Calgary and Edmonton, Alberta		
April 2	Toronto, Ontario		
April 16	Regina, Saskatchewan		

SOURCE: Adapted from Dallas Johnson and C. W. Gilchrist, "*Challenge Science Against Cancer: A Project Report on Promotion and Distribution*," c.1950, NCI archives, AR-4900-010785.

local organizers managed to get the local television station—KSTP-TV—interested in the film. As an unknown correspondent explained, there were 80,000 television sets in the Twin Cities area, with an average of five people per set: with only two stations in the area there was a maximum viewing audience on a Friday evening of 200,000 people. "If only 10,000 people see the picture," the correspondent noted, "we have really started the ball rolling."[43] The main problem was that the film ran two and a half minutes longer than the thirty-minute slot open on March 24 when the film was due to be broadcast, which meant it would overlap with Friday night wrestling. However, the unknown correspondent had good news: KSPT-TV would delay the broadcast of the wrestling matches to allow the screening of the entire film, and it would rebroadcast the movie on March 29.

In Canada, provincial premieres were held in Calgary and Edmonton in Alberta (last week of March/first week of April), Regina, Saskatchewan (April 16), Montreal, Quebec (last week of March/first week of April), Moncton, New Brunswick (last week of March/first week of April), Halifax, Nova Scotia (March 26) and St. John's, Newfoundland (last week March).[44] In addition, there was another premiere in Toronto (April 2), where the NCI director, John Heller spoke.[45] There is less information on these premieres than on the US ones, but some were tied to local events and all were dependent on local organizers, often juggling many different demands. The organizer of the Toronto event, the president of the Toronto Branch of the Canadian Cancer Society, seems to have had a particularly busy time: "With my daughter's wedding and a trip to Europe in the offing, plus the campaign, you can imagine how jumbled my thoughts are, but not too jumbled to recall your kindness to me while in New York City."[46] The last letter was written to Dallas Johnson, thanking her for her help with the then forthcoming Toronto event: Gilchrist was not the only one to help with the Canadian provincial premieres.

With the New York and Ottawa premieres done and the regional premieres underway, Johnson's and Gilchrist's major organizational work seemed to be over. Gilchrist had other work to complete, and Johnson was still familiarizing herself with her new job at the Public Affairs Committee. Both would have welcomed an end to the affair, but it was not quite over for either. Attention was beginning to shift to efforts to capitalize on the media reception of the movie.

CHAPTER 11

Receptions and Responses

F OR JOHNSON AND GILCHRIST, the initial responses to the premiere were disappointing. While many reports praised the film, others were quite critical. Crucially, criticism came from within sponsoring organizations including the NCI and the Department of National Health and Welfare, and the AAMC, and from colleagues—information officers—who were supposed to promote the film. Some critics suggested that most audiences could not follow the film: it was pitched at too high a level for the average moviegoer, was ill-focused, or better at dramatic presentation than in getting across a focused educational message. The problem facing Johnson and Gilchrist was how to manage such criticism.

Part of the issue was that the film's intended audience had changed at the last moment. The film had been made with an audience of high school and college science students in mind, but in the months before the premiere the intended audience expanded to include the general public. Yet it was quite unclear how a film aimed at one audience would work with another. The film assumed that the audience would have some knowledge of the sciences involved, at least as much as high school or college science students might be expected to have. Critics doubted that the general public had the necessary experience of the science to understand *Challenge*, and that the fantastical elements of the movie were confusing, and work had not even begun on the version of the film that was to be targeted at the public, eventually called *The Fight: Science Against Cancer*. No small wonder then that some critics claimed that the film was pitched at the wrong level.

But the problem was not simply one of confusion over the intended audience. Critics also suggested that the film might be too difficult for the audience it was supposed to reach: high school and college science students. They argued that it lacked educational punch: the message was vague, and the package that was supposed to drive the message home—the Lester Grant book, the teaching guide, and the filmstrip –was not ready at the time of the premiere. Until the supplementary materials were available it was unclear how the film was to be used in the classroom. Such criticisms suggested that the filmmakers and the information officers did not know their audience, had not thought about it, or at best had delivered only a partial product; the film without the package that would enable *Challenge's* use in the classroom. While the filmmakers agreed with some of the criticisms of *Challenge*, however, both they and the information officers who sponsored them had in fact given considerable thought to these issues. No one suggested that it was a perfect film, but they disagreed with their critics as to its suitability in the classroom, even allowing for the missing teacher's guide.

At the heart of such claims about the value of the film was the question of how filmmakers imagined the audience they sought to reach. Grierson had long argued for the need to tailor films for specific audiences.[1] *Challenge's* filmmakers echoed such views, but the problem for them was that no matter how an audience was divided, there would always be divisions with the groups they sought to target. Thus, they imagined an audience of school and college students not as a homogenous whole, but as a collection of individuals of differing abilities, knowledge, and curiosity. As they saw it, their task was to devise strategies to appeal to students across the spectrum, attempting to excite the less advanced or incurious students without losing the more advanced or curious. It was perhaps in part for this reason that critics were able to attack the film for failing even to reach its target audience, for the target audience was itself diffuse and difficult to characterize.

Imagined audiences

Efforts to work out how to reach an audience of high school and college students had started even before the film was commissioned. Johnson's remit to figure out how to persuade young scientists to think of cancer research as a career meant that, almost from the start of her appointment, she began looking at the existing classroom materials available to the NCI. Much of this material was then provided by the American Cancer Society (filmstrips, booklets, pamphlets, and other printed materials), and Johnson started to work out how best to turn these materials to her target audience and what else was needed. Her initial impressions were not positive. She had somehow to fit cancer into existing science classes and, except for *Youth Looks at Cancer*, there was not much on the biology of cancer that could fulfil this task. So she began to look for other materials. She was aware that the ACS was beginning to think of a film as a way of generating student interest in cancer. Thus when she met with Dryer in July 1948, she quickly came to see film as a key to expanding the range of materials available to students. Film, from her point of view, could reach students in ways that books and pamphlets could not.

But she never imagined film as a stand-alone project. Learning from the ACS experience of trying to reach children and students in the 1940s with *Detectives Wanted!* and *Youth Looks at Cancer* (chapter 1), she also saw a need to ensure that teachers knew how to use the film in the classroom. Many did not have the specialized knowledge to teach about cancer and needed materials to allow the students to delve deeper into the subjects and issues raised in the film. Ideally, she would have liked a training program for teachers, along the lines previously organized by the ACS in the 1940s. But it was not to be, and instead she planned to develop an educational package that included the teaching guide and Lester Grant's book to facilitate the use of the film in the classroom and recruited Prince George's County, Maryland, science teachers to work on the guide. Moreover, once the film was commissioned Johnson also began to search out other advice on reaching students, notably from the science educator Morris Meister. It was Meister who helped to cement the idea of the student audience as a group that needed to be challenged and inspired.

That image of the audience, however, did not originate with Meister. Johnson had been thinking along these lines long before, as had Lester Grant, the author of the *New York Herald Tribune* cancer articles and the companion book. So too the filmmakers. While the title *Challenge* was late in coming to the film, the idea that audiences needed to be challenged and inspired had been there from the beginning, when Constant wrote his first script in 1948. Guy Glover and Morten Parker had built upon these ideas, trying to figure out how far audiences could be challenged and where to draw back. For them, the audience was not homogeneous. It was made up of people of mixed ability and knowledge, and the trick was to work out how to target the higher-level students without losing their lower-level ones. There is little documentary evidence on how such thinking shaped the film, but Parker and especially the animator Colin Low were quite explicit about it in conversation with this author.[2]

It is not known exactly when the two animators, Colin Low and Evelyn Lambart, began the task of figuring out the best way of addressing an audience that included people with very different levels of knowledge about the inner world of the cell and the body. But there were discussions in the planning meetings especially with Glover, and perhaps with Norman McLaren and Morten Parker, as they sketched out the storyboard before filming began. In these meetings, they agreed to begin by using a range of visual references to images that students would have been familiar with from their textbooks, other films, and their own lived experience—the cell, the human embryo, and parts of the human body such as the hand, the eyes, the beating heart, among others. Some of this was already there in the 1948 script, which the scientifically-trained Constant had written, and during the revisions he helped figure out what students might be expected to know and how this changed as a student progressed through high school and college.

With Bazilauskas and perhaps Ruhe to advise them, they created what might be described as a visual thread. This meant that for the less advanced student, the film moved from something visually familiar to something unfamiliar or vice versa, with the unfamiliar aspects of these processes sandwiched between the familiar, and given their place by the chronological order of sequence. By the same token, more advanced students, the animators hoped, would be able to fill in more of the gaps than their lower-level brethren, since fewer parts of the visual thread should be unfamiliar to them. The trick for the animators was to determine what students at each level might know and recognize, and then to figure out how to create a visual thread that worked for students across the spectrum.

But Low and Lambart were not only interested in targeting students of different levels of knowledge, they were also interested in stimulating curiosity. To this end the mix of the familiar and unfamiliar served another purpose. Situated within the visual thread, the familiar images helped to frame the unfamiliar, providing a context for the latter, and—the animators hoped—raising questions in the minds of less advanced students about what they represented biologically and how they fitted into the animated narrative. More advanced students might know more about what was going on the animation, but the plan was to include much in the animation that even they did not know. In this way, the hope was that students might begin to ask questions about the events on screen that they did not understand, perhaps figuring out the answers for themselves, or with their teachers, their parents, or friends, or through a trip to the library or their classroom textbooks.

The risk with all of this was that the animators might misjudge their audience. They might pitch it at such a level that students would be frustrated in their efforts to work out what was going on visually, even with the help of the narration. It was no easy task to devise solutions to this issue, and there seem to have been regular discussions as to what aspects of the biology of the cell should be included in the film, countless revisions of sketches, a stream of paint, broken chalk, and discarded black cards, before they settled on the final set of images for the animation. The hard fact of sponsorship was that the NCI and the DHNW did not want every student, especially low-achieving or incurious students, as future cancer researchers. Yet the filmmakers could not ignore those these students. How would the film work in the classroom if they lost part of their audience?

For this reason, Low and Lambart turned to another means of stimulating student interest and curiosity—spectacle. Spectacle had been a part of the animation since the earliest version of the script, back in June 1948, even before the animators had been appointed, and it was to be crucial to efforts to rise above the details of biology. For example, Constant and his cowriters had wanted the animation of the inner world of the cell to convey something of the vast scale of the cancer problem by conjuring up a parallel with the immensity of interstellar space. For Low and Lambart, this requirement also promised a way of generating curiosity and interest in their student audience. They wanted to leave their audiences open-mouthed at the events on screen, impressed with the sheer wonder and awe of it all—the vastness of the inner world of the cell, the beauty of a functioning organism, the marvel of a dividing cell, the terror of cancer, and the spectacle of time-lapse photography, for example. What is more, this requirement also meant that they did not have to worry too much if students did not understand everything on screen and were occasionally lost in the details. The animators might never capture the intellectual curiosity of less-advanced students, but they could capture their eyes and attention.

In such ways, the animators sought to challenge and tantalize students (as Morris Meister urged, even if he had his reservations about their success in doing so), prompting their curiosity and interest in the biology of the cell and the body. They also sought get them to think about the difference between the world of biology and the imaginative world of the film. Thus they included in the movie many images that bore only a tenuous relationship to biology, fantastical improvisations on a biological theme: sugar-storing liver cells that blink, cancer cells that glow compared to the surrounding normal cells they overwhelm, the Tchelitchew-esque network of semi-transparent blood vessels and clear flowing blood, the mysterious light in the darkness of the intestine that illuminate the swaying villi, the mysterious swirling biomorphic effects of Bazilauskas' cinemotifs. Such improvisations served to direct the eye to certain parts of the body and cell. They also served to impress students, visually, with the scale of the problem, its excitement, the beauty of the functioning body, and the opportunities the fields of cancer and cell biology opened to them. But they also blurred the boundary between the imaginative world of film and biology. The animators sought to focus inquiring minds not only on the biology they brought to life, but also where it drifted into fantasy.

If the animators tried to appeal to a mix of students by using a combination of spectacular events grounded in biology (some with a fantastical riff) so did the authors of the narration. It will be recalled that Constant, Parker, and Dryer wanted to introduce what they called oversimplifications into the commentary. In their view, there was a virtue in leaving much unsaid, because it ensured that the narration did not act as a drag on the film by trying to describe everything, and because it encouraged curiosity among students as to what the narration omitted, or at least offered the teacher the chance to raise the question. The commentary provides viewers with a general orientation to the events they are watching and helps to construct a temporal sequence, but it does not explain every biological event on screen. There are many silences that the viewer/listener is left to fill; details in the animation—the bank holiday of frenzied biological events—to which the commentary makes no explicit reference. So a problem facing the authors of the narration was very similar to that faced by the animators: how to address the more advanced student without losing the less advanced, and how to ensure that the more advanced student was not bored by a narration pitched at too low an intellectual level.

Much of this was worked out in the writing and rewriting as Constant, Parker, and Dryer juggled the text, sought to remove unwanted details, added allusions, and kept the commentary to time. As they scribbled their changes to the text, they also inserted judgments as to what would work best for the range of students they were seeking to address. Bazilauskas likely provided advice on this, as he had to the animators, and David Ruhe may well have added his suggestions. All the while the writers struggled to find the right word, the suggestion of detail, the correct orientation, and to evoke the spectacular and the fantastical: think of the "the birth crisis" when the "astral body" separate in a "quiver of creation" in the heredity sequence (chapter 8).[3] In phrases such as this and many others, the writers gave Massey and Dauphin, the narrators, words to soar poetically above the events (biological/fantastical) depicted on-screen and so to invoke the themes of wonder, scientific opportunity, and concern about cancer.

Inside criticism

Once the premieres were over, it was clear that the filmmakers had not assuaged their critics. To the promoters of the film, the disheartening fact was that much of it came from within the organizations that were sponsoring the film. Johnson's move to New York meant that there was no one among the information specialists at NIH and NCI with a personal investment in the movie, and the disquiet over

Johnson's handling of the premiere gave their criticism added edge and allowed them to distance themselves from the former director of the NCI's Cancer Reports Section. But criticism was not limited to the NIH and NCI. Critics could also be found in other organizations such as the American Association of Medical Colleges and even within the NFB itself. A worry for those who supported the film was that much of the criticism came from those whose job it was to promote it. Information specialists were particularly critical of the movie, and if these individuals were not convinced of its value, how was it to be promoted effectively?

The point can be highlighted by criticism within the NIH's Office of Special Reports, created in 1948 under Judson Hardy (formerly chief, Scientific Information Section of the PHS Venereal Disease Division) for much the same reasons as Johnson's Special Reports Section had been created the year before: to deal with the overwhelming flood of public inquiries after the war, cultivate support for the expansion of NIH, and promote public education about biomedicine.[4] Hardy was to be responsible for the accuracy of most information coming out of the NIH, and it was possible that the NCI's efforts could have been subsumed under Hardy's office. Yet as the biggest institute of the NIH, the NCI opted to create an independent section, as did the National Heart Institute, the second biggest institute after the NCI, a development that set the stage for friction between Hardy and Johnson, as he sought to challenge her independent line on the release of the film. *Challenge* for Hardy would not only be about the challenge of cancer, but the challenge of reining in the NCI.

Hardy's office would under normal circumstances have been expected to provide Johnson (and Hugh Jackson, her successor) with help in promoting the film, especially as its director of public information and public relations, John E. "Jack" Fletcher, was an early advocate within the agency of using motion pictures in health education.[5] But after the problems over the involvement of the Federal Security Agency in the premiere, and the general feeling that Johnson was sidelining the NIH, the branch was less than willing to be generous in its assessment of the film. Fletcher himself was critical of the movie, as were others such as Donald R. Reed (head of the Color Reproduction Section of the Special Reports Branch). "After seeing the movie this noon I was quite aware of the deficiencies of which you spoke this morning," Reed wrote to Fletcher, sharing his disquiet about the film and the fantastical elements so carefully introduced by Low and Lambart.[6] "In addition I can only add that if such expenditure of funds by way of aesthetic vaporizings in the field of abstract art (with quite a superfluity of SCHMALTZ thrown in to boot) is justified then we surely have reached a sorry day for the poor taxpayer."

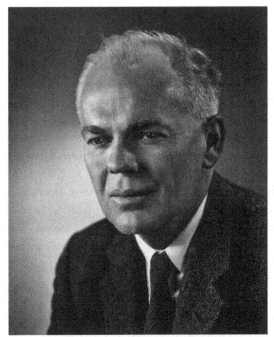

FIGURE 11.1. Judson Hardy, no date.
Source: Images from the History of Medicine, National Library of
Medicine, NLM Unique ID 101442545. NLM Image ID B010477.

Reed had attended a presentation of the film a few days after the New York premiere, probably the special screening for scientists, laboratory workers, and other NIH personnel held at NIH's Bethesda campus on March 16 and 17.[7] In his view, the audience reaction did not bode well for the film. People were confused and uncertain how to respond. "By the faces on the audience at the conclusion of the film I should judge that they were not quite sure whether they had seen a medical film or 'The Lost Week End'"[8] *The Lost Weekend* was Billy Wilder's 1945 film that followed a chronic alcoholic through a long drinking bout, and won four Academy Awards. The meaning of the reference to this film in the quotation is not clear. Perhaps Reed also found it schmaltzy? Or objected that *Challenge* fell between the stools of a medical education and public health or entertainment film? Whatever the meaning of the Billy Wilder reference, Reed hoped for an opportunity to demonstrate the waste of time, opportunity, and money that this film represented to him. "Let us hope for the day soon when we can prove our point,"[9] he concluded.

Other criticism came from the AAMC, which had supported the film through its Medical Film Institute. Dean F. Smiley, the secretary and editor of the Association's journal, *Medical Education*, wrote to David Ruhe at the MFI. Smiley had published several books on health aimed at children and general audiences and had been an educational collaborator for Coronet Instructional Movies on at least two public health education movies, *Attitudes and Health* and *Rest and Health*.[10] His letter began on positive note. He thought the film highly successful in helping viewers to visualize cancer research and what was being done. In his view, the film would work best if it were accompanied by a good introduction and followed by good discussion. In such circumstances, it could be useful for high school and college biology students, and in hygiene classes for lay groups, such as Parent-Teacher Associations and service clubs.[11]

But that was about all he had to say that was good about it. Smiley noted that he had seen *Challenge* twice, and that he had been confused at the first showing (not so much after the second) because so much was packed into the film. "In general, I felt that the film was long on artistic and dramatic presentation, imaginative treatment and scientific content, short on organization from the educational angle."[12] In his view, it did not move plainly from the simple to the complex, nor did it make its main points obvious. Nowhere, he complained, was any main point "punched out"[13] so that the student could carry at least that one important thought away with him [*sic*]. He felt it would not mean much to those without some education or training in biology.

As seriously, Smiley repeatedly interpreted the film in ways that the ways that the filmmakers had not intended. Where the filmmakers wanted the opening (sequence 1) to situate the challenge of cancer within the calm assurance of a hospital and the past triumphs of medical science, Smiley questioned the "sinister atmosphere"[14] created by the appearance of the patient with the cancer "while he had this mask-like hard look on his face."[15] Where Louis Applebaum sought to imitate growth and multiplication musically in sequence 2, Smiley argued that "the synchronized sound"[16] showing the structure and multiplication of the cell "seemed unreal and cheaply dramatic."[17] The music was not "inaudible" to this viewer/listener as Applebaum seems to have hoped; Smiley brought it to the foreground, not the background. The picture of the cell (perhaps that in sequence 10) "looking for all the world like a coiled cobra was confusing"[18] to Smiley; he could not identify it. Where the tea-making scene (sequence 9) was intended to show the character of the scientist, Smiley found the conversation of the laboratory workers too loud to be written off as atmosphere and too blurred to be understood. The process of metastasis was shown (sequence 2) but inadequately explained, Smiley noted. Bazilauskas' cinemotifs— "upsurging bubbles" [19] and so on inside the cell left him confused as to what was real and what was imaginary. And, finally, Smiley did not like the credits at the end that gave the film a "Hollywood flavor."[20]

Reviews produced for the Medical Film Institute itself were themselves divided. "This film is recommended for use by the Department of State,"[21] noted one report. "The film is not recommended for distribution by the Department of State,"[22] noted another. The former described the film as a "beautifully produced documentary film"[23] that appeared to target the viewers it wanted effectively: "students in high schools and colleges are impressed with its message of motivation, challenge and hope."[24] Nevertheless, even this positive report was cautious about its ability to reach some audiences: "the story continuity depends upon the idea of the cell, an idea difficult to sustain interest in those who have not had scientific training or bents."[25] The animation was "at once imaginative and skillful but also unreal to the untrained."[26] (The fantastical here was not simply the creation of the animators, but also that of the untrained viewer.) The narration might be "accurate and poetic," [27] but it was "dissociated from the visual continuity in a number of important places."[28] It was also "couched in a high scientific verbiage which makes it less intelligible than was often demanded by the complex science, equipment, and operations seen at all points."[29]

The other review started with praise but was much more damning. There were two versions of this report; one short, one long. "Photographically excellent, but far too long and confused," noted a short version of the report. [30] "Makes unnecessary atristic [artistic] trials unsuccessfully. Information and emotion admixed to detriment of each." The longer report noted that while the film covered much scientific ground, too much was inadequately explained, and too many topics mentioned by the narrator were given too little attention in the visuals. Anyone, the review claimed, who was not well-versed in science—at least to the high school level—would have problems understanding the film, and some of the laboratory sequences might not be adequately understood even by those who had achieved such a level of education. The film to this reviewer was inspirational in nature, more a glorification of cancer research than a clear explanation of the problems and methods of the field. "It was originally designed to attract students to a career in cancer research," it noted, conceding that it[31] "may be effective in this respect."

Reviews in professional journals echoed some of these criticisms. For some authors, it was not clear that the artistry of the movie served its educational objectives. As Caroline Keller, a reviewer in the *American Journal of Nursing* put it, questioning the movie's suitability for an audience of high schoolers.

"Technically it is a beautiful piece of photography," she noted.[32] "Throughout the film many highly dramatic effects are secured." But its tone was depressing for a movie about cancer, which undermined any message of hope the film might have been intended to provide: "However, the atmosphere which seems to permeate the film is gloomy, eerie, even mystic—long, dark laboratory corridors, rain, and an assortment of somber patients who appear in the film sustain the feeling of impending doom."[33] Keller also echoed the point about the lack of educational punch. She thought it comprised "a disjointed series of scenes, following no pattern or continuity of thought."[34] And she also wondered whether it offered a positive view of science: "At its conclusion one is left with a vague impression that much work is being done in the fight against cancer but that very little has been accomplished."[35] For these reasons, she felt that the film was not suitable for high school students, though she felt that for nurses, it might be used in conjunction with the other films on cancer.[36]

According to Bill McClelland at the NFB, the "feeling that <u>Challenge</u> is too much of a strain on the average intelligence has been the most persistent criticism."[37] He was prompted to make this remark following criticism from Alberte Sénécal, of the Information Services Division of the Canadian Department of National Health and Welfare who thought that the French version of the film, *Alerte*, was too technical for the average lay audience. McClelland noted that he had heard similar comments from friends who had seen the film. Yet these friends never themselves admitted to being baffled, and he wondered if there was a tendency to underestimate the average intelligence of Canadian audiences. Sénécal had also been particularly critical of the use of French subtitles, something that the NFB representative at this screening felt that no one else shared (they are used during Mr. Davis consultation and the tea-making sequence, not in the narration). Sénécal also echoed the points that the film was too scientific, that the conclusions drawn from the film were not precise enough, and that it did not get across the menace of cancer.[38]

Even among the filmmakers there was some feeling that the film was not all that it could have been. For example, Guy Glover, the film's producer, was worried about the response of the British to *Challenge*. It will be recalled that he had trained in the UK, and the NFB's approach owed much to the documentary film tradition there. Glover noted: "I have not heard any details of its reception in England or Scotland, and I would not be surprised if that reception were disappointing. I feel the original film has many faults which the British film-makers would rightly be extremely severe with."[39] Glover did not elaborate on what these faults might be. But his comments highlight a pessimism about the response to the film even among those who had been closely involved in its production, though Glover would change his view of the film later, coming to regard *Challenge* as one the better films produced by the NFB.[40]

The media

Such doubts and criticism raised a problem for Johnson and other promoters of the film. They had invested a huge amount of money, time, and reputation in this film, and they could not allow it to fail whatever its limitations. For the NFB it was perhaps its most important film of 1949, a key example of a coproduction effort (important even after Ralph Foster left) and its most prominent international collaboration, and a failure would not help its efforts to extricate itself from its postwar political problems. A failure would also have been problematic for the Medical Film Institute, then trying to establish itself as an arbiter of what counted as a good medical/public health educational film: how could it support such efforts if it was associated with a film that failed to do the work its sponsors wanted? Nor could the NCI or the Department of National Health and Welfare afford such a spectacular failure. Austin Deibert had been involved in the film since the beginning, and his Cancer Control Branch, then losing influence within the NCI to the research side, might suffer if the film was perceived as a failure. The information officers at the NCI and the NIH were also in a bind. Johnson had noted earlier, these offices were particularly vulnerable, constantly dependent on the good will of other groups within the organization they served. Despite their criticism of the film, they also realized that it had support from scientists at the NCI who had signed off on it, and the NCI was still committed to the broader effort to recruit high school and college students into cancer research and biology. The failure of the film would have removed a centerpiece of this campaign, and would have embarrassed the NCI in a major international collaboration with the Department of National Health and Welfare in Canada. Whatever their real feelings about the film, it would be a problem if it did not succeed.

The media campaign provided an opportunity for Johnson, Gilchrist, and other supporters to turn things around. It will be recalled that this had begun in early 1949 and had been ratcheted up for the New York and Ottawa premieres. Johnson, Gilchrist, and their colleagues realized that any internal and professional criticism was likely to be muted by a positive response from the media, and to this end they provided the media with enormous amounts of information, what Johnson had called "press handling" during the planning for the premieres.

Press handling was essentially an effort to structure the media's response to the film by providing newspapers, magazines, radio, and television with readymade stories they could use. The media, always desperate for copy, it was hoped, would take these up and reproduce them.

This is not to say that there were no risks with this strategy. The media was a fickle partner, sometimes supportive of the NCI and sometimes not, always bent on its own agendas. The NCI had, for example, long complained about the tendency of the media to exaggerate the promise of research, so that public expectations were unduly raised, only to be dashed when the expected results did not materialize or did not materialize in time. The problem only got worse with the expansion of funding for research after the war. Commentators complained that media interest in cancer and cancer research had grown as cancer research expanded, and that successful wartime programs such as the Manhattan Project or the efforts to develop penicillin had generated an expectation that cancer would soon succumb to the assault of science. Scientists came to dread the reporter's call, fearful that an innocent word would be misrepresented. It had been in part to handle such demand for news that the NCI had created the Cancer Reports Section, and Johnson was more than aware that the media did not always respond in ways that its handlers hoped. It was always possible that the media might be hostile to the movie or take the story and run with it in ways that had not been anticipated, or that it might ignore the film altogether. Aware of these potential problems, Johnson began to plan a media campaign.

Johnson's main concern was to get wide coverage, and she felt that this meant getting the attention of the Associated Press (AP) and similar news-gathering organizations that distributed stories to member newspapers. So she went fishing for an AP reporter and soon seemed to land one: the AP's science correspondent, Alton Blakeslee, was interested in producing an article.[41] As educational director of the Public Affairs Committee, Johnson had recently published Blakeslee's pamphlet *Polio Can Be Conquered* and she had plied him—and other reporters at the Hunter College premiere—with booze and "good speeches."[42] Blakeslee's first offerings, however, cannot have been quite the sort of report that she wanted: they were more about the discovery that rat glands could be grown outside the body to yield adrenocorticotropic hormone (ACTH) than about the film.[43] Blakeslee had picked up on a story mentioned by Leonard Scheele in his talk at Hunter College on the "By-Products of Cancer Research."[44] As noted in the previous chapter, Scheele had included this story among a number examples of research undertaken at the National Cancer Institute that had

had unexpected outcomes outside of cancer. Blakeslee took this one example, ignored the others, and made it, rather than the film, the main story.

There were good journalistic reasons to focus on ACTH, but they had little to do with cancer.[45] In the early 1950s, ACTH and cortisone were lauded as wonder drugs that would transform the treatment of hitherto incurable rheumatoid arthritis among other conditions. The problem was that both drugs were extremely expensive and in short supply. The NCI's new ability to grow pituitary glands outside of the body raised the possibility of addressing these problems. Scheele had warned that the research was still in an experimental stage, and that the results would not transform into meaningful treatments for rheumatoid patients for many years. But Blakeslee suggested that the research was already "yielding cheap harvests of scare, expensive hormones,"[46] and also held out the promise of a "harvest" of hormones that stimulated sex glands to make sex hormones. The only qualifier was in the longer of the two versions of the article, which mentioned that Scheele had cautioned against "undue optimism"[47] as to the help these developments may provide to cancer patients. The script of Scheele's talk contained no such caution for cancer patients.[48] Johnson boasted that these stories (one a morning release, the other an evening release), were carried in papers throughout the US and Canada, but it did her no good that the story of cancer had lost out to that of arthritis.[49]

If Blakeslee's early reports buried the story of the film in the broader enthusiasm for wonder drugs for rheumatoid arthritis, his later reports, which appeared as Sunday features the following weekend, were much more appealing to Johnson and her colleagues. Her efforts to use the Associated Press to capture the Sunday features market seemed to have paid off. She and Gilchrist reported that the AP story went to 500–600 papers and had largest pickup of any AP feature on April 2, 1950, appearing in 300–350 papers.[50]

In the movie, the narrator briefly refers to cancer cells as "outlaws" (animation sequence 2), and Blakeslee expanded on this metaphor. The cancer cell started life as a law-abiding citizen, Blakeslee explained, but turned into an outlaw, villain, thief, gangster, "a Jesse James of biology."[51] This metaphor had recently been used in the ACS campaigns to target children in the 1940s: recall how in *Detectives Wanted!* (1942) children had been invited to fight cancer the gangster by joining the FBI (Family Bureau of Investigation) as G-men (chapter 1). The rest of the article echoed the themes and structure of the film, highlighting the nature of the cancer problem and what science was doing to address it, and concluding with a discussion of the intended audiences for the film. Given the criticisms then emerging about the ability of the film to reach a general audience, Johnson and her colleagues may have been relieved to note that the review said little about the quality of the film itself other than that it was "dramatic." [52] His article is also noteworthy in that it used images that were not from the film. Johnson and her colleagues did not restrict themselves to the NFB-supplied stills from the film, but offered a variety of images for an article, many of which had little or nothing to do with the film.

If Blakeslee was the mainstay of the Sunday features, a 30-year-old freelance science writer, Morton M. Hunt, was the mainstay of the Sunday magazines. Despite early hopes of roping in *Parade, This Week,* the *New York Times Sunday Magazine,* and *American Weekly,* only *Parade* came through with a feature on cancer research.[53] Hunt, however, opted not to write about the film, but published a more general piece on cancer research instead. He was interested in the social sciences including psychology and framed his account of cancer research with the story of how Curt Richter at Johns Hopkins University was seeking to apply the principles of the lie detector to locate hidden cancers. In between the Richter bookends, Hunt argued that new research on hormonal and chemical interventions sought to attack cancers not amenable to surgery or radiation, and that research into finding a suitable test for cancer would help therapists improve their ability to treat the disease. The only mention of the film was that that the article used two stills from it. Nevertheless, Johnson and Gilchrist presented it as a success in the broader objective of bringing the latest cancer research to a wide general public, an audience that the film itself was increasingly being used to target. They pointed out that *Parade Sunday Magazine* was distributed by thirty-one newspapers in thirty-one cities to 4,937,493 subscribers.[54]

The good news for Johnson and her colleagues was that film and school magazines, including those that targeted educational films, reviewed the film positively.[55] *Educational Screen* and *See & Hear* gave broadly positive reviews of the film, describing it as "dramatic and vivid"[56] and an "important new visual interpretation of . . . [the cancer] problem and an inspiring message to all young students of science."[57] *School Life* devoted three pages to the film (and the forthcoming booklet, teaching guide, and filmstrip), explaining how cancer was now a teachable subject for the young.[58] In the past, it claimed, cancer education material had tended to emphasize symptoms and dangers, and also had tended to be more appropriate for older age groups and for youngsters in elementary and high schools. By contrast, this package made it possible to introduce the subject of cancer into school programs, not as a health education subject but as a fascinating aspect of scientific research. The article may have overplayed the claim that health education did not appeal to children, because as noted in chapter 1, the

ACS and others had attempted since the 1940s to recruit children who might be persuaded to encourage their parents to seek early detection and treatment. Nor was it correct about the novelty of the cinematic presentation of cancer as a research subject: recall that in 1950 the ACS also released *From One Cell* targeted at school biology students, though reports to the MFI about the ACS film were if anything even more damning than for *Challenge*—"an excellent example of a bad instructional film,"[59] according to one review.

Particularly important in addressing internal criticism of *Challenge* were reviews in the *Saturday Review* and *Film News*. In the *Saturday Review*, the filmmaker, producer, and commentator on educational film, Cecile Starr, acknowledged that the film was not organized and edited as precisely as it could be, and that it could have done with a less obtrusive musical score (for her, as for Smiley, Applebaum's efforts to make the music "inaudible" had not worked). Nevertheless she noted that by "allying fears rather than aggravating them, by being specific rather than vague, and by relating the problem of cancer to many other problems, the film achieves an overall excellence which earns for it the highest praise. . . . More than any other film yet produced this one is an inspiring account of science at work for the good of all,"[60] and she recommended it for high school and college students. The review in *Film News* was, if anything, more effusive:

> This film not only succeeds in being a remarkably lucid presentation. It is also a remarkably beautiful piece of work which we predict will take international cinematographic awards—for its contribution to both applied and research science; for its special music, perhaps a shade on the dramatic side but of unusual quality; for its excellent photography and special effects; for its particularly thrilling animation sequences of "the quivering world" of the cell; for its finely worded and spoken narrative.[61]

Other reviews also helped to counter internal criticisms and doubts. It will be recalled that Morten Parker had had doubts about Raymond Massey's narration, and that others had found some of the scientists' chatter, especially in the tea-making sequences, a distraction from the narration and difficult to follow. W. Ward Marsh's review in the *Cleveland Plain Dealer* that followed the premiere at the Cleveland Health Museum dealt a blow to such criticisms. In his view, Raymond Massey's narration was clear, concise, and informative, and he made a virtue of the "often hollow and echoing"[62] dialogue usual among doctors and scientists. In his view, the dialogue in the film seemed to be "a purposeful recording so that the narrator may tell the spectator all he need know while those working in the field of research may seem mysterious, possibly a little supernatural."[63]

Press handling and the public

"Press handling" was not only about responding to internal criticisms of the film. It was also about structuring public responses. In part, its function was simply to let people know about the film, what it sought to achieve, and who was behind it. It also sought more generally to raise public awareness of cancer research. Indeed, the prevalence of articles on cancer research in general (rather than about the film itself) suggests that the briefings and press releases that Johnson and the Canadians gave to the media did not restrict themselves to the film. Johnson had long seen her Cancer Reports Section as the choke point through which all NCI dealings with the media should pass. The irony of the broad range of the promotional campaign is that it came about *after* she had resigned from the NCI and was only working for the organization part-time as a consultant. Quite how Hugh Jackson or other information specialists in Bethesda felt about this is not known, though it is likely that Johnson's expanded role fed into their general concern that she was sidelining them. Now it seemed that the old regime at the Cancer Reports Section was not only in charge of the promotional campaign for the film, but also the NCI's handling of broader public information about cancer. Still, they could do little to stop her, at least until the promotional campaign was over.

Johnson and Gilchrist collected the many media responses to the film in a scrapbook called *A Project Report on Promotion and Distribution*.[64] It probably confirmed the fears of information specialists at NCI and NIH that Johnson's promotional campaign was about much more than the film. While some of the periodical articles limited themselves to the film, most did not. Indeed, those that did covered much the same ground as the Hunt article (albeit without the Curt Richter bookends) about how research on hormones and chemicals and for a cancer test promised to overcome the limitations of surgery and radiotherapy.[65] Moreover, Johnson was also using images—some from the film, but many from elsewhere—to expand her activities. Despite the disappointment that the *New York Times Sunday Magazine* had not taken up the article, Johnson noted that the Sunday *New York Times* retained some of the pictures for use on occasion with credit to the film, as did the International News Service.[66] Six pictures and a story were also sent to the Acme picture service.[67] The State Department used the pictures to accompany a feature photo story that was distributed to magazines and newspapers in seventy-eight countries as part of their overseas information program on "American science." And some fifty to sixty others were in the hands of the editors for use as a filmstrip to be sent "to the more backward areas of the world"[68] and in an exhibit that could be sent to major population centers worldwide. Some of the publicity stills are from scenes that do not appear in the film, such as a scene in which Mr. Davis, the cancer patient, is seen shaving with his cancer prominently displayed in the mirror.[69] Others had nothing to do with the film. It is unclear whether these images were distributed by Johnson or others associated with the film, and some were erroneously credited to the film itself.

Thus, after a shaky start, the propaganda campaign seemed to have done its work. The early criticisms of the film seemed to have been countered, and the movie was about to enter classrooms. It was in this context of that on May 5, 1950, Austin Deibert, the NCI's head of cancer control, showed the movie to a senior biology class at the nearby at Bethesda–Chevy Chase High School. Immediately after the screening he sent a letter to David Ruhe in New York: "A hasty note to let you know that I finally have given a deep sigh of relief!"[70] The students were enthralled by the movie. "During its presentation," he told Ruhe,[71] "I could not see any evidence at all of squirming in the seats, weaving or nodding of heads. In fact, the entire class was frozen in watching and hearing the film. Brother, I surely gave a sigh of relief!"[72] He further noted that after the show there followed a lively discussion of the merits and shortcomings of the movie. A few students grumbled about the extent and elaborateness of the animation, and some were irritated by the scene in which scientists took a tea break in the laboratory and felt it could be cut. But in general, the responses were positive. Deibert summed up his thoughts: "I firmly believe that it is just what we want for science high school classes."[73]

This assessment and his relief at the students' enthusiastic response had much to do with the attacks on the film that had surfaced over the previous few months, which seemed to undermine all the work of the past year. Critics in the sponsoring agencies had finally gotten behind the film, but the aftertaste remained. At times critics had seemed intent on portraying it as a failure for internal reasons and had only backed away from this course to avoid public embarrassment for the agencies. It was clear to Deibert and other promoters of the film that the idea of failure had been pushed for political and institutional reasons, and it left a bitter feeling, forcing the promoters of the film to respond. Failure, in other words, had been manufactured, in turn prompting Johnson and Gilchrist to manufacture its success with their media campaign. In the end, the internal critics of the film had backed away, and come to embrace— at least publicly—the idea that the film was success. But the struggle was not yet over, and without the other versions of the film, Lester Grant's book, the teaching guide, or the filmstrip it could all yet fall apart. Attention would now turn to these.

CHAPTER 12

The Package

I
T WAS INEVITABLE THAT Johnson's efforts would end. The demands of her beautiful new job were beginning to take more of her time, the promotional campaign for the film was beginning to wind down, and the NCI's information officers were reasserting control over the agency's public information programs. Johnson had taken the NCI and the NIH in directions that its information officers were unhappy about in the three to four months after her resignation, but from about April 1950 they slowly took charge again and began to ease her out. With no resources and no support back in Bethesda, and anxious to move on, Johnson turned her attention to her new life in New York. Her brief tenure at the NCI, and its ghostly afterlife in the early months of 1950, was over.

This meant that Johnson was only partly involved in the other parts of the package—the book, the teaching guide, the filmstrip, and the other versions of the movie. Indeed, she was really only involved in the book and the teaching guide. These two publications had been commissioned to make the film more usable in the classroom, and (in the case of the Grant book) perhaps to broaden the audience. But in fact what they tended to do was to raise questions about the centrality of the film to efforts to both educate the public and recruit scientists to cancer research.

As regards educating the public, the brief flurry of efforts to target *Challenge* at a general audience dissipated after the regional premieres were over. The NCI sent copies of the film to its regional offices, and Austin Deibert asked regional directors to ensure that all state and city public health departments in their region be given a screening, and be encouraged to purchase a copy.[1] Deibert seems to have taken some responsibility for in the film after Johnson's departure: recall (chapter 1) that in 1949 the Medical Film Institute (MFI) of the Association of American Medical Colleges (AAMC) had applied to the NCI for a grant to make the movie, and that this money had come from the Cancer Control Branch, of which Deibert was the head. But apart from such efforts *Challenge* received only limited public distribution, while the sponsors, makers, and

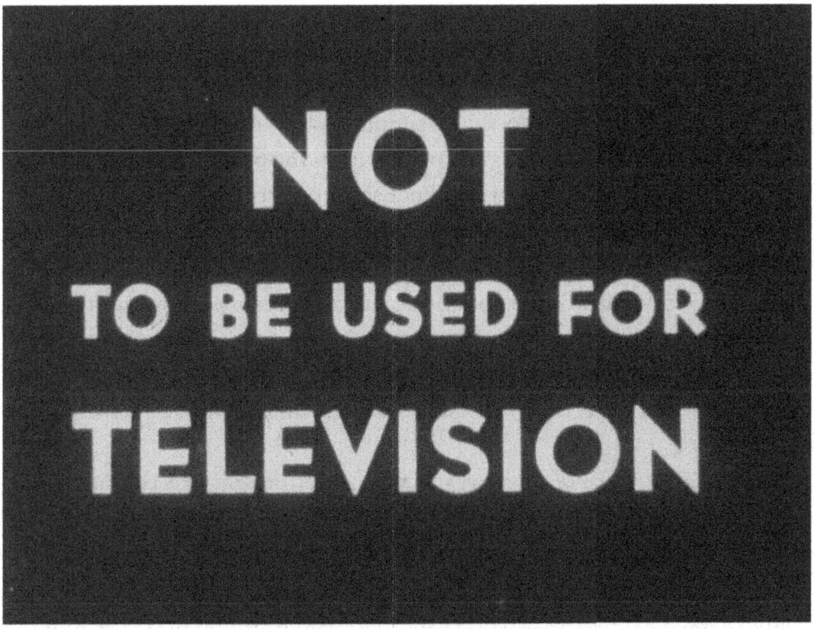

FIGURE 12.1. Not for Television: from the National Library of Medicine's copy of *Challenge*. Source: Frame grab from *Challenge*.

promoters awaited the promised theatrical version, which was intended from the start for a broader audience. Earlier plans to show *Challenge* on television were canceled because of plans for the theatrical version, what Deibert called a "featurette," and he worried that the distribution of the featurette might be harmed.[2] "As you probably know," he wrote to NCI regional directors,[3] "there is such competition between television and the movies that once a film has been used over television the movies won't touch it." Some copies of the film were marked not for television (figure 12.1).

Instead, *Challenge* was increasingly aimed at classroom audiences, but even in the classroom, the film seems to have been sidelined. The teachers who produced the teaching guide focused most of their attention on the book and gave very few indications as to how the film might be used in the classroom beyond a few generalities. They saw the book as ideally suited to teaching students about biology, chemistry, and physics, something that the recruitment film was not well suited for. The package, in other words, had shifted focus from recruitment and public education to supplementing the school curriculum, and it was not clear what role the film had now that the spotlight had moved away.

The irony of the fate of *Challenge* cannot have been lost on Johnson. She had spent much of her time for the past year promoting a movie targeted at high school and college science students, only to find that the teachers she had recruited to ease its way into the classroom had changed the goalposts. As a recruitment film, it had a marginal place within the broader package that was now aimed at supplementing the school science curriculum. The early hopes that *Challenge* would be the center of a major recruitment drive seemed to have dimmed, in part because the recruitment picture was rapidly changing. If in 1948/9 the NCI had worried about the paucity of recruits to cancer research, by the early 1950s its pessimism about recruitment seems to have diminished. Indeed, it seems to have concentrated most of its efforts at reforming the school curriculum, and in getting teachers, students, and their families enthused about science.

The marginal place of *Challenge* in school recruitment and education programs should not, however, be interpreted as meaning that the NCI or the DNHW had lost faith in film as a tool of education, for in 1951 they released a theatrical version of *Challenge* aimed at a general audience. This film, *The Fight* (and to a lesser extent the two other shorter versions) would make the film the center of educational efforts, but in ways that Johnson had not anticipated.

The book and teaching guide

There was some pressure for the publication of the book and teaching guide to coincide with the premieres of *Challenge*. It will be recalled that Johnson had recruited the journalist Lester Grant to write the book, and that the NCI had secured permission from the *New York Herald Tribune* to use his articles for that publication as the basis for the book *The Challenge of Cancer*. But Johnson's early hopes that the book would be ready by the time the film was released were dashed, as were her hopes that the teaching guide would also be ready on time. The result was that it was difficult to deflect criticism that the film failed to reach either the general public or its intended audience of high school and college science students. The book and teaching guide should have dented such criticism. With the premiere out of the way, and the film ready to enter the classroom, these anxieties gained urgency.

Why the book was so delayed is not entirely clear from the surviving records. Likely part of the reason was that Johnson wanted a high-quality production so as to make the publication appealing to its audiences of science students and the interested public, and this would take time and negotiation. In the first place, she wanted her close friend from Occidental days, the Californian fine book designer Ward Ritchie, to design the book. Johnson had worked with Ritchie on several projects, including during her time for the Institute of Consumer Education in the 1930s. He had gained a reputation as a leading figure in modernist book design, one of the major individuals of the fine-printing movement in Southern California.[4] He had left the Ward Ritchie Press (incorporated 1932) on the outbreak of World War II to produce technical manuals for Douglas Aircraft, and returned to the press full time only in 1950, about the time that Johnson approached him for help with the Lester Grant book. In Ritchie's recollection, this commission was an interesting distraction from his work for the press that bore his name.[5]

According to Ritchie, his involvement began when Johnson invited him to work on several projects she had going at the time for the ACS and the NCI: "She [Johnson] had an abiding interest in my work and a certain reliance upon my ideas whenever she got into a new job."[6] Johnson, he recalls, arranged for him to come East, first to New York, to lay out the proceedings of the First National Cancer Conference jointly sponsored by the NCI and the ACS, and then to Washington and Bethesda to work on several other projects including Grant's book.[7] In Washington he worked directly with the Government Printing Office (GPO), which was to print the book, where he recalls he had the only air-conditioned office in the building, and access to people at the top of the agency: "Ordinarily you don't have the opportunity to work with the chiefs. I was taken in; I was shown everything that was available. The chief designers were at my beck and call if I wanted them."[8]

It was a hot summer; so hot, he remembers, that they closed the government offices at 2 p.m. every day. Ritchie, however, had air conditioning not only at the GPO but also in his room at the Statler hotel. So when he was not at the GPO people would come to his hotel room, refreshments would be ordered, and they would work until 10, when it would be cool enough to go out for dinner. He would be back in his room at midnight, where he would go to his drawing board and work for hours to have graphic solutions to the day's problems to present at the 9 a.m. session the next morning. "A week of this left me a complete wreck and most happy to go home."[9]

The problem facing both Ritchie and Johnson was that the GPO did not have a reputation for the high quality of its publications in terms of design, paper quality, or feel. Quite the opposite. Most of its publications were printed on paper of poor quality, and the GPO generally did not give its publications the attention to detail and design that Richie would give to a book. Yet Johnson did not regard the situation as without hope. She had worked with the GPO on earlier publications—including William Hueper's 1948 booklet for the NCI, *Environmental Cancer*[10]—and knew how to get around some of its limitations.

To Johnson, the key was to secure the backing of Frank H. Mortimer, the director of GPO's Division of Typography and Design. In her 1949 memorandum to Heller on the relationship between the Cancer Reports Section and the research side of the NCI she had outlined some of the problems they faced in working with Mortimer.[11] While Mortimer was an excellent designer, she explained, his options were highly restricted. He was limited in the number and extent of typefaces available to him, in the amount of high-quality paper he could use, and in the grade and weight of cover stock that he could allocate. So he compromised where he could, and the better typefaces went to those who specifically requested them, as did the better grades of paper and the better cover stock. The GPO could do an excellent job, she noted (citing Hueper's *Environmental Cancer* as an example), if presented with a challenging typographical design, complete with specifications as to typefaces, paper stock, color selection and so on. The issues facing the Lester Grant book were the same as those she had earlier faced with the Hueper booklet. Mortimer would have to be persuaded that this book was worth it.

Johnson's correspondence with Frank H. Mortimer has not survived, but it is likely that her earlier work on the Hueper booklet and the fact that she had persuaded Ritchie to design the Grant book helped ensure Mortimer's support. Not only was Ritchie extremely well regarded among book designers (and not only by his own estimation as set out in his comments above), but he could give Mortimer the sorts of specifications for the book in a way that would appeal to a fellow book designer. Having produced technical manuals during the war, Ritchie knew where to compromise and where not to, and could empathize with the limitations that Mortimer faced at the GPO. By the time the proofs were being created, Mortimer was fully on board according to Johnson. "I crept into the GP & O yesterday with your letter and I can't even begin to tell you, this late in the day, how the Mortimers reacted," she wrote to Ritchie, regarding the book and a review by three unnamed gentlemen.[12] "They drooled, bowed, kissed the hem of my gahment [*sic*] and practically went out of their minds. The three gents involved pored over your epistle with Mortimer standing there shouting 'Give him anything he wants.' They plum adore you." The GPO was having problems with the proofs and the ink "but God knows they're trying," Johnson reassured Ritchie. "They are so nervous for fear they will do something you won't like."[13]

If the issue of negotiations with the designer and printer complicated publication, so too did Johnson's resignation from the NCI. After mid-December 1949 she could no longer allocate NCI funds to the book but had to go through her successor, Hugh Jackson. Jackson was supportive of the publication, and the associated teaching guide, especially as the Grant book had the backing of John Heller (NCI director) and Austin Deibert and made liberal and positive references to the NCI and to NCI researchers. But the publication also gave him some control over Johnson at a time when he and others at NIH worried about her tendency to sideline them. So Johnson's requests were used as pretext to rein her in, and the book slowly fell behind schedule with Johnson almost overwhelmed with her new job in New York and struggling to stay abreast of the demands of the promotional efforts associated with the premiere of the film. Johnson herself acknowledged that the marketing of the film was exhausting. She confided in Ritchie during one of her stays in the Washington area, "after a muscle and marrow shattering month or so in N.Y. promoting the research movie - . Jeepers, it fragiled me."[14]

Meanwhile, there was another issue to sort out at the NCI. The plan was to print 10,000 copies, and Johnson wanted practically the entire distribution to go to people and institutions on lists provided by the Office of Education and others, including approximately 5,000 copies to members of the National Association of Science Teachers. Jackson was uneasy. "Personally, I think the book is too expensive a one to throwaway on a grand scale, although it is certainly a worthwhile book, and won't do any good on the shelves, either here or at the GPO. My only question is, is the book going where it will do us the most good."[15] How this issue was resolved is unknown. But the cost was to be substantial. At US$4,475, the book was one of the largest expenditures of the Cancer Reports Section in 1950, second only to the costs of the *Journal of the National Cancer Institute*.[16]

The book was near to going to press, with a launch date set for April 15, 1950, a little over a month after Hunter College premiere. Johnson seems to have gotten some of her wishes about fonts and paper and cover-stock quality. Mortimer allocated the typefaces 11/13 Intertype Baskerville for the text, and Monotype Baskerville, Bauer Weiss (for the display). Printing would be by letterpress technique, using two colors on a heavy vellum-like paper stock with a rich feel, often used for publications with a significant amount of text, and but also suited to the sorts of images Ritchie wanted, with line engraving in two colors by Cas Duchow, his in-house artist. The cover would be paper, glued, and preprinted in two colors. "Aren't we going to have a beautiful book?" Johnson enthused to

Ritchie about the upcoming launch.[17] "On April 15th why don't you flee here for its birthing and we'll have us a bender."

The bender, however, had to wait (the celebratory bender, that is: I cannot vouch for the absence of others). Production deadlines slipped and Johnson struggled to push the book forward: flirting with Ritchie, monitoring Mortimer, and pleading with Jackson to move things along. The scientists at NCI seemed behind the project, and she appears to have gained the (sometimes grudging) acceptance of some of her information officer colleagues. But it was slow work, with many technical hitches along the way, and frequent trips to Washington, all on top of the increasing demands of her new job in New York. Then, on June 12, the advance copies arrived.[18] The waiting was over, and one can hope that Johnson and Ritchie had their bender (no record of it has survived), and perhaps a second the following year—1951—when the book was named as one the fifty best books of the past year by the American Institute of Graphic Arts. One delighted cancer researcher wrote congratulating Johnson on the award, stating that it came as no surprise to him: "A great guy wrote it and a pretty swell gal had much to do with its production."[19]

If the book was a struggle for Johnson, so too was the teaching guide. Like *The Challenge of Cancer*, the guide involved much negotiation with Mortimer and Jackson and as well as some new partners: the US Department of Education and the Prince George's County public school system: Prince George's County is northwest of the Washington DC border, adjacent to Montgomery County, where the NCI is based in Bethesda. The Prince George's system appointed a committee of local science teachers to develop the guide, headed by Howard B. Owens (1909–71), a biology teacher at Hyattsville High School, who had recently emerged as a prominent local advocate of science teaching.[20]

Owens and his committee met several times in the next few months. Johnson had directed Joan P. Karasik (1918–2021) a member of the Cancer Reports Section, who had recently authored an NCI pamphlet on how pharmacists might help detect stomach cancer for publication in pharmaceutical journals, to write the story line in 1949.[21] Owen and his committee (all local science teachers in Prince George's County) worked out how to evaluate and adapt Karasik's text among themselves. Then there was the rewriting, discussion, and internal revisions, before the manuscript went out for review and clearance. In this case a whole raft of organizations had to approve the guide, including the National Education Association, the United States Office of Education, NCI staff members, the NCI Editorial Board, the National Institutes of Health, the Public Health Service, and the Federal Security Agency. The guide went out to all these organizations, comments came back, and revisions were made before final clearance.

Few details of this process have survived, but it too was likely complicated by Johnson's leaving for New York and the Jackson succession. Ritchie is not mentioned in the correspondence on the guide, but its design—including the print font, paper quality, and colors—matched that of Grant's book, and so its production was probably also dependent on the timing of the design of the other book. Johnson planned a print run of 10,000 copies for the guide (the same number as for Grant's book), hoping that it would be ready in time for the premiere of the movie in early March 1950, but approval for printing came through only on March 30, 1950, after the national premieres were over.[22] Even so, production seems to have gone more quickly than with Grant's volume, and the teaching guide appeared slightly before the book. Both were ready for the fall 1950 semester, and likely made their way into the schools over summer. A supplement to Grant's book was produced in 1955.[23]

Learning from film?

The book and guide might have been intended to counter criticism that the film did not reach its intended audiences, but they proved as much a liability as a help. The movie had started as a tool for recruiting college and high school science students into cancer research and biology. Then, especially during the promotional campaign in early 1950, it had been transformed into a vehicle of public education about cancer research, beyond the classroom. Now, with the publication of the book and teaching guide, it became part of a package for educating students about cancer and biology. That role was not inconsistent with its other role as a recruitment device: educating students about cancer and biology could be used to enthuse them about these fields as career possibilities. But the package was about much more than recruitment. It also aimed to teach students about cancer, biology, and medicine. "The subject of cancer can be worked into a course of study in many places and for various purposes," the authors of the guide noted.[24] "Sometimes it can be used to motivate a lesson; sometimes to indicate a practical application of a scientific principle; sometimes to illustrate a research method; sometimes to dramatize the progress of a science." The problem was that the writers of the teaching guide seemed to have few ideas about how the film might be used for such purposes. Its title, *A Teaching Guide to "The Challenge of Cancer,"* picked up on the title of the book rather than the film.

This is not to say that the teachers saw no use for the film. In their view it was a "jumping-off point":[25] a stimulus to discussion, a means of exciting students, and a way of drawing them into these subjects: "Interest in the disease, aroused by the film or by many news stories which announce each scientific advance, can be channeled into new interest in the study of biology, chemistry, and physics."[26] But beyond this they seemed to be at a loss to know what to do with it, and gave no specific instructions on its use, just some general suggestions that it might be used for class discussions and projects related to medical research. The *Teaching Guide* thus tended to marginalize the film and focused on Grant's book.

The centrality of Grant's book can be highlighted by the two main chapters of *A Teaching Guide*, which account for almost half the publication. The guide begins with a summary of the main points of Grant's book and indicates the chapters in which they occur.[27] There follows a chapter on how cancer might be used in the curricula at elementary, junior high, and senior high school levels (but not college level courses, one of the target audiences for the film).[28] The last section includes summaries of biology, chemistry, and physics topics covered at the senior high school level in *The Challenge of Cancer*, along with discussion questions on each subject. The film is not mentioned in either chapter until the section on senior high level curriculum where there is a vague mention that it might be used to stimulate interest in the subject and classroom discussion.[29] The film is mentioned only three more times in the nineteen-page booklet—once in a further reading/viewing section, once in the introduction to the volume where it is mentioned as part of the package, and once on the title page.

Grant's book itself did not marginalize the film in quite the same way as the teaching guide. Indeed, Grant described the book and the film as a "dual presentation,"[30] and his book can be read as an expansion on many of the themes of the film, with chapters developing subjects it raised (the world of the cell, tissue culture, the role of heredity, viruses, and so on). In general, it portrayed cancer research as an effort to unravel the mysterious laws that shaped the growth of the cell, the basic unit of life; a challenge that was intended to stir the imagination of readers much as Morris Meister, the school science educator, had suggested. Cancer research emerges as a sort of detective story, in which "clews"[31] as to the nature of cancer and its cure were slowly and painstakingly put together (albeit a different sort of detective story than that imagined in *Detectives Wanted!* [1942)] where children were invited to follow the clues left by cancer the gangster to determine whether it might be present in their families.) The book also gave considerable attention to NCI scientists (and American scientists more than Canadian[32]), and allowed them to silently correct some of the problems with

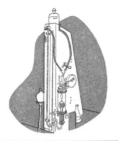
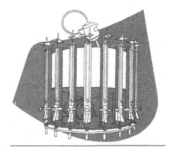

The Van Slyke apparatus is used in enzyme studies of cancer. For example, the enzymes of a tumor extract are allowed to act on peptides and the rate at which amino acids are formed is measured by this instrument.

The Warburg apparatus is used in enzyme studies of cancer. The manometer measures the enzymatic activity in terms of gas exchange in a closed vessel submerged in the circular tank. Water in the tank is kept at body temperature to simulate natural conditions.

FIGURE 12.2. Illustrations of Van Slyke and Warburg apparatuses by Cas Duchow. Source: Grant, *The Challenge of Cancer*, 45 and 55. Collage created using Photoshop.

the film—the industrial metaphor that Jesse Greenstein disliked was replaced with his metaphor of the cell as factory (albeit absent the administrator gone haywire).[33] The role of sunlight in skin cancers, which had been raised by the NCI's environmental scientists, is also given greater emphasis than in the film, through there is no mention of its effects on farmers, which the scientists had once proposed as a subject within the film.[34] Tissue culture, which environmental scientists had felt was overrepresented in the film, was reduced to little more than a page in the book.[35]

Thus, a teacher reading the book and watching the film could use both to discuss some of the questions raised in the teaching guide. But in general teachers would have found the book provided them with more detailed information than the film could, and much that was unexplained or alluded to in the film was explained or illustrated in the book. For example, each chapter of the book begins with a Duchow two-color line engraving, often illustrating technologies shown in the film, some of which the film did not identify.[36] Thus if teachers wanted to use the film to discuss the use of these technologies in science, they would have largely relied on Grant's book and other course textbooks. Cas Duchow's images included lengthy captions detailing their use in relation to the subject of the chapter (figure 12.2).

It is possible that teachers may have found other uses for the film. But no evidence of its use in the classroom has survived, apart from the sample comments of high school students sent by the librarian at the Gary Public Library described in chapter 10 and Deibert's test screening at the Bethesda–Chevy Chase High School described in chapter 11. The fact that the teaching guide gave few directions as to how it might be used cannot have helped its deployment in the classroom. Indeed, the limited mentions of the film in the teaching guide reinforce the criticism of some reviewers that the movie was ill-adapted to the task of pedagogy and failed to get its educational points across. The film might have started as the center of the package that Johnson put together (and indeed it was the center as measured in terms of the amount of work she had to put in compared to the book and the guide). But by the time the book and teaching guide had been published its place, at least in the school classroom, was unclear. No one seems to have suggested that the film should not have been part of the package (with perhaps the exception of some of its harshest critics among NIH information officers). But its place at the center of the educational campaign was not as secure as it once had been.

Different versions

All this would change in the coming months as the Americans and Canadians began to plan the filmstrip and especially the other versions of the film. But for a while in 1950 the future of the film project seemed uncertain. The danger was that it would disappear or fail to achieve its goals, and that questions would be raised about the huge expenditure on the film, and those that had backed it. With Johnson leaving, it was likely that she would have been blamed for its failure. Increasingly the NCI began to regard the whole undertaking as a legacy project, and few people wanted to touch the legacy.

The filmstrip

The filmstrip was the first to suffer the neglect of a legacy project. It will be recalled that plans for the NFB to produce a filmstrip had been mooted in early 1949 with hopes that it would be produced by the time of the national premieres in March 1950, but delays prompted revisions of the timetable. Hugh Jackson noted in March 1950 that he did not know the status of the filmstrip, or who at NCI had seen or approved it. It seemed to be languishing somewhere in the NIH, he did not know where, and no one seemed to be pushing its production. "Sometime ago I saw a proposed script, upon which Joan Karasik was supposed to have been working, the last I heard of that, Ummie Booth was checking it with Deibert, but I have heard no more concerning it."[37] As mentioned in chapter 9, Ummie Booth may have been Florence H. Booth of Johnson's section and Judson Hardy's Scientific Reports Branch.

In 1949, Johnson had assigned Karasik—who had written the first draft of the *Teaching Guide*—to write the script.[38] The initial plan called for three filmstrips on biology, physics, and chemistry, using stills that the NFB already had in its film library and animation artwork or, preferably, making the strips by a blowup process. The three-filmstrip idea seems to have been abandoned early on and, with Johnson leaving the NCI and beginning her tenure as an NCI consultant, the project fell behind schedule. In January 1950 Johnson reported that Karasik was having a difficult time on the story outline: most of the still pictures taken with the film were not suitable for the strip (they had not received the animation stills yet—recall that the animation sequences were late in coming), and they were waiting for an entirely new set of stills to be shot. In addition, it seemed that there was little enthusiasm among the Canadian health authorities for the strip. Johnson noted that Gilchrist was lukewarm about the idea and seemed to Johnson to want more encouragement before deciding to invest his $1,500 ($1,000 for the English version; $500 for the French version). Johnson noted that she practically guaranteed him a sale of at least 1,000 copies and that this seemed to encourage him.[39]

With the Canadians now on board, Karasik produced a draft script, which Johnson sent to the NFB on January 23, 1950.[40] The Karasik script (called *Challenge: Science Against Cancer*) comprised forty-nine slides, too long for use in one class period according to Johnson. "Accordingly, the strip is divided in two parts, and this solution seems to work out quite well. Part I is essentially presentation of the problem and Part II is the research story."[41] The first part of the filmstrip concentrated, as Johnson suggested, on the scale of the cancer problem and the ways cancer could currently be treated and prevented. Its focus was on the supposed two-thirds of cancers that could be treated and set up the problem of the remaining third and how science investigated them. The second part explored the scale of the scientific endeavor, and the ways in which biologists, chemists, physicists and biostatisticians were tackling the problem of the cell.[42] As Johnson pointed out "no effort was made to follow the film but rather to make a film strip that could be used by itself, either with or without a previous showing of the film, as the nucleus of a class discussion of cancer."[43] Johnson herself later reported in 1950 that the filmstrip was developed separately from the film so as to use color, but other reports suggest that they used sections from the film itself.[44]

If the filmstrip had been slow to get off the ground, it really began to slow down in January/February of 1950. Karasik left the NCI for a post at the National Institute of Mental Health;[45] Johnson was increasingly focused on organizing the premieres of the film and could devote little attention to the filmstrip; and when she finally stopped her consulting work it took some time before people at the NCI took up the idea again. A second substantially revised draft of the script is dated February 11, 1950. Deibert wrote to the NFB to say he liked the rough draft very much but suggested that it might "pack too much information into each frame."[46] It might need cutting, and he felt that cuts might best be made in the slides dealing with therapy to create more space for the sections on fundamental cancer research.But beyond this no one at the NCI or NFB seems to have followed up, nor at the Department of National Health and Welfare, nor the Medical Film Institute.[47] The plans for the filmstrip were momentarily abandoned. No wonder that Jackson had little idea what was happening.

Things started up again later in 1950, when on May 16 the Canadian Embassy in Washington teletyped the National Cancer Institute to inquire about progress.[48] The NFB quickly organized a panel to review the script for the filmstrip, which met May 25 and gave a mixed review of the original script.[49] The filmstrip had originally been intended for high school and college students who might think of biology and cancer as careers—the same audience as the film. Now Gilchrist wanted a change of focus. He felt that they should proceed with the filmstrip as a university level production, with a high school version to follow.[50] There followed a rewrite of the outline for the filmstrip dated June 13.[51] Then came a further mixed evaluation of the June script, and further revisions.[52]

With Karasik and Johnson gone, much of the revision was carried out by the Canadians with little or no consultation with the Americans, who were also funding the project. Then on June 28, the NFB received an inquiry about the filmstrip from David Ruhe, and on July 26 the NFB sent the new storyboard and script to the NCI. The new script was quite different from the original Karasik script, but the NCI seems to have been content with the revisions, and an agreement was reached to have separate introductory frames, one for use in Canada, the other for use in the US.[53]

But things continued to move slowly, and trouble began to brew. By March 1951, the Department of National Health and Welfare had become concerned that things were getting out of hand. Costs were rising, the script had been revised a half-dozen times following the comments of experts, and the normal "technical vetting" procedures of the department seemed to have been abandoned.[54] The NFB's Filmstrip Unit disagreed with the last point, noting that they had followed Gilchrist's guidelines, and that they had sought technical help from the Canadian Cancer Society since the department did not have an expert on cancer.[55]

If the Canadian sponsors were unhappy, so too were the Americans, who were feeling increasingly sidelined. It will be recalled that the Canadians had long complained about having to Canadianize American public health movies about cancer; now the Americans complained that the filmstrip was too Canadian—despite the earlier agreement for US and Canadian versions of the filmstrip. Thus, in June 1951 Raymond F. Kaiser, who had replaced Austin Deibert as head of the NCI's Cancer Control Branch in February that year, raised the question of the absence of US statistics in the chart frames of the now renamed *What We Know about Cancer*.[56] Kaiser's question prompted one NFB official to "anticipate some trouble with the US version of this strip insofar as deletions having been made in the visuals and commentary without consultation with our American friends."[57]

A second issue was the French version, which was sometimes on and sometimes off. Johnson had budgeted $500 for a French version in late 1949/early 1950.[58] In March 1951, the Department of National Health and Welfare noted that it expected to be billed for a French version.[59] But the NFB still seems to have done nothing, and by June 1951 the NFB's Filmstrip Unit believed itself to be "relieved of the necessity of making a special French edition."[60] All this changed by the end of the year, and the idea of a French version was revived. The NFB now seemed keen to learn from the lessons of the French version of the film. With memories of the criticism of French subtitles in the film in mind, the NFB was hesitant about simply releasing a captioned version for the French market: "a second-class way of handling the job, and [which] might result in considerably more trouble and inconvenience later than that caused by attempting to produce a French version at this time."[61] The NFB began work on translating the script into French and figuring out the cost of changing the nine frames bearing English lettering in the script to produce a French version negative.

The English version (thirty-nine frames) seems to have been published about October 1951, and the French version—*Ce Que Nous Savons du Cancer*—was released shortly after in early 1952.[62] In 1952, Leonard Scheele recommended *What We Know About Cancer* as suitable for illustrating lectures in high school and junior college courses (a lecturer's reading script accompanies the filmstrip.)[63] It could be borrowed from the National Cancer Institute and purchased from the National Film Board of Canada for US$2.50.

The Fight: Science Against Cancer

The theatrical version of the film was also delayed. The idea of a theatrical version had been mooted by the Canadians before the Americans got involved and had periodically been dropped and reinstated. By 1949 the plan was to begin production of the movie very soon after production of *Challenge* began. In the event, however, this did not transpire, and the delay meant that *The Fight* happened largely without Johnson's involvement. Yet the theatrical version of the film did something that Johnson and her allies did not expect. The book, the teaching guide, and the filmstrip had marginalized the film component of the package to varying extents. *The Fight*, however, reestablished its centrality (at least the theatrical version of the film) in ways that those producers and sponsors could not have imagined.

Planning for a theatrical version of the film seems to have gotten underway in March 1950, shortly before the premiere of *Challenge*: a sketch of it is dated March 3, 1950.[64] At this stage it was not clear what length the film would be, nor how it would be distributed, nor what the market might be. So to test the waters, the recently appointed head of theatrical distribution at the NFB, Ralph C. Ellis, began putting out feelers to theater distributors shortly after the American premiere of *Challenge*. He noted that he had talked to another NFB figure, Wilfred Jobbins, about the reaction of Famous Players—the largest theater chain in Canada—to the cancer film (*Challenge*). "It seems," he noted, "that [J. J.] Fitzgibbons [president of Famous Players] feels that a 15-minute version is just what the Doctor ordered."[65] Given Ellis's involvement there may have been hopes that this was to be a part of *Canada Carries On* (1940–1959), a documentary series modeled in part on the *March of Time*. However, Ellis noted that there was no immediate prospect of using *Challenge* for this series.[66]

With this positive reaction from theatre owners, in April 1950 Arthur Irwin—the NFB commissioner—authorized the production of a theatrical version of *Challenge*, provided that the estimated cost was not more than CAN$5,000. Irwin asked for work to start as soon as possible, and he also urged Glover to plan for a French-language version.[67] Glover immediately contacted David Ruhe at the Medical Film Institute informing him of the decision and seeking his advice. Ruhe had already sent him numerous letters setting forth the different reactions of professional people to *Challenge*. These letters do not appear to have survived, but they likely included some of the mixed responses discussed in the previous chapter. Glover noted that he would take these into account as he began to think about the theatrical version.[68]

Production began later in April.[69] By this stage, plans for a French-language version had been postponed, since there was a possibility that the theatrical distribution of the French version of *Challenge* would be achieved in Quebec.[70] (In the event no French-language version of *The Fight* was made, though there were still thoughts of a French version as late as September 1950[71]). The estimated budget now rose from the authorized CAN$5,000 to CAN$6,053.50. The hope was that a test print would be ready by the end of May 1950.[72]

Most of the estimated costs of the new movie were to be gobbled up by reediting the existing film stock. But the new movie was also to be quite different in emphasis than *Challenge*. Aimed at a theatrical audience rather than potential recruits to science, it was to be more focused on therapeutics than on science, the wonder of the body, and the environmental causes of cancer. Where *Challenge* had ended on the theme of science the endless quest, *The Fight* script called for Mr. Davis to return to the hospital waiting room with his tumor healed. So, one of the tasks for the new production team was to order a simulated healed carcinomatous lesion for CAN$18 from the same company that had produced the original simulated tumor for Mr. Davis's cheek, cheaper than the original unhealed simulated lesion (CAN$50).[73] A new photograph of Mr. Houghton, the actor playing Mr. Davis, was taken—a still to check make up—at a cost of CAN$5.[74]

The new script also meant undertaking some additional location shooting, including the scene when Mr. Davis returns to the hospital waiting room. Soon after the board authorized production, plans were afoot for a return to Toronto, this time by train, not car. In April 1950, shortly after production began, the NFB ordered four first-class return tickets from Ottawa to Toronto for Parker, Grant McLean (the cameraman), and Jean Roy (who had acted as assistant cameraman in *Challenge*) and J. M. Cots.[75] They did not take a soundman, as all the new shots were to be done in silence with sound added later. They also hired the Ontario-based theater actor Ross Millard for services on April 18 for CAN$25.[76]

The additional location shots seem to have been completed in April, and all seemed set to produce a test print by May 1950 as called for in the early budgets. But then production seems to have slowed. The reasons for the delay are not entirely clear, though there were innumerable discussions with the expert advisers over aspects of the movie—the dripping faucet scene, the tea bag scene, the projector and growth rings scene, an animation sequence, the student sequence, a scene with an old lady, even the presence of two men at the pillar in the opening waiting room scene—all were discussed with the experts: Should they be removed, modified, or retained?[77] The animation sequences in *Challenge* were cut from five to two sequences, and the surviving sequences—sequence 1 (growth and pathology) and 2 (the scientist as explorer)—were shortened. Whereas in *Challenge* they had served to set up the work of science, the animation sequences have a reduced role in *The Fight*.

Then there was the question of the title of the movie—something still under discussion in September 1950. One option for the title was to call it *Advance*—perhaps *Advance: Science Against Cancer*. Parker wrote to Ruhe, however, to say that the NFB found this quite unsatisfactory "in that it hasn't enough force as a word."[78] The NFB wanted the title *The Fight* but encountered objections from Ruhe. As an alternative Parker suggested *The Attack*, "which is both more vigorous and more active,"[79] than *Advance*. Ruhe's objections to *The Fight* are unknown, and he eventually relented. Shortly after Parker's letter, and after further consultation with David Coplan, who was "midwifing" distribution, *The Fight* had been chosen as the title.[80]

Since this was to be a theatrical version there was also a problem of how to allow for a proper lead-in to the film. Parker suspected that any distributor would attach as a prefix their own credit at the beginning of the film, which would read something like "Warner Brothers presents."[81] For this reason the opening title card was to read "A Progress Report on Cancer *from* the Department of National Health and Welfare, Canada *and* National Cancer Institute, United States Public Health Service." The versions I have seen do not include the prefix Parker expected, so the film begins as *A Progress Report*.

There was also the issue of the narrator—should they approach Raymond Massey again? Glover himself preferred to use another commentator, but he felt under pressure from the theatrical side of NFB, who felt Massey was important for the success of a theatrical version. The problem was that the NFB could not offer commercial rates, so the only way to do it would be to get Massey to perform as an act of charity for a good cause, for which he would accept only a nominal fee. (As he had with *Challenge*.) The difficulty was that the Department of National Health and Welfare was unwilling to approach Massey again, since the new film would be a commercial undertaking, and Glover wondered about the possibility of getting the Canadian and American cancer organizations to help.[82]

In the end the Department of National Health and Welfare reversed itself. Paul Martin—the minister—tried to persuade Massey to do the commentary, but he turned him down. Massey wrote to Martin that he was leaving for Hollywood at the time the new narration was to be recorded and would not be available.[83] Given his criticisms of Massey's earlier commentary, Parker may not have been too dismayed at this turn of events, though it meant the film would lose the publicity of Massey's name. Besides, as an unidentified NFB official put it later, the NFB could not afford him financially.[84] So the search was on to find a replacement commentator. Parker enlisted the help of Ralph Foster, now at the United Nations, who also consulted with Bernard Dryer.[85]

By September, the NFB—perhaps because of concerns about Massey's earlier commentary—planned to go with a commentator "whose performance we can rely on completely."[86] This reliable commentator was the Canadian actor John Drainie (1916–1966). Drainie was "the greatest radio actor in the world" according to Orson Welles. He had previously narrated Morten Parker's 1948 film, *The Home Town Paper.*[87] He was paid CAN$120 plus expenses and CAN$60 a reel. The recording was to be done on October 16, 1950.[88] The new commentary was dated October 12, 1950.[89]

All these negotiations took time, and there were other delays as well; for example, in getting the approval of the American sponsors. As Glover noted in September 1950: "we have been delayed in matters of finalizing the actual film itself with the international experts."[90] He hoped for a completed film by October 15, but the delays were impacting the distribution, and were beginning to annoy some of the film's sponsors.

The original plan had been for a speedy theatrical release after *Challenge*. *Challenge* had not received any general distribution, neither the English nor the French version, despite the earlier hopes that the French version might receive theatrical distribution in Quebec. Copies of *Challenge* had been sent to the regional offices of the cancer societies in the US and Canada for use in their promotional campaigns, but the general distribution of the film was deliberately held back in favor of the theatrical version. In other words, Glover noted, *The Fight* was to be the first of the films to be given widespread theatrical coverage. One option might have been to distribute this film as part of the *Canada Carries On* series, but the NFB decided against this. Instead, it favored distribution by a major distributor in the US and Canada, with other plans for international distribution and for the still hoped-for French version.[91]

By September it was clear that there had been a substantial delay. The American cancer organizations were now looking forward to a release in March 1951, their next cancer campaign. Glover envisaged working toward peak coverage of *The Fight* in March, with *Challenge* distributed sometime after for use in nontheatrical venues. (There remained to be discussed whether it was to be televised: *Challenge* had generally not been, apart from the premieres.[92]) But the Canadian Cancer Society was increasingly exasperated. The Department of Health and Welfare had promised them immediate nontheatrical use of *Challenge* in the spring of 1950, and they were annoyed when the NFB told them that it had to be held up for theatrical distribution. At that time, the hope was that the theatrical version would be released in September 1950, and the CCS was promised use of the nontheatrical version for their campaign in the coming April. With the

Americans wanting a delay in the release of the theatrical version, the NFB was in a difficult situation. As one NFB official put it: "We are hardly in a position to go to them again and say that they can't have the film,"[93] especially since the Canadian Society was sponsoring prints of their trailer—A Message from the Canadian Cancer Society—for attachment to *Challenge*.

By February 1951 publicity was beginning to build for *The Fight*. The US surgeon general, Leonard Scheele, had seen the film and liked it, and he and Paul Martin had wired the influential gossip columnist Walter Winchell, urging him to see it and give it his support: Winchell had been a key to Johnson's and Gilchrist's efforts to promote *Challenge*. "This is part of the publicity campaign to pave the way for a theatrical deal through the M.P.A.A. [Motion Picture Association of America],"[94] one NFB official noted.

Then in February the NFB was advised that *The Fight* had been selected for final balloting for an Academy Award, the winner to be announced at the awards ceremony on March 22—actually March 29.[95] The announcement prompted a flurry of plans to attend the Oscars ceremony, and likely much dusting off of dinner suits or tuxedos. At the NFB, Arthur Irwin planned to accept the award as Canadian government's film commissioner; at the NCI, John Heller planned to accept the award as the NCI's director, and at the MFI, David Ruhe also began to make plans. They were all to be disappointed. The Academy of Motion Pictures wrote back to say that if *The Fight* won the award, they could not give it to three individuals, unless they were specially credited on the film, which Heller and Irwin were not. They suggested that Guy Glover, the producer, or his representative, might accept.[96] The NCI's response is unknown, but the NFB was unable to decide what to do, prompting an urgent telegram from Los Angeles asking for a response.[97] Glover was unable to attend, since he had recordings in Ottawa on March 30 and 31. So the NFB suggested the award should be accepted by on behalf of the National Film Board by V. E. Duclos, the Canadian trade commissioner in Los Angeles.[98]

The omens seemed good. Shortly before its release *Challenge* had won first place at international film competitions in Venice (category: scientific films. Mostra Internatzionale del Cinema, August 20 to September 10, 1950) and New York (category: scientific. Annual Documentary Film Competition, January 1, 1951). But in the end, the nomination for *The Fight* did not turn into an Oscar. *The Fight* was released in May 1951. A downside was an echo of *Challenge's* earlier problems with the FSA. The FSA was not credited in the titles. No record of the FSA's response has survived.

The Outlaw Within and Cancer

By early 1951, the NFB reversed its earlier decision and determined that it wanted another ten-minute theatrical version of the movie for the *Canada Carries On* series. The series had been established by John Grierson and Stuart Legg to boost national morale during the war.[99] With the end of the war, the series lost its financial backing from the Wartime Information Board but continued under Sydney Newman (from 1945 to 1952) as the board's principal theatrical series. The style of these postwar movies was less propagandistic that those produced before 1945, but the format changed little: each film in the series was about ten to twenty minutes in length and employed voiceover commentary and minimal dialogue, in part to facilitate translation for the French-language version of the series, *En avant Canada*.

When Arthur Irwin took over as film commissioner in 1950, the series enjoyed a brief revival. Irwin introduced an "international programme" designed to propagate Canadian ideals of democracy and promote the Canadian image abroad. Given its internationalist perspective, *Challenge* or *The Fight* were soon identified as fitting very well into this program, possible candidates for the series. They also served the objective of calming CCS annoyance about the delay in arranging nontheatrical distribution of *Challenge*.

Once again, the NFB started by getting approval for the new version from the American and Canadian sponsors of the original film. In February 1951, David Ruhe at the AAMC and the Canadian Cancer Society agreed to the release, the latter hoping that it would inform the public of the meaning and difficulties of laboratory research in relation to cancer.[100] The Department of National Health and Welfare was at first noncommittal, and referred the matter to the CCS.[101] When it became clear that the CCS and the Americans were on board, the department wrote to say that it did "not object to such a project, provided, of course, that we are not involved in any further expenditure, for production, distribution, promotion, or otherwise."[102] The NCI does not seem to have been directly contacted; David Ruhe acted as a go-between.

Perhaps with the CCS annoyance in mind, the plan was to have the movie ready for April 1951—Cancer Month in Canada. This meant a very rushed schedule. The NFB's director of production, Donald Mulholland, told Ruhe that the movie would have to be in the hands of the distributors by March 10—which meant that the entire movie would have to be produced in just over two weeks. Ruhe promised twenty-four hour clearance on the commentary (which would be reviewed by him, Raymond Kaiser at the NCI, and Dr. O. H. Warwick at the CCS), and that they would not have to review the visuals.[103] Mulholland reported this to Arthur Irwin the same day as his conversation with Ruhe, with a recommendation that they go ahead with production—the *Canada Carries On* series needed a film, and this would "make a very good one."[104] Ruhe confirmed the substance of his conversation with Mulholland in a letter to Arthur Irwin, asking that the omission in the credits to *The Fight* of any acknowledgement to the US Federal Security Agency be rectified in the new short.[105] Irwin agreed.[106]

As soon as the new version was given the go-ahead the film was reedited by Nicholas Balla,[107] with the help of a negative cutter, Meta Bobet.[108] At the same time, Morten Parker quickly rewrote the commentary.[109] Ruhe seems to have been true to his word; approval for the commentary seems to have come through quickly, and production continued on time. When the commentary and reediting were complete, the next task was to match the two. A cue copy of the script was produced, slightly adapted from the version approved by Ruhe, to fit the film.[110] The screenwriter, director, and producer, Jacques Bobet, who had earlier been involved in the production of the French version of *Challenge* (chapter 8) produced a translation for *Cancer*, the French-language version of the film.[111]

On March 10, 1951—the date the film was supposed to be ready for distribution—the English-language commentary was recorded by the Canadian radio personality and satirist Max Ferguson (1924–2013), best known for his long-running program *Rawhide* for the Canadian Broadcasting Corporation (CBC).[112] The French-language commentary was recorded the same day by the Montreal-based radio announcer Gérard Arthur. Both men were paid CAN$60 each plus expenses for their work.[113]

The only hint of a problem was the publicity for the film. The florid prose of an early version of the publicity release cause minor consternation. An unidentified NFB office scrawled "Not good" across the text and asked for the text to be redone. "He's going to re-write," the unidentified official noted of the unnamed writer.[114]

Like *The Fight*, *The Outlaw Within* and *Cancer* have an optimistic outlook. They start with the appearance of Mr. Davis (now given the first name Charles) with a cancer on his cheek, and includes his return to the hospital waiting room, his cancer cured. In between viewers are treated to a brief account of the body (Low and Lambert's animation) followed by a quick tour of different types of research (basic research in tissue culture, biochemistry, genetics etc; clinical research on x-rays, radium, and surgery) before we return to the cured Mr. Davis. "Today—Charles Davis is cured";[115]"Aujourd'hui, nous pouvons guérir monsieur Davis,"[116]the narrators tell us, and "Each year more people are cured. And the power of our attack on the mystery of cancer mounts steadily." [117] But whereas *The Fight* ends with Mr. Davis's return to the hospital, this version of the movie ends with research. Mr. Davis's cure provides the reassurance necessary to conclude with a discussion of the continuing mission of scientists to understand cancer, and—with a view of the chemist/actor James J. Rae's back as he walks down a corridor—"bringing the promise of life;"[118] "des hommes qui redonnent espoir dans la vie."[119]

Endings

B Y 1951, THOSE WHO had promoted *Challenge* had succeeded in branding the film (and the package of which it was a part) a success. *The Fight* had been nominated for an Academy Award, *Challenge* had won film competitions in Venice and New York, and Lester Grant's *The Challenge of Cancer* had won a prestigious book design award on top of the prize for the original series of newspaper articles. Given such outside recognition, critics of the project within the sponsoring agencies were silenced, at least for a while.

But so too were many of the main promoters of film and its package. Johnson's consultancy with the NCI had ended in 1950, leaving the film in the hands of her successor in the Cancer Reports Section, Hugh Jackson. Jackson was in turn succeeded in 1951 by James F. Kieley, a former journalist and newscaster who worked previously as an information officer for several government agencies.[1] Jackson, and perhaps his successor, were eager to overcome the disquiet Johnson had created among information officers at the NIH and the FSA. Lt. Col. Gilchrist left the DNHW in 1954, so that his minister, Paul Martin, with whom he did not have an easy relationship, was free to appoint a successor more attuned to his ideas.[2] These departures meant that none of the main advocates of the film were left in the sponsoring agencies. With the ructions of 1950/51 behind them, those left in the NCI and the DNHW were happy to take credit for whatever good came from the package, and they also ensured its storage and distribution. But no one was there to advocate for it, and the enthusiasm soon diminished. Other projects took its place, and by the 1960s the package was rarely mentioned.

Such a fate within the sponsoring organizations was not uncommon. As people left, priorities changed, or the political winds shifted. Projects that had once absorbed time, money, and attention could be abandoned or neglected. In these circumstances, all the work that went into them—the countless meetings and visits, the form-filling, the telephone calls and letters, the politics and administrative bother—could be forgotten, buried under the weight of new priorities, projects, and agendas. The concerns that had prompted the film—about a shortfall of recruits to cancer research—did not disappear overnight, but they diminished somewhat in the 1950s, so that their urgency also diminished. *Challenge* and its package were put on a backburner, and the burner eventually went out.

The gradual disappearance of *Challenge* was caused in part by the budget process. In both organizations, budgets had to be submitted each fiscal year, with some projects carrying over to a new year and others left without a budget line or included among others in a general budget line, such as for the distribution of educational materials. This was the case for *Challenge* and its package. The initial Canadian and American funding for the film meant that it had its own budget lines, but the budget covered only the production and early promotion of the package. After that, both organizations buried *Challenge* and its package in the general budget for the storage, promotion, and distribution of educational materials, one package among many, and an increasingly small part. The budget was enough to ensure that the stock of films and books were stored properly and distributed to those who requested it but provided little beyond that, aside from special monies for the 1955 supplement to Grant's book.

While stocks remained, and demand continued, the film and its package continued to receive support from the general budgets for distribution and storage, including the supply of free loan copies of *Challenge* by the NCI. But it was a tiny sum. There was little for publicity after the rush of 1950/1951, except that parts of the package continued to be listed in the reports and catalogs of the two agencies for several years. The package now had to compete for attention with newer educational materials and newer projects. The records do not make clear when the film and package stopped receiving funding, but it probably began to fade in the 1960s.

The NFB did not experience the sorts of controversies around the film that had at times engulfed the sponsoring agencies. It is true that the filmmakers harbored certain concerns about critics' responses to the film, most notably pessimism from Glover about the how the British would react, but also concerns about reactions to the French versions and general anxieties that the film might be too technical for some audiences. But such qualms were nothing compared to the internal fights in the NCI and NIH, and they were soon swept away in the euphoria over the prizes and nominations for prizes that the films received. These provided a powerful validation of the work of the filmmakers, attracted positive attention from those higher up the NFB hierarchy, and ensured that a warm glow settled over the films in the memories of those involved in them. In later years, Glover, Low, and others would mention *Challenge* as among the best of the NFB films of the period.[3]

For the NFB, *Challenge* also came to be a harbinger of future triumphs. Many of those who made the film went on to important roles in film and the arts. Low was to be a key figure in documentary filmmaking and animation and an important contributor to the development of the IMAX technique of widescreen cinematography. His co-animator Evelyn Lambart became one of McLaren's closest collaborators as well as having a distinguished animation career of her own. The Oscar-winning composer Louis Applebaum was to become one of Canada's leading modernist composers and music educators. He was the first music director of the internationally renowned Stratford Festival, an annual theater event in Stratford, Ontario, and in 1955 he established the Stratford Music Festival as a spin-off of the main festival. Guy Glover, Colin Low, and Morten Parker went on to work on other Oscar-nominated NFB shorts: Glover produced *The Romance of Transportation in Canada* (1952), which Low directed, and *The Stratford Adventure* (1954), which Parker directed, about Applebaum's festival. Even the science adviser to the animators gained later prominence in 1968, albeit in more tragic circumstances. Bazilauskas was the first physician at Central Receiving Hospital in Los Angeles to see Robert F. Kennedy after he was shot. In more ways than one this was a movie that brought the worlds of film and medicine together.

Low himself saw *Challenge* as a beginning of his later involvement with the director Stanley Kubrick's *2001: A Space Odyssey* (1968). He noted that Lambart's use of a curved movement in the cell-as-universe sequences was an early example of the sort of curved movement that he would later use in another NFB Oscar-nominated film and Low's second, *Universe* (1968), which prompted Kubrick to try to recruit Low to work on *2001*. "Plotting curved movement is very hard to do mathematically," he noted,[4] "Sine curves and three-axis movement get very complicated." But there were also other techniques that filtered through to *Universe*. *Universe* created its animation with motorized movement, a further development of McLaren's technique of overlapping zooms, which had employed motorized movement. There may also have been adaptations of Bazilauskas' cinemotif technique, for the film created some of its portrayals of the cosmos by filling tanks of clear paint thinners with suspended inks and oil paints, filmed under bright lights and at a high film rate.[5] Others have suggested that *Universe* anticipated the stargate sequence from *2001*.[6] The stargate-like sequence in *Universe* presents an imaginary journey through a corridor of clouds to the edge of the solar system, an image that could be traced back to similar images in *Challenge* and perhaps to McLaren's *C'est l'aviron*.

As the foregoing suggests, once *Challenge* and its companion films were released, those involved in them at the NFB moved on. The man who had started it all, Ralph Foster, left the NFB in 1949, the crew that Glover and Parker had assembled dispersed to other projects, and some left the NFB. The films remained

in the NFB catalog for many years, and *The Fight* and *Challenge* would occasionally be bought out among the polished silver for special screenings of NFB films.
But after the 1950s, the films were not screened often, and increasingly rarely in
the places where they had been intended to be screened: the classrooms (*Chal-
lenge/Alerte*), film theaters (*The Fight*) or in the film circuits where *the Canada
Carries On* series was shown (*The Outlaw Within* and *Cancer*). The NFB kept
the film stock in its vaults, and in the late twentieth century some versions were
made available for purchase as VHS tapes and later DVDs. Today it is possible to watch copies of some of the films for free on the NFB website (and the
US National Library of Medicine website). But between the 1960s and their
recent video, digital and online presence, the films were largely hidden from
view, kept in some libraries but not widely available. By 1970s the films were
rarely mentioned.[7]

Their brief runs were not atypical of educational movies, which were often
screened only for a short while. Eventually audiences would tire of the films,
newer ones would replace them, and copies of the original films would get damaged with use. Copies that survive in film collections show signs of such damage: the NLM's copy is missing part of its leader, replaced with a piece of film
stock from a US Army training film, and there are broken sprockets, scratches,
and dust. In other libraries, copies were deaccessioned at some point, so that
they were no longer available for screening, their fate unknown. Some may have
ended up in private hands; others will have gone to the dump. Such is the fate of
many educational movies and all the work that went into them.

Recruitment and education

Did *Challenge* achieve its recruitment goals? Concerns about recruitment to
cancer research did diminish after its release, but it is almost impossible to dis-
entangle the effect of the film on this change from that of the package of which
it was a part, the broader recruitment efforts by the sponsoring agencies, the
general shift in school science education toward sustaining the professional science community, or changes in the job market and economy. The film seems to
have been widely used in the 1950s, but one film could not turn things around.
Its sponsors would not have expected it to, and critics implicitly suggested that it
was unlikely to help recruitment. Thus when, as noted in chapter 11, some commentators argued that the film failed to reach its intended audience of school
and college science students, they also—obliquely—suggested that it was unlikely to serve the goal of attracting science students to the field of cancer. How

could it, when it failed even to reach the audience the sponsors hoped it would reach? Even those tasked with ensuring that it was used in the classroom seem to have had their doubts about the value of the film: as mentioned in chapter 12, the teachers who were asked to develop the teaching guide seemed unsure how to make use of the film, except as general inspiration.

The best that can be said is that the film may have contributed to some students becoming aware of cancer research as a career. But even this statement must be treated with caution. Virtually nothing has survived on how the film was used in classrooms (other than screenings in Bethesda–Chevy Chase High School, and Gary, Indiana), there seem to be no scientific memoirs that cite *Challenge* as an inspiration for a turn to cancer research, and it receives no mention in oral histories of scientists who entered cancer research in the 1950s and 1960s.

The film, however, tells us much about how sponsoring organizations perceived and responded to the problem of recruitment. Both sponsoring agencies made efforts to expand research facilities, establish training fellowships, cultivate career structures for cancer researchers, and reform how research grants were administered and how they could be used. The film and its package were only one small part of this broader effort, and a part that capitalized on and promoted the shift in science education toward sustaining professional scientific development. It also represented an accommodation between the Americans and Canadians, given that the latter were fearful that Canadian scientists were being tempted to better paid positions in the United States, which was undermining Canadian cancer research efforts.

The story of the film's sponsorship also tells us something about the changing focus of public education about cancer. Since the early twentieth century, cancer education had sought to bring (adult) patients into programs of early detection and treatment. Beginning in the 1930s, the traditional focus of educational efforts for adults was supplemented with a focus on children, and the traditional stress on patient recruitment was joined with efforts to educate the public (children, students, and adults) about the biology of cancer, to recruit scientists into the field, and to ensure that expectations of cancer research were not unrealistic. To the extent that Canadian public education efforts regarding cancer were dependent on American materials, this shift also had an impact north of the international border. Still, educational efforts in both countries remained overwhelmingly focused on patient recruitment. Early detection and treatment continued to be the heart of cancer education, and adults remained the major audience.

The growing focus on research and on children and students gained additional impetus in the mid-to-late 1940s as planning for a huge increase in cancer research took off. But there was an additional concern that the huge media interest in cancer research might generate unwarranted expectations of research and put pressure on researchers to deliver a cure long before they were ready to do so. Public education efforts were increasingly aimed at countering such expectations. Although research remained subordinate to patient recruitment, it accounted for a growing part of American and Canadian cancer education materials and was increasingly included within materials that were primarily about early detection and treatment. Concerns that a focus on research might undermine efforts to promote early detection and treatment by highlighting the limitations of medical and scientific knowledge began to dissipate.

Challenge and its package were part of this new emphasis in public education on research. For the Canadians, it was also part of an effort to distance public education efforts about cancer from their historical reliance on American educational materials. *Challenge* marked an extraordinary turnaround. For the first time, the Americans were reliant on a Canadian educational effort.

Information offices and officers

Challenge and its package also illuminate the role of a hitherto unacknowledged group in the well-known story of the dramatic expansion of cancer research in the 1940s and 1950s: information or public affairs officers. In the traditional story, the focus of attention has been on the activities of influential individuals such as the philanthropist Mary Lasker, on legislators and policymakers, and on scientists and scientific administrators involved in cancer and biomedicine.[8] But these individuals tended to rely on information officers or public affairs specialists to generate support for the expansion. It is true that some of the effort to expand cancer research was carried out behind closed doors, in conversations between advocates and those with political influence or control of financial purse strings. Advocates of expansion, however, also wanted to generate public support for growing cancer research, to recruit young men and women into the field, and to counter media reports that might diminish faith in research. It was here that the information officers were so important, for it was they who would create the media campaigns to address these goals.

The significance of public affairs specialists to the story of postwar cancer research is highlighted by the organizations for which they worked. In the United

States, both the NCI and the NIH created information offices in the 1940s as part of their efforts to get the message out about the need for more cancer/biomedical researchers, to address the more general problem of managing the growing media interest in cancer and biomedicine, and to fulfill new mandates for public education after the war.[9] The Canadian DNHW did not have to create a new office for this purpose, since its Information Services Division could trace a history back to 1919. But the division was not the organization that it had been at the beginning. It was reorganized after the Second World War to promote the health care reforms of the Mackenzie King (and from 1948 the Louis Stephen St. Laurent) government, and to manage its ever-changing policies on reform, including efforts to promote Canadian cancer services and research. The creation and reorganization of these various offices suggests a growing recognition by the American and Canadian agencies that managing public attitudes toward cancer and cancer research would involve expertise that the scientists, physicians, and administrators who ran these agencies did not have.

All these offices—together with those in campaign organizations such as the American and Canadian cancer societies—were to focus considerable attention on cultivating public support for research in the 1940s and 1950s, and *Challenge* was to be a key part of this story. It is true that the ACS declined the Canadian invitation to support the film, but it seems to have done so because it was already planning its own effort to encourage recruitment through the release of *From One Cell* (1950), together with other educational materials (see chapter 1). Thus, while *Challenge* might have been in competition with *From One Cell* for funding (and probably for school audiences), the two movies together represented an unprecedented use of film both to recruit science students into cancer research and to educate audiences about the biology of the disease. The NIH and the FSA seem to have come late to *Challenge*, and they might have had misgivings about the film and the way that its promotion was handled by Johnson. But they too were keen to recruit young scientists to biomedicine and to educate students about the biology of the cell. Their misgivings about *Challenge* did not distract from these goals.

What sorts of expertise were involved? These offices were populated by (or drew upon the skills of) specialists who are generally not mentioned in histories of cancer. Science writers, book designers, typographers, printers, graphic artists, photographers, and journalists—to say nothing of the filmmakers hired to make *Challenge* and its companion films. Many of these specialists portrayed themselves as the mouthpieces of the agencies that employed them. They brought to these agencies a range of ways of getting their messages out. But they often did much more than echo the concerns of their agencies. These specialists had particular views on how best to communicate the messages of their employing agencies, what to emphasize and what to cut, and some—especially the filmmakers, and perhaps book designers such as Ritchie—were involved only in a specific project and had no interest in their sponsors beyond it. Thus, the messages of these agencies were always shaped by information specialists, who wrote and rewrote them for different publics, chose the graphic and typographic designs, and decided how best to ensure that they got to their intended audience. It follows that the educational efforts of the NCI, the NIH, and the DNHW should never be portrayed as the unadorned messages of the scientists and physicians who staffed them.

The offices might have employed a diverse group of specialists, but they were all led by journalists and former journalists. Dallas Johnson had a background in journalism and consumer activism; Gilchrist was a former journalist, as were Hugh Jackson and Judson Hardy at NIH. The involvement of journalists or former journalists meant that information officers often came to their organizations with contacts in the media that they could exploit to get a story out or to counter ones that they wanted to challenge. And even when they did not have direct contacts themselves, they often knew enough people with enough contacts to make a connection. In addition, their general knowledge of how the press, radio, and television worked could be applied to the problem of marketing. As Johnson's and Gilchrist's efforts to promote *Challenge* indicate, such knowledge allowed them to tailor their promotional efforts to the demands of the different media, at least as they saw them. Finally, it might be noted that their experience in journalism may have given them something in common with staff members at the NFB who were involved in the film and were also journalists by training. They included Ralph Foster and Morten Parker, while others such as Arnold Schieman and Gordon Petty had worked as news/documentary cameramen earlier in their careers.[10]

Scientists and administrators could be suspicious of journalists, fearful that they heightened public anxieties about disease, raised unrealistic hopes, or simply got the science wrong. In their view, the role of information officers was to counter such tendencies in the media; they were to distinguish themselves from their colleagues in the newspapers, radio, or television, and also to compensate for the problems in the media, at least as scientists and administrators saw them. For such reasons, information officers were often keen to dissociate themselves from their journalistic background. Judson Hardy allegedly told his subordinates, "Don't describe yourself as a reporter,"[11] because an irate NIH scientist had let all his colleagues know that he was embarrassingly misquoted in a newspaper article. Information officers thus cultivated images of themselves defined by their relations to the outside media, the public they sought to reach, and colleagues within the organizations that employed them.

Information officers might have been hired to deal with the growing media interest in cancer health and biomedicine after the war. They might also have been an essential part of the efforts by the American and Canadian health authorities to grow cancer research by tempting recruits into the field. Yet they were often in a vulnerable position within their organizations. At the NCI, Johnson's anxieties over *Challenge* were partly a reflection of her concern that her Cancer Reports Section depended for its effectiveness on the approval of scientists and administrators within the NCI that it was struggling to achieve. Her pleading with Foster to pay attention to the scientists was a product in part of her concern that she had been unable to secure a central place for her section within the NCI. She worried that the NFB—which did not rely on such approval—would worsen the situation by ignoring scientific recommendations. Her political missteps over invitations to the premiere added to the problems. By that stage she had left the Cancer Reports Section, so it was her successor who had to deal with the fallout, this time not from scientists but from other information officers at the NIH and FSA who saw it as an opportunity to rein in the NCI office. All these information officers were constantly looking over their shoulders trying not to generate the ire of those upon whom they depended for support.

Less is known about the situation in the DNHW, except that Gilchrist did not always see eye to eye with his minister, Paul Martin. His Information Services Division had a longer history than the equivalents at NIH and NCI and was likely not subject to problems of the sort that faced the start-ups at the American agencies. But even Gilchrist had to step carefully. He could not—and probably did not want to—antagonize either his minister or the scientists in the Canadian Cancer Society or the National Cancer Institute of Canada. The Information Services Division had only recently been reorganized, and it was always possible that with the constant changes in government health policy it would be reorganized again. *Challenge* likely helped Gilchrist in his relations with his minister, given its high visibility and the international nature of the venture, which gave Martin an opportunity to promote his ideas and himself on an international stage. Gilchrist too had constantly to turn to Canadian scientists both to ensure scientific approval and to counter any possibility that the film might elicit a negative reaction from them.

For scientists in the various agencies, these information officers played several roles. They were to cultivate patient confidence in programs of early detection and treatment along the educational lines first established by the ASCC/ACS in the 1910s. They were also to cultivate support for research and to provide basic information on what was known about the biology of cancer and the major areas of research, much like the small group of science writers working in newspapers, radio, and television, which meant that information officers had to take on something of the role of a science writer. They were to inform the public about the latest developments in science, to explain their implications, and plead for patience in waiting for basic research, which promised results only in the long term. However, they were also to advance the agendas of the organizations for which they worked, the NCI, NIH, FSA, or Department of National Health and Welfare. This meant much more than simply informing the public about the latest science and its implications. It also meant protecting those organizations from the misconceptions of the media, much as former journalists such as Edward Bernays had sought to protect and promote business corporations through the then new field of public relations.[12] Their role was to shape public opinion and to manufacture support for their organizations and their missions. The boundary between education and public relations could be thin. *Challenge* and its package served as both an educational and recruitment effort and a public relations effort that aimed to manage public expectations of science and what the sponsoring agencies could achieve.

Why film?

So why did they turn to film to tempt people into the field? It was a risky move given its expense and the long history of doubts about the medium. Surely a campaign using books, pamphlets, inspirational lectures, filmstrips, and a well-thought-out educational program in the schools would do the job, with less expense and less risk. Part of the answer is happenstance. Several elements had to fall into place: the enthusiasm for film as a tool of education among Canadian cancer experts; their desire to reverse years of dependence on American motion pictures; Gilchrist's need to promote his minister; Ralph Foster's hope of using the Canadian commission to rope in the Americans; the decision to show the 1948 Constant script to American cancer agencies; Johnson's struggle to figure out a campaign to recruit scientists, and her desire to establish her Cancer Reports Section at the heart of NCI educational and informational efforts. All these factors fed into the decisions to fund the film, ensured that doubts about its cost and effectiveness could be sidelined, and that other arguments gained ascendency: notably that film had a power to transform beliefs and behaviors that other media did not. Thus the decision to commission *Challenge* was not a simple reflection of the enthusiasm vested in film, but the outcome of a broader struggle between such enthusiasm and concerns about costs and effectiveness that had to be fought out each time a film was commissioned.

Indeed, the story of *Challenge* is also about how such concerns did not disappear once the film was commissioned. Johnson, for example, worried that the film might turn into a liability, especially if the NFB ignored the advice of NCI scientists. We saw that in her letters to Foster outlining her concerns that the filmmakers might alienate scientists, and her efforts to recruit the MFI as a mediator between the filmmakers and the scientists. Gilchrist probably had similar concerns (though they are unrecorded), since the film offered him an opportunity to ensure that Paul Martin was a presence on an international stage, and any disquiet among scientists could have harmed such ambitions. Both Johnson and Gilchrist had to fight constantly against the threat that the film might pose to their ambitions, and against those within their respective agencies who continued to doubt the value of the film.

A further issue was that Johnson, Gilchrist, and other supporters believed that the film would not sell itself. It had to be packaged and promoted in particular ways if it was to do its job, and promotion was a seemingly never-ending task since the initial reactions to the film were not what its promoters wanted. Its eventual characterization as a success was likely because neither the Canadian or American agencies could stomach a flop, the embarrassment that this might cause with their international partners, and the unexpected boost of prizes and the nominations for prizes, including an Oscar. After that, the project could be allowed slowly to die, with a tiny part of the budget set aside for the storage and distribution of educational materials, until demand for it disappeared.

Filmmakers

For their part, the filmmakers do not seem to have had the sorts of anxieties that their sponsors had. Where the latter constantly worried about their dependence on filmmakers, the filmmakers expressed less concern about their dependence on the outside sponsors. Part of the reason was that the sponsorship of Canadian and American health agencies gave the NFB enormous resources, promised to open the door to future coproduction deals, and allowed the NFB to produce a film of a quality that would have been difficult with their own funding. In addition, the filmmakers found that the NCI and the DNHW generally had a hands-off approach to sponsorship. Having set the goals for the film, they generally left it up to the filmmakers to get on with turning it into a workable movie.

Foster's enthusiasm for coproduction approaches to filmmaking provides a clue to the relaxed attitude of the NFB. Such deals were seen as a solution to the political and funding problems facing the NFB after the war, and Foster accepted that coproduction meant that there was an expectation that films would have to bend to their sponsors' desires. Indeed, for Foster, commissioning a script became a way of bringing in sponsors, and of addressing their concerns and agendas before filming began. In the case of *Challenge*, as we saw in chapters 3 and 4, Foster had used the DNHW commission to develop a script which he then hawked to the Americans. Then when the NCI came on board, Foster had the script rewritten in part to reflect the new international nature of the sponsorship. It is likely that this rewrite was carried out after detailed discussions with the sponsors, but once the script was ready, and reviewed by the sponsors, the filmmakers found themselves relatively free in how they turned it into a film.

Foster might have had political and financial reasons for his flexibility, but the producer and director—Guy Glover and Morten Parker, respectively—seem to have been equally relaxed about the sponsors. Both men had been involved in the rewrites after the Americans came on board, and any concerns they might have had about interference from the sponsors soon were put to rest. Once the script was complete, they found themselves more or less free to interpret it as they liked. It is true that Dallas Johnson constantly sought to ensure that the film had NCI scientists' approval, and that Gilchrist probably did the same for NCIC scientists, and they—Glover and Parker—worried about reactions to the film from the sponsors at the screening of the rough cut. But Glover and Parker were also aware that a mechanism was in place to keep the scientists at bay; the involvement of the Medical Film Institute, which was to act as a mediator between the filmmakers and the scientists. Parker latter recalled with approval the hands-off approach of the MFI, and its involvement in the appointment of Bazilauskas as a scientific consultant reaffirmed this positive view. "Baz" not only provided scientific input into the animation sequences but also contributed his own cinemotif technique to the production.

But there were limitations to the filmmakers' willingness to have the sponsors and scientists involved. As deadlines loomed, and pressure mounted to finish production, the filmmakers were increasingly worried about such involvement. They constantly struggled with the exigencies of filmmaking—the variable skills of the actors, the dull visual palette of the laboratory, the choice of locations, the problems of recording ambient sound, the juggling of the various representations of the scientist, the patient, the cell, the work of science, and much more —and their judgments had generally found approval from the scientists in the sponsoring agencies, even if they did not always follow their advice (such as the factory metaphor to describe biochemical processes within the cell). But at some point the advice had to stop, and the fear was that it would not, even at the last minute: recall how Constant, Parker, and Dryer pleaded against scientists' demands for strict accuracy as they rushed to compete the commentary.

Works in progress

It should be clear from the above that the film—in each of its five versions—was a product of three projects—sponsoring, film production, and packaging—each a work in progress that involved a variety of groups and individuals, with different interests, skills, and agendas, distributed across a variety of organizations. The meaning of the film differed for each group and individual, and it also changed for each over time. Part of the work involved in each project was an attempt to address these differences, and this often meant that that the projects were not self-contained but overlapped, each with the others, and across the many organizations involved with the film.

Thus the work of sponsorship did not stop once the filming began. Sponsors continued to have a say in how the film was made, almost up to the time of release, sometimes to the consternation of the filmmakers who had to figure out when to follow the demands of the sponsors and when to resist, and how to address the different goals of the two main sponsors. It was also the case that the work of sponsorship involved more than the activities of the NCI and the DNHW. The NFB—and Ralph Foster in particular—actively cultivated sponsorship and saw the film as a malleable entity that could be molded to meet the concerns and agendas of the two sponsors as well those of the NFB itself at a time when it was struggling politically and financially in the early Cold War. Finally, sponsorship also overlapped with packaging, in that neither of the two main sponsors felt that the film could stand alone. In their view, it had to be packaged and promoted. They sought to attract the attention of the media (so briefly changing *Challenge* from a recruitment to a public education film), and to ensure that teachers were aware of the film and that they were given guidance on how to use it in the classroom. All this meant developing a media campaign, ensuring that other films were developed for public education purposes, and creating a teacher's guide and a book about cancer to be made available with the film.

The work of making the movie also overlapped with the other projects. Not only did the filmmakers cultivate sponsors and expect the film to change to meet their requirements; not only did sponsors constantly proffer advice and criticism to the filmmakers on how the film might be made; but production and packaging overlapped considerably. Soon after filming began the sponsors began trying to harmonize promotional efforts with production. Thus, sponsors sought to ensure that the media had access to the filmmakers. We might recall the general excitement surrounding the prospect of a *Life* magazine spread and how the magazine was provided with the storyboards and offered the opportunity to document the making of the film. To sponsors, the film was never to be separated from its package, and Johnson and Gilchrist both sought to ensure that the filmmakers coordinated with Lester Grant's book and the teaching guide. They also sought to accommodate the fact that the audiences for the different versions of the film were quite distinct (even if the marketing of *Challenge* meant that at times—notably around the time of the premieres—it trespassed on audiences more properly the target of *The Fight*). At times the boundary between production and promotion was quite blurred.

The end of the universe

All this jostling came to an end sometime after 1951 as the last of films were completed and the promotional efforts began to dissipate, leaving finally only small publicity efforts and modest funding put toward storage and distribution. "This film tells the story of a great adventure—science's effort to conquer a universe so small that it cannot be seen with the naked eye, so huge that it contains the entire mechanism of life,"[13] noted a 1951 advertisement in *Popular Photography*, just as the cinematic adventure was beginning to wind down. It would be all but forgotten in a decade or so, as would its striking vision of a microscopic universe encompassing the wonders of life.

This imagined universe was shaped, as this book has shown, by much more than science. To be sure, with Bazilauskas' help, the film made ample references to the world of the cell as documented in school science textbooks. But mixed in with the biology were other visual and aural references: the Apollo Belevedere, the paintings of Pavel Tchelitchew and Salvador Dalí, tone paintings of cell division, and musical references to the otherworldly, among other fantastical elements. If the foregoing narrative has done anything, it should show how representations of the body and cell—and the character of the scientist and the patient—were actively constructed during filmmaking, and how their meanings and uses within the film changed over time. Some representations were visual, others were metaphors invoked during the narration, still others were tone paintings or musical gestures toward themes such as the uncanny in science fiction movies. Sometimes these images worked together, at other times they drifted in parallel, and at others they may have clashed. Thus while the filmmakers sought to marshal all these references and images into an argument—for making the body and cancer objects of science and of enrolling would-be scientists and the public to this project—the film was such a complex of layers of imagery that its meaning was rarely stable, and the sponsors, makers, and viewers of the film could come to very different views as to its value.

Central to the creation of these representations was the Griersonian approach to filmmaking, which—alongside the animation and live-action film techniques—was a key to the transformation of the sponsors' ideas into something that the filmmakers thought would work on screen. Grierson's belief in subordinating naturalism to symbolic expression allowed the filmmakers to create the bigger themes of the film about the wonder of the body and cell, the work of science, the character of the scientist, and the humanitarian needs of the patient. Symbols such as the patient and scientist, or the darkness of outer space and the inner world of the cell and body, were refined during the revisions of the script, and continued to be refined as filming got underway, and in the editing, music composition/performance, and narration. But such symbols also blurred the boundary between fact and fantasy for some viewers. In the animation sections especially, symbolic expression opened the possibility of readings other than the factual, even as it allowed the filmmakers to rise above the mess of details on the screen and produce a visually interesting and coherent movie. While tensions within these representations were never entirely resolved, they provided the key symbols that sought to meet the sponsors' hopes of recruiting more students into cancer research.

Such dynamic complexities were not confined to this film but were common features of representations and arguments in educational films. For the historian of medicine, such complexities should act as a caution against ascribing to medical and health education films a simple meaning or argument, as if these meanings remained stable over the years and across the many groups that sponsored, produced, and viewed a film. Arguments could be fleeting (think of the argument in Constant's script about the need to keep Canadian scientists from moving abroad, or the long sequence on the fables and phantasms of the past in the same script), and the meanings of arguments that survived though the various scripts, the shooting schedule, and the edits could change dramatically over time and from one stakeholder to the next. In addition, it should be clear that health education films were rarely just about health or illness. As my discussion of *Challenge* has shown, they could draw on a considerable range of visual and aural references. Thus the image of the scientist as "ordinary man" drew on postwar discourses that Shapin suggests sought to humanize scientists, and filmmakers turned it to the particular concerns of the sponsors of this film. The image of the scientist as "hero" drew on a long tradition of media portrayals of scientific heroes that Bert Hansen traces back to media representations of Pasteur, which he suggests helped to cultivate public interest and support for medical science. The difference here is that *Challenge* sought to cultivate such interest and support by melding the biologist or medical hero with the postwar enthusiasm for space exploration. The theme of space travel also appeared in the cell-as-universe sequences (as the filmmakers sought a visual portrayal of the huge scale of the problem of understanding the cell), while the image of cell-as-factory (a fleeting image absent from the final version of *Challenge*, but which returned in Lester Grant's book) drew on postwar concerns about inefficient business management. Films such as *Challenge* are thus cultural objects that illuminate how filmmakers, sponsors, and viewers sought to mobilize representations to their own (sometimes conflicting) ends. Yet, as this book has suggested, the mix of images sometimes worked in harmony and sometimes in tension (such as between the scientist as ordinary man and someone exceptional, a hero, much as ordinary men had been portrayed as heroes during the war). *Challenge* had a bigger budget than many educational films of this period, and its filmmakers had more resources to figure out the problems with a film. Nevertheless, making an argument that the body and cancer should be objects of science was a complex task that could come together, fall apart, or wander off in other directions at any time during the creation and release of this film. So could the associated argument for encouraging would-be scientists and the public to support this project.

In the case of *Challenge*, it is clear that sponsors, makers, and viewers of the film sometimes came to very different interpretations of its meaning. For sponsors, for example, the film might have been about making the body and cancer objects of science, but for the NFB it was also about making the body and cancer filmic objects, and especially objects—creations—of the NFB, keen to rope in American sponsorship, develop cosponsorship schemes, and to make more health and science-based films. Here was an advertisement for the filmmakers and for the NFB, its animators and composer, and a means by which the NFB sought to counter its political and financial problems of the 1940s and 1950s.

Thus arguments for science and film merged. Information specialists had still other interpretations. For Johnson, and to a lesser extent Gilchrist, filmic arguments were also about securing the place of information specialists within their agencies; and, for Johnson especially, these arguments were helpful in showing the scientists and physicians who ran the NCI that her newly created Cancer Reports Section had value in recruiting scientists into the field. Arguments for science and film were thus also arguments for the emergent role of information specialist; hence the concern of the NCI Special Reports Section when colleagues questioned the value of the film. Such questions threated their claims to expertise. Recall also the delicate calculations that NIH critics of the film had to make. They were not willing to completely undermine it, for while failure might have allowed them to seize back control of public educational efforts about cancer at the NCI, failure would also have been an embarrassment to their agencies participating in a high-profile international collaboration.

A more general point arising from this book is the malleability of film as a tool of health education. A close look at the making of *Challenge* demonstrates how sponsors with overlapping agendas and conflicting goals sought to shape a film in ways that fitted their interests. We have seen how the film changed during the rewrites, the filming and editing, the composition of the narration, the performance of the musical score, and the consultations with sponsors. Also evident is how malleable a film remains long after its final production and release. Consider further the role of the public relations campaigns, what Dallas Johnson called the "press handling," and the classroom educational materials developed to accompany the film, all of which were intended to shape audience responses and prepare the ground for the arguments projected on the screen. In addition, the release of other versions of the film for other audiences shows how the sequences used in one film might be repurposed in another, as when sequences in *Challenge* intended to recruit young students into cancer research were reused in *The Fight* for a theatrical audience. Films are intrinsically malleable, with sequences that can be cut out, reordered, transposed, and adapted from one film to another. And this book has indicated how the key representations deployed in a film—here, the scientist, the patient, the work of science, the cell, and the body—were also malleable. The filmmakers struggled to control this malleability so that the imagery made the arguments they wanted. However, the aural and visual imagery could distract some viewers, and the arguments themselves had multiple meanings and uses for different stakeholders—the sponsors, professional groups such as information specialists, the filmmakers, and viewers.

And finally, there is the ephemeral nature of these films. The administrative struggles, the filmmaking, the propaganda campaigns, and other activities mainly happened in the three to four years from 1948 to 1951. Over time, sponsors, producers, exhibitors, and viewers moved on. *Challenge* and its package came to be used less and less, and the imaginary universe that the film had conjured disappeared. The dust settled within the American and Canadian sponsoring agencies within a couple of years, and they moved on to other projects, as did the NFB, leaving the welcome glow of the film's successes and prizes. In the classroom, teachers eventually abandoned *Challenge/Alerte*, and theatrical screenings of *The Fight, The Outlaw Within,* and *Cancer* also eventually ended, as did the few television screenings. Each time the projectors rolled, the arguments in these films burst into life once again, a universe brought into being briefly, only to dim again when the lights came on. The messages and images lingered on for the few viewers who heeded the film's call: the teacher who wanted to inspire a young scientist, or the anticancer advocate looking to make a statement. But as the 1950s and 1960s wore on, the projectors rolled less and less often. Increasingly the reels remained confined to their canisters, filed away, the frames sometimes scratched, the leaders torn, and sprockets broken. The arguments of *Challenge* were splashed across the screen less often; students, teachers, and other viewers engaged with them less and less, and then not at all. The classrooms emptied. The theaters went dark. And the film faded from memory.

Introduction

1. Breslow, Wilner, Agran et al., *A History of Cancer Control*, vol. 3, book 2, 556–57. Breslow erroneously claims this was a joint American Cancer Society/NCI project. Graham, *Canadian Film Technology*, 116; Barnouw, *Mass Communication*, 140; Spottiswoode, *Film and Its Techniques*, 383.

2. There is a huge literature on the NFB. See, for example, James, *Film as National Art*; Evans, *In the National Interest*; Jones, *Movies and Memoranda*; Jones, *The Best Butler in the Business*; and Druick, *Projecting Canada*. More generally on Canadian ephemeral films, see Druick and Cammaer, *Cinephemera*. Other references can be found in the chapters on the NFB's involvement in *Challenge*.

3. LoBrutto, *Stanley Kubrick*, 273; Glassman and Wise, "Filmmaker of Vision Pt.1," 24, 29–30.

4. Rettig, *Cancer Crusade*; Strickland, *Politics, Science, and Dread Disease*; Patterson, *The Dread Disease;* Rushefsky, *Making Cancer Policy*; Scheffler, *A Contagious Cause*; Hayter, *An Element of Hope*; Clow, *Negotiating Disease.*

5. Patterson, *The Dread Disease*, chap 7; Robinson, *Noble Conspirator*; Mary Lasker Papers, National Library of Medicine.

6. On postwar films see Cantor, "Uncertain Enthusiasm"; Cantor, "Choosing to Live"; Cantor, *Man Alive! (1952)*; Cantor, "*Inside Magoo* (1960)"; Reagan, "Projecting Breast Cancer"; Reagan, "Engendering the Dread Disease."

7. Harrison, "In the Picture of Health."

8. Beaulieu, "L'incursion de l'ONF dans la thérapie psychiatrique." More generally see Low, *NFB Kids;* Brian, "'The New Generation.'" The Mental Mechanisms series included *The Feeling of Rejection* (1947), *The Feeling of Hostility* (1948), and *Feelings of Depression* (1950).

9. Bonah, Cantor, and Laukötter, "Introduction." On early-twentieth-century cancer education campaigns see Cantor, "Cancer Control and Prevention in the Twentieth Century"; Aronowitz, *Unnatural History*; Wailoo, *How Cancer Crossed the Color Line*; Gardner, *Early Detection*; Lerner, *The Breast Cancer Wars*; Hayter, *An Element of Hope*; Clow, *Negotiating Disease.* On other health education films in the context of health campaigns see, for example: "Thomas Edison's Tuberculosis Films"; Pernick, "More than

Illustrations"; Posner, "Communicating Disease"; Posner, "Prostitutes, Charity Girls, and *The End of the Road*"; Colwell, *"The End of the Road"*; Kuhn, *Cinema, Censorship, and Sexuality*, 49–74; Schaefer, *Bold! Daring!* 17–41; Marsh, "Visual Education in the United States"; Ostherr, "Cinema as Universal Language"; Ostherr, *Medical Visions*. 28–47; Cantor, *The Reward of Courage (1921)*; Cantor, "Uncertain Enthusiasm"; Cantor "Choosing to Live"; Cantor, *"Inside Magoo* (1960)"; Cantor, *Man Alive! (1952)*; Pernick, *The Black Stork*; Parry, *Broadcasting Birth Control*, 12–44; Parry, "'Pictures with a Purpose'"; Sumpf, "Film and Anti-alcohol Campaigns"; Lebas, *"'Where There's Life, There's Soap.'"*

10. *Challenge* (1950); *The Fight* (1951); *The Outlaw Within* (1951); *Cancer* (1951); Grant, *The Challenge of Cancer*; National Cancer Institute, *A Teaching Guide: What We Know About Cancer* (1950); *Ce Que Nous Savons du Cancer* (1950).

11. Hediger and Vondrau, "Introduction," esp. p.10. For other histories of educational and training film see Acland and Wasson, *Useful Cinema*; Orgeron, Orgeron, and Streible, *Learning with the Lights Off*; Boon, *Films of Fact*. For an application of the idea of the utility film to health educational films see Bonah, Cantor, and Laukötter, *Health Education Films*.

12. Aitken, *Film and Reform*. More generally on Grierson, his approach, and influence see Evans, *John Grierson and the National Film Board*; Williams and Druick, *The Grierson Effect*; Winston, *Claiming the Real*; Winston, *Claiming the Real II*; Ellis, *John Grierson*.

13. Bonah, Cantor, and Laukötter, "Introduction."

14. Hansen, *Picturing Medical Progress*.

15. On scientists as advisers in Hollywood films see Kirby, "Scientists on the Set"; Kirby, *Lab Coats in Hollywood*.

Chapter 1

1. Patterson, *The Dread Disease*, chap 7; Robinson, *Noble Conspirator*, 2001; Mary Lasker Papers, National Library of Medicine.

2. Scheele, "The Cancer Problem of the United States Health Service," 241.

3. Scheele, "The Cancer Problem of the United States Health Service," 241.

4. Bernays, *Biography of an Idea*; Tye, *The Father of Spin*. More generally on the history of public relations see Tedlow, *Keeping the Corporate Image*, 27–51; Tedlow, *New and Improved*; Ewen, *P.R!*

5. Ora Marshino, "A Short History of the National Cancer Institute: July 1, 1946–June 30, 1947," NCI archives, AR005179, 38.

6. *Annual Report, National Cancer Institute, Fiscal Year 1949 (July 1, 1948–June 30, 1949)*, NCI archives, AR-4900-010824, "Technical Services," section 4. *Annual Report, National Cancer Institute, Fiscal Year 1950 (July 1, 1949–June 30, 1950)* NCI archives, AR-5000-005987, 3–9.

7. National Cancer Institute, "National Cancer Act of 1937."

8. Ora Marshino, "Early Relations Between NCI and the American Cancer Society," NCI archives, AR010104, March 11, 1949.

9. Cantor, "Uncertain Enthusiasm"; Cantor, "Choosing to Live."

10. Reagan, "Engendering the Dread Disease"; Reagan, "Projecting Breast Cancer."

11. On the ACS film unit see "Adelaide Brewster is Cancer Victim." On UPA and cancer see Cantor, *Man Alive! (1952)*; Cantor, "*Inside Magoo* (1960)"; Cantor, "Uncertain Enthusiasm"; Cantor, "Choosing to Live."

12. American Society for the Control of Cancer, *Catalog of Educational Material*.

13. For example, see Johnson and Little, *Facing the Facts about Cancer*, 1947. This was a revised version of an ACS educational leaflet, Little, *The Fight on Cancer*.

14. Johnson and Golding, *Don't Underestimate Woman Power*.

15. See, for example, Dallas, *The Consumer and the Anti-Chain Taxes*.

16. Meader, Ray, and Chalkley, "The Research Grants Branch"; Mider, "Research at the National Cancer Institute."

17. "Cancer: The Great Darkness," *Fortune*, 114.

18. Transcripts of the first meeting of the National Advisory Cancer Council, November 9, 1937, National Archives Record Group 443, box 6, p.48.

19. "Cancer: The Great Darkness," 114.

20. Scheele, "The Cancer Problem of the United States Health Service," 241. On the shortage more generally see Steelman, *Science and Public Policy*.

21. Shapin, "Who is the Industrial Scientist?" 339–40.

22. Louis H Seagrove, testimony, US Congress, Senate Committee on Foreign Relations, *Cancer Research*, 179.

23. US Congress, Senate Committee on Foreign Relations, *Cancer Research*, 180. For an article comparing industrial and cancer research and urging industrialists to become interested in the subject to increase life expectancy and so to "prolong man's **purchasing power**," see Brinkley, "Industrial Research vs. Cancer Research," 2, emphasis in original.

24. Johnson and Little, *Facing the Facts about Cancer*, 1947, 27; Johnson, *Facing the Facts about Cancer*, 1951, 28.

25. Kaiser, "Cold War Requisitions"; Kaiser, "The Postwar Suburbanization of American Physics"; Kevles, *The Physicists*.

26. Failla testimony in US Congress, Senate, Joint Hearings, *Cancer Research*, 114.

27. Failla testimony in US Congress, Senate, Joint Hearings, *Cancer Research*, 114.

28. Dallas Johnson, Undated and unattributed MSS, 1950[?], 1. [Listed as "Cancer Research Educational Program/Challenge: Science Against Cancer Documentary Film/Challenge of Cancer Book" in the finding aid], NCI archives, AR-5000–010683.

29. Scheele, "The Cancer Problem of the United States Health Service," 242.

30. Scheele, "The Cancer Problem of the United States Health Service," 242.

31. Bayard H. Morrison, "NCI History," typescript, n.d., NCI archives, AR-0000-010718, 43. See also "Dr. Leonard A. Scheele," typescript, April 1, 1948, NCI archives, AR-4804–004584.

32. National Institute of Health. *The U.S. Fights Cancer*; Meader and Payne, "Cancer Research Facilities Construction Grants"; "The Program of the National Cancer Institute."

33. *Cancer Control Letter* 19 (July 1, 1949): 2.

34. Marshino, "The Expanded Federal Cancer Program."

35. National Institute of Health. *The U.S. Fights Cancer*; "The Program of the National Cancer Institute."

36. On the ASCC/ACS school campaign see [Little], "Schools and Cancer Education"; Charlton, "Taking Cancer to School"; Fish, "The Situation Confronting"; [Little], "Development of the Society's Secondary School Educational Program"; "Secondary Schools." See also Stewart, "A Psychological Approach," esp. 9–10.

37. Gerster and Wood, "Cancer Education in New York City"; "A Project in Cancer Education"; Westchester Cancer Committee, *Youth Looks at Cancer*.

38. Westchester Cancer Committee, *Detectives Wanted!* [2].

39. Westchester Cancer Committee, *Detectives Wanted!* [2]

40. Westchester Cancer Committee, *Detectives Wanted!* [2]

41. Westchester Cancer Committee, *Detectives Wanted!* [5]

42. Westchester Cancer Committee, *Detectives Wanted!* [6]

43. Westchester Cancer Committee, *Detectives Wanted!* [6]

44. "Cancer Committee Opens Drive to Raise $40,000."

45. "90,000 Letters Carry Appeal of County Cancer Committee."

46. "Face the Facts about Cancer."

47. See, for example, these pamphlets: American Cancer Society, *Suggestions on What to Teach About Cancer*; American Cancer Society, *Why Learn About Cancer*; American Cancer Society, *A Statement of Principles as a Guide to Cancer Education in the Schools*: Early editions of some of these are listed in the article "You Can Teach about Cancer." See also Wells, "Science Teachers Join the Fight Against Cancer," 145.

48. American Cancer Society et al., *Teaching about Cancer: Thoughts for School Administrators*.

49. American Cancer Society, *1952 Annual Report*, 25.

50. On *From One Cell*, see also "Learning to Live" and "Next Step—Teacher Training." A Spanish-language version was also released; see "Spanish-speaking Vets See ACS Films."

51. See, for example, Moon, Mann, and Otto, *Modern Biology*, 571–72.

52. Rudolph, *Scientists in the Classroom*.

53. Dallas Johnson to Ralph Foster, July 23, 1948, *Challenge: Science Against Cancer*, production file 02-130, vol. 1, NFB archives.

54. Gittings, *Canadian National Cinema*; Evans, *In the National Interest*; Evans. *John Grierson and the National Film Board*; Jones, *Movies and Memoranda*; James, *Film as a National Art*; Morris, "After Grierson"; Acland, "National Dreams, International Encounters." A clue to NCI reading on the National Film Board comes from an article stuffed into a project report on the movie, Hill, "The Canadian Way of Life," 26. The project report is in NCI archives, AR-4900–010785.

55. *"Challenge: Science Against Cancer,* Elgin Theatre, Ottawa 3.00 p.m., Sunday 19th March. Under the distinguished Patronage of His Excellency the Governor-General," produced by Information Services Division, Department of National Health and Welfare, c.1950, NCI archives, AR-4900-010785, 4. On the Mental Mechanisms series see Brian, "'The New Generation.'" On the NFB films in the context of Canadian health education see Harrison, "In the Picture of Health"; one of the versions of *Challenge* is discussed on pp.151, 161. Beaulieu, "L'incursion de l'ONF dans la thérapie psychiatrique." More generally, see Low, *NFB Kids;* Brian, "'The New Generation.'" For other Canadian published reports on the origins of this program see "New Educational Film"; Maurice, "Cancer Research in Pictures"; Lawrence, "Challenge: Science Against Cancer"; "Challenge! Science Against Cancer"; Ellsey, "What Science is Doing to Combat Cancer"; "Cancer: Health Education Film Shows Battle Being Waged." Gilmour, "Cancer Battle Film Draws Top Praise"; "Unusual Film is Screened in Ottawa" *(Evening Citizen);* "Cancer Research Film is Studied"; "Unusual Film is Screened in Ottawa" *(Ottawa Citizen);* McLaughlin, "Films Reveal How Science Winning Fight Against Disease."

56. Dallas Johnson, Undated and unattributed MSS, 1950[?] [Listed as "Cancer Research Educational Program/Challenge: Science Against Cancer Documentary Film/ Challenge of Cancer Book" in the finding aid] NCI archives, AR-5000-010683, 1.

57. Johnson interview, March 23, 2005.

58. Dallas Johnson to Ralph Foster, November 28, 1948, and December 27, 1948, NFB archives, *Challenge Science Against Cancer,* production file 02-130, vol. 1, The drafts and final application are in Ross McLean, Canadian Government Film Commissioner, "Proposal for a Joint project to Combine Facilities and the funds of the Responsible authorities in the United States and Canada in the production of an educational film to dramatize the story of cancer research in order to attract scientific students to the field," c. December 1948, *NFB archives, Challenge: Science Against Cancer,* production file 02-130, vol. 1.

59. More generally on such concerns about a tension between control and research see David Cantor, "Uncertain Enthusiasm".

60. MFI, AAMC "Application for Grant to Cancer Control Project," received February 28, 1949, NCI archives, AR-4900–010785.

61. Ruhe and Stubbs, "A Method for the Curriculum Integration."

62. Bloedorn, Markee, and Walton, "Report of the Committee on Audiovisual Aids"; Elias, "Principles of Scientific Teaching Film Production."

63. Bahaikipedia, "David Ruhe"; "David S. Ruhe, 1914–2005"; "Dr. David S. Ruhe." Note the discrepancy in his birthdate, sometimes given as 1913 and sometimes 1914.

64. "Association of American Medical Colleges Opens Its Medical Film Unit."

65. Morten Parker interview, March 26, 2008.

66. Morten Parker interview, March 26, 2008. Johnson interview, March 23, 2005.

67. "Memorandum of Agreement," c. February/March 1949, NCI archives, AR-4900–010785.

Chapter 2

1. Macbeth, "The Origin of the Canadian Cancer Society."

2. For accounts of Canadian/American relations see Stuart, *Dispersed Relations*; Thompson and Randall, *Canada and the United States*; Von Heyking, "Talking About Americans." On the NFB and Canadian identity see Druick, *Projecting Canada*; Payne, *The Official Picture*. More generally on Canadian films and national identify see Edwardson, *Canadian Content*.

3. "Report on Films Available in Canada," attached to Jean E. Pierce (secretary, Canadian Society for the Control of Cancer) to Maj. Gen. G. B. Chisholm (Deputy Minister of National Health), Library and Archives Canada, National Health and Welfare, RG 29, volume 189, file 311-C1-29, July 20, 1945.

4. "Cancer Conference: Proceedings of Proceedings of Committee A," Monday, January 27, 1947, Library and Archives Canada, National Health and Welfare, RG 29, volume 191, file 311-C1-37, part 2.

5. For a showing in Canada of *The Reward of Courage*, the first cancer education movie produced by the ASCC, see Macdonald, "The History of Cancer Treatment in Nova Scotia." On this film see Cantor, *Reward of Courage*.

6. Hayter, *An Element of Hope*, 105. A few trailers may also have been produced in Canada; see "Public Health Speech Delivered by the Honorable J. J. Uhrich, Minister of Public Health and Provincial Secretary in Saskatchewan." Legislative Assembly, *Journals and Speeches*. In general on Saskatchewan cancer campaigns, see Shephard, "First in Fear and Dread." A one-minute trailer produced by the CCS in April 1946 is mentioned in Jean Pierce to General Brock Chisholm, telegraph, March 6, 1946, Library and Archives Canada, National Health and Welfare, RG 29, volume 189, file 311-C1-29.

7. The existence of technical and semi-technical movies is mentioned in "Report of the British Columbia Branch Canadian Cancer Society to Grand Council, Winnipeg 21st, 22nd & 23rd June, 1947," Library and Archives Canada, National Health and Welfare, RG 29, volume 1180, file 311-C1-29, part 1.

8. Cantor, "Uncertain Enthusiasm."

9. Hayter, *An Element of Hope*, 105.

10. "Report on Films Available in Canada," attached to Jean E. Pierce to Maj. Gen. G. B. Chisholm, July 20, 1945, and Isabel Oliver (Secretary, Ontario branch CSCC) to Jean E. Pierce, July 18, 1945, Library and Archives Canada, National Health and Welfare, RG 29, vol. 189, file 311-C1-29; "Ontario," 322; McCorquodale, "A Nurse Looks at Radiology"; McCorquodale, "The Patient and Radiotherapy."

11. "Report on Films Available in Canada."

12. Alice K. Smith to Jean E. Pierce, March 7, 1945, Library and Archives Canada, National Health and Welfare, RG 29, vol. 189, file 311-C1-29.

13. Jean [E.] Pierce to Gen. Brock Chisholm, telegraph, March 6, 1946, Library and Archives Canada. National Health and Welfare, RG 29, vol. 189, file 311-C1-29.

14. Canadian Cancer Society, *Newsletter*, no 8 (February 10, 1947): 2–3, Library and Archives Canada, National Health and Welfare, RG 29, vol. 189, file 311-C1-29.

15. Canadian Cancer Society, *Newsletter* (February 10, 1947).

16. "Report of the British Columbia Branch Canadian Cancer Society to Grand Council, Winnipeg 21st, 22nd & 23rd June, 1947," Library and Archives Canada, National Health and Welfare, RG 29, vol. 1180, file 311-C1-29, part 1.

17. Hayter, *An Element of Hope*.

18. "Report on Films Available in Canada," attached to Jean E. Pierce to Maj. Gen. G.B. Chisholm, July 20, 1945, Library and Archives Canada, National Health and Welfare, RG 29, volume 189, file 311-C1-29.

19. "Proposed Educational Campaign for Canadian Cancer Society; Films, Film Strips & Stills," January 17, 1947, Library and Archives Canada, National Health and Welfare, RG 29, volume 1180, file 311-C1-29 part 1, p.4. More generally on Canadianization and national identify see Edwardson, *Canadian Content*. On Canadianization in film and academia, see respectively Dorland, *So Close to the State/s*; Cromier, *The Canadianization Movement*.

20. Comments of Dr. MacDonald in "Cancer Conference: Proceedings of Committee A. Monday, January 27, 1947," Library and Archives Canada, RG 29, National Health and Welfare, volume 191, file 311-C1-37, part 3, p. 5.

21. Isabel Oliver to Jean E. Pierce, July 18, 1945, Library and Archives Canada, National Health and Welfare, RG 29, volume 189, file 311-C1-29.

22. Isabel Oliver to Jean E. Pierce, July 18, 1945, Library and Archives Canada, National Health and Welfare, RG 29, volume 189, file 311-C1-29.

23. Alice K. Smith (public health nurse, Division of Rural Education) to Jean [E.] Pierce, March 7, 1945, Library and Archives Canada, National Health and Welfare, RG 29, volume 189, file 311-C1-29.

24. Hayter, *An Element of Hope*, especially chap. 9.

25. On Canadian interest in health films see Harrison, "In the Picture of Health," 100–120.

26. Jean E. Pierce to Maj. Gen. G. B. Chisholm, July 20, 1945, Library and Archives Canada, National Health and Welfare, RG 29, volume 189, file 311-C1-29. See also minutes of meeting of the board of directors of CSCC, June 29, 1945, Library and Archives Canada, National Health and Welfare, RG 29, volume 189, file 311-C1-29.

27. Evans, *In the National Interest*.

28. Harrison, "In the Picture of Health," 66–72.

29. Finkel, *Social Policy and Practice in Canada*, chap. 6. On the 1945 proposals see p.135.

30. Harrison, "In the Picture of Health," 66–72.

31. Quoted in Harrison, "In the Picture of Health," 112.

32. Quoted in Harrison, "In the Picture of Health," 112.

33. Macbeth, "The Origin of the Canadian Cancer Society"; "The King George the Fifth Silver Jubilee Cancer Fund."

34. Jeff Hurley (director, Division of Information Services, DNHW) to Jean [E.] Pierce, July 25, 1945, Library and Archives Canada, National Health and Welfare, RG 29, volume 189, file 311-C1-29.

35. On the complex relationship between Canada and the British Empire see, for example, Buckner, *Canada and the British Empire.*

36. Macbeth, "The Origin of the Canadian Cancer Society"; "The King George the Fifth Silver Jubilee Cancer Fund."

37. Comments of Jean [E.] Pierce, in "Cancer Conference: Proceedings of Committee A, Monday, January 27, 1947," Library and Archives Canada, National Health and Welfare, RG 29, volume 191, file 311-C1-37, part 3, p.61.

38. "Report of the British Columbia Branch Canadian Cancer Society to Grand Council, Winnipeg 21st, 22nd & 23rd June, 1947," Library and Archives Canada, National Health and Welfare, RG 29, volume 1180, file 311-C1-29, part 1. The BC branch, however, noted that other provinces had produced technical or semi-technical movies before this.

39. For minutes and other documentation of the conference see Library and Archives Canada, National Health and Welfare, RG 29, volume 191, file 311-C1-37 parts 1-4, and National Health and Welfare, RG 29, volume 1183, file 311-C1-37 parts1-2.

40. From 1939–1945, close to 80,000 men and women had died of cancer, compared to 38,834 killed or missing during the war. "National Cancer Institute of Canada."

41. "National Cancer Institute of Canada," 325.

42. "National Cancer Institute of Canada," 325.

43. "Proposed Educational Campaign for Canadian Cancer Society; Films, Film Strips & Stills," January 17, 1947, Library and Archives Canada, National Health and Welfare, RG 29, volume 1180, file 311-C1-29, part 1.

44. "Proposed Educational Campaign for Canadian Cancer Society; Films, Film Strips & Stills," January 17, 1947, Library and Archives Canada, National Health and Welfare, RG 29, volume 1180, file 311-C1-29, part 1.

45. "Proposed Educational Campaign for Canadian Cancer Society; Films, Film Strips & Stills," January 17, 1947, Library and Archives Canada, National Health and Welfare, RG 29, volume 1180, file 311-C1-29, part 1.

46. On alternative cancer medicine in Canada see Clow, *Negotiating Disease.*

47. "Proposed Educational Campaign for Canadian Cancer Society; Films, Film Strips & Stills," January 17, 1947, Library and Archives Canada, National Health and Welfare, RG 29, volume 1180, file 311-C1-29 part.1, p.3.

48. "Proposed Educational Campaign for Canadian Cancer Society; Films, Film Strips & Stills," January 17, 1947, Library and Archives Canada, National Health and Welfare, RG 29, volume 1180, file 311-C1-29, part 1, p.3.

49. "Proposed Educational Campaign for Canadian Cancer Society; Films, Film Strips & Stills," January 17, 1947, Library and Archives Canada, National Health and Welfare, RG 29, volume 1180, file 311-C1-29, part 1, p.4.

50. "Proposed Educational Campaign for Canadian Cancer Society; Films, Film Strips & Stills," January 17, 1947, Library and Archives Canada, National Health and Welfare, RG 29, volume 1180, file 311-C1-29, part 1.

51. Patterson, *The Dread Disease*, 175.

52. "Proposed Educational Campaign for Canadian Cancer Society; Films, Film Strips & Stills," January 17, 1947, Library and Archives Canada, National Health and Welfare, RG 29, volume 1180, fFile 311-C1-29, part 1, p.4.

53. "Proposed Educational Campaign for Canadian Cancer Society; Films, Film Strips & Stills," January 17, 1947, Library and Archives Canada, National Health and Welfare, RG 29, volume 1180, file 311-C1-29, part 1, p.4.

54. Goetz, "The Canadian Wartime Documentary." On the problems of the documentary see Jones, *The Best Butler in the Business*, 67–68.

55. "Proposed Educational Campaign for Canadian Cancer Society; Films, Film Strips & Stills," January 17, 1947, Library and Archives Canada, National Health and Welfare, RG 29, volume 1180, file 311-C1-29, part 1, p. 3.

56. "Proposed Educational Campaign for Canadian Cancer Society; Films, Film Strips & Stills," January 17, 1947, Library and Archives Canada, National Health and Welfare, RG 29, volume 1180, file 311-C1-29, part 1, p. 3.

57. "Proposed Educational Campaign for Canadian Cancer Society; Films, Film Strips & Stills," January 17, 1947, Library and Archives Canada, RG 29, National Health and Welfare, RG 29, volume 1180, file 311-C1-29, part 1, p. 3.

58. Cantor, *Man Alive! (1952)*.

59. Cantor, "Uncertain Enthusiasm."

60. Adolf Nichtenhauser to Louis J. Neff, March 22, 1944, Nichtenhauser Papers, MSC 277, box 4, folder "Cancer 1948."

61. "Lieut.-Col. C. W. Gilchrist."

62. "Maple Leaf Appears on German Streets."

63. Gilchrist, "Canada Sees New Horizons"; Gilchrist, "Health Education in Canada." See also "3 New Health Movies."

64. This point and the list of Canadian icons come from Harrison, "In the Picture of Health," 113.

65. Cantor, "Uncertain Enthusiasm."

66. Hayter, *An Element of Hope*.

67. "National Cancer Institute of Canada," 325.

68. "Brief Presented by the Directors of the Canadian Cancer Society," attached to the agenda of a Joint Conference of the boards of directors of the CCS and NCIC, February 4, 1948, Library and Archives Canada, National Health and Welfare, RG 29, volume 1180, file 311-C1-31, part 1.

69. C. W. Gilchrist to Ralph Foster, November 4, 1948, NFB archives, *Challenge: Science Against Cancer*, production file 02-130, volume 1.

70. Comments of Dr. Cameron, in "Minutes of the First Annual Meeting of the National Cancer Institute of Canada," September 20, 1947, Library and Archives Canada, National Health and Welfare, RG 29, volume 1181, file 311-C1-32, part 1, p.16.

71. Motion moved by Dr. Hall, in "Minutes of the Interim Committee of the National Cancer Institute of Canada," May 11, 1947, Library and Archives Canada, National Health and Welfare, RG 29, volume 1181, file 311-C1-32, part 1, p.11.

72. "Minutes of the Interim Committee of the National Cancer Institute of Canada," May 11, 1947, Library and Archives Canada, National Health and Welfare, RG 29, volume 1181, file 311-C1-32, part 1, pp.10–12.

73. Comments of Mr. J. G. Parker, NCIC, in "Minutes of Fund-raising and Cancer Education Conference Convened by NCIC," June 6-7, 1947, Library and Archives Canada, National Health and Welfare, RG 29, volume 1181, file 311-C1-32, part 1. "National Cancer Institute of Canada," 325.

74. Ralph Foster to Alan Field, January 31, 1950, NFB archives, *Challenge: Science Against Cancer*, production file 02-130, vol. 1.

75. "Report of Board of Directors: First Year's Activities of National Cancer Institute of Canada," Library and Archives Canada, National Health and Welfare, RG 29, volume 1181, file 311-C1-32, part 1. NCIC scientists were to be advisers to the Department of National Health and Welfare in the preparation of the film. See press release, "National Cancer Institute of Canada," February 18, 1948, Library and Archives Canada, National Health and Welfare, RG 29, volume 1180, file 311-C1-31, part 1.

76. "Brief Presented by the Directors of the Canadian Cancer Society," attached to the agenda of a Joint Conference of the boards of directors of the CCS and NCIC, February 4, 1948, Library and Archives Canada, National Health and Welfare, RG 29, volume 1180, file 311-C1-31, part 1.

77. "Minutes of the Second Annual Meeting of the National Cancer Institute of Canada," May 7–8, 1948, Library and Archives Canada, National Health and Welfare, RG 29, volume 1181, file 311-C1-32, part 1, p.2.

78. See Chapter 3 of this book.

79. *Cancer Control Letter*, October 22, 1948.

80. *Cancer Control Letter*, September 1, 1948.

81. "Memorandum of Agreement., c. February/March 1949, NCI archives, AR-4900–010785.

82. Ralph Foster to Bernard Dryer, October 29, 1948, NFB archives, *Challenge: Science Against Cancer*, production file 02-130, volume 1.

Chapter 3

1. For biographical information on Foster see Pratley, "Close-Up on Ralph Foster"; "Sympathy for Chief"; Ralph Foster biographical file, NFB archives.

2. [Ralph Foster], memo, "The Part Played by the National Film Board of Canada in the Development of the National Film Board of Australia," in Ralph Foster biographical file, NFB archives. See also Kuo, *Migration Documentary Films*.

3. Connolley, "Ralph Foster."

4. Druick, *Projecting Canada*, 93–99, esp. 96.

5. An earlier, more controversial coproduction was *The People Between* (1947), produced for the United Nations Relief and Rehabilitation Agency.

6. He was briefly loaned to the MFI in 1949. American Association of Medical Colleges, *Minutes of the Proceedings of the Sixtieth Annual Meeting*, 31.

7. Biographical information on Constant comes from Sugarman, "Jews Who Served"; "Idealists Fought the Good Fight". Constant, Maurice. Interview by Linda Kellar. June 7, 1999, in Waterloo, Ontario. Digital file. University of Waterloo Archives, Waterloo, Ontario. Information on Maurice Constant's time at the University of Toronto from Lagrimas Ulanday, records archivist, University of Toronto Archives and Records Management Services, email to the David Cantor, January 30, 2008. Constant was allegedly inspired to go to Spain on hearing a speech by André Malraux in Toronto. On the Malraux connection see Clarkson, "MacKenzie-Papineau"; Howard and Reynolds, *The Mackenzie-Papineau Battalion*; Ervin, "Men of the Mackenzie-Papineau Battalion"; Zuehlke, *The Gallant Cause*; Beeching, *Canadian Volunteers, Spain*; Petrou, *Renegades*, 44–47, 82, 103, 186–87.

8. Ralph Foster to Alan Field, January 31, 1950, NFB archives, *Challenge: Science Against Cancer*, production file 02-130, vol. 1.

9. Bernard Dryer to Ralph Foster, August 14, 1948, NFB archives. *Challenge: Science Against Cancer*, production file 02-130, vol. 1.

10. Ralph Foster to Bernard Dryer, September 13, 1948, NFB archives, *Challenge: Science Against Cancer*, production file 02-130, vol. 1.

11. Maurice Constant, First Draft Suggested Treatment for Script on "Cancer Research," June 1948, NFB archives, *Challenge: Science Against Cancer*, production file 02-120, vol. 2, p. 1.

12. Maurice Constant, First Draft Suggested Treatment for Script on "Cancer Research," June 1948, NFB archives, *Challenge: Science Against Cancer*, production file 02-120, vol. 2, p. 1.

13. Maurice Constant, First Draft Suggested Treatment for Script on "Cancer Research," June 1948, NFB archives, *Challenge: Science Against Cancer*, production file 02-120, vol. 2, p. 3.

14. Maurice Constant, First Draft Suggested Treatment for Script on "Cancer Research," June 1948, NFB archives, *Challenge: Science Against Cancer*, production file 02-120, vol. 2, p. 4.

15. Maurice Constant, First Draft Suggested Treatment for Script on "Cancer Research," June 1948, NFB archives, *Challenge: Science Against Cancer*, production file 02-120, vol. 2, p. 4.

16. Maurice Constant, First Draft Suggested Treatment for Script on "Cancer Research," June 1948, NFB archives, *Challenge: Science Against Cancer*, production file 02-120, vol. 2, p. 7.

17. Maurice Constant, First Draft Suggested Treatment for Script on "Cancer Research," June 1948, NFB archives, *Challenge: Science Against Cancer*, production file 02-120, vol. 2, p. 9.

18. Maurice Constant, First Draft Suggested Treatment for Script on "Cancer Research," June 1948, NFB archives, *Challenge: Science Against Cancer*, production file 02-120, vol. 2, p. 9.

19. Maurice Constant, First Draft Suggested Treatment for Script on "Cancer Research," June 1948, NFB archives, *Challenge: Science Against Cancer*, production file 02-120, vol. 2, p. 9.

20. Maurice Constant, First Draft Suggested Treatment for Script on "Cancer Research," June 1948, NFB archives, *Challenge: Science Against Cancer*, production file 02-120, vol. 2, p. 10.

21. Maurice Constant, First Draft Suggested Treatment for Script on "Cancer Research," June 1948, NFB archives, *Challenge: Science Against Cancer*, production file 02-120, vol. 2, p. 11.

22. Maurice Constant, First Draft Suggested Treatment for Script on "Cancer Research," June 1948, NFB archives, *Challenge: Science Against Cancer*, production file 02-120, vol. 2, p. 18.

23. Maurice Constant, First Draft Suggested Treatment for Script on "Cancer Research," June 1948, NFB archives, *Challenge: Science Against Cancer*, production file 02-120, vol. 2, p. 18.

24. Maurice Constant, First Draft Suggested Treatment for Script on "Cancer Research," June 1948, NFB archives: *Challenge: Science Against Cancer*, production file 02-120, vol. 2, p. 19.

25. Maurice Constant, First Draft Suggested Treatment for Script on "Cancer Research," June 1948, NFB archives: *Challenge: Science Against Cancer*, production file 02-120, vol. 2, p. 19.

26. Maurice Constant, First Draft Suggested Treatment for Script on "Cancer Research," June 1948, NFB archives, *Challenge: Science Against Cancer*, production file 02-120, vol. 2, p. 19.

27. Maurice Constant, First Draft Suggested Treatment for Script on "Cancer Research," June 1948, NFB archives, *Challenge: Science Against Cancer*, production file 02-120, vol. 2, p. 22.

28. Maurice Constant, First Draft Suggested Treatment for Script on "Cancer Research," June 1948, NFB archives, *Challenge: Science Against Cancer*, production file 02-120, vol. 2, p. 22.

29. Maurice Constant, First Draft Suggested Treatment for Script on "Cancer Research," June 1948, NFB archives, *Challenge: Science Against Cancer*, production file 02-120, vol. 2, p. 23.

30. McCurdy, *Space and the American Imagination*, chap. 2; O'Donnell, "Science Fiction Films." See also Evans, *Celluloid Mushroom Clouds*. One of the first major space adventures, George Pal's *Destination Moon*, was released in 1950. Loosely based on a Robert Heinlein story, it echoes Heinlein's suspicion of government. When a government agency fails to launch a rocket (there is a suspicion of sabotage), a general and a scientist turn to an industrial aircraft magnate to finance a spaceship. As part of his sales pitch to potential investors the magnate notes that only American industry can do this, though the US government will foot the bill. There is also a film within a film, an industrial recruitment film starring Woody Woodpecker, who explains the principles

of rocketry and how easy it is to get to get to the moon. The (patriotic) financiers are persuaded, and there follows a race to build the rocket and get it into space.

31. Cantor, "Uncertain Enthusiasm"; Cantor, *Reward of Courage*.

32. Lederer, *Subjected to Science*; Beers, *For the Prevention of Cruelty*, chap. 6; Gaarder, *Women and the Animal Rights Movement*; Landsbury, *The Old Brown Dog*; Elston, "Women and Anti-Vivisection."

Chapter 4

1. Morris, "After Grierson."

2. James, *Film as National Art*, 126–34.

3. On Gouzenko and the beginnings of the Cold War see Knight, *How the Cold War Began*; Duflour, "'Eggheads' and Espionage"; Whitaker and Marcuse, *Cold War Canada*.

4. Kristmanson, "Love Your Neighbor"; Forsyth, "The Failures of National and Documentary."

5. For a survey of the problems of the NFB after Grierson, see Evans, *In the National Interest*, chap. 1; Jones, *Movies and Memoranda*, chap. 4.

6. On internationalism as an aspect of Canadian cultural life see Tippett, *Making Culture*, 180, 187.

7. On the problems of internationalism within the NFB see Jones, *Movies and Memoranda*, 50–51; Jones, *The Best Butler in the Business*, 45–50.

8. More generally on internationalism in the NFB see Druick, *Projecting Canada*, chap. 4.

9. Cantor, "Uncertain Enthusiasm," 57.

10. Dallas Johnson to Ralph Foster, July 23, 1948, NFB archives, *Challenge: Science Against Cancer*, production file 02-130, vol. 1.

11. Probably Dr. Harry Eagle, the scientific director of the Research Branch and Dr. David E. Price (chief) or Dr. Ralph G. Meader (scientific director) of the Research Grants Branch.

12. Bernard Dryer to Ralph Foster, August 14, 1948, NFB archives, *Challenge: Science Against Cancer*, production file 02-130, vol. 1.

13. Ralph Foster to Bernard Dryer, September 13, 1948, NFB archives, *Challenge: Science Against Cancer*, production file 02-130, vol.1; Ralph Foster to Bernard Dryer, October 29, 1948, NFB archives, *Challenge: Science Against Cancer*, production file 02-130, vol. 1.

14. Ralph Foster to Bernard Dryer, October 29, 1948, NFB archives, *Challenge: Science Against Cancer*, production file 02-130, vol. 1. See also Ralph Foster to C. W. Gilchrist, October 29, 1948, NFB archives, *Challenge: Science Against Cancer*, production file 02-130, vol. 1.

15. Bernard Dryer to Ralph Foster, November 2, 1948, NFB archives, *Challenge: Science Against Cancer*, production file 02-130, vol. 1.

16. C. W. Gilchrist to Ralph Foster, November 4, 1948, NFB archives, *Challenge: Science Against Cancer*, production file 02-130, vol. 1.

17. Dallas Johnson to Ralph Foster, November 28, 1948, and December 27, 1948, NFB archives, *Challenge: Science Against Cancer*, production file 02-130, vol. 1. The drafts and final application are in Ross McLean, Canadian Government Film Commissioner, "Proposal for a Joint Project to Combine Facilities and the Funds of the Responsible Authorities in the United States and Canada in the Production of an Educational Film to Dramatize the Story of Cancer Research in Order to Attract Scientific Students to the Field," c. December 1948, NFB archives, *Challenge: Science Against Cancer*, production file 02-130, vol. 1.

18. Ralph Foster to C. W. Gilchrist, December 10, 1948, NFB archives, *Challenge: Science Against Cancer*, production file 02-130, vol. 1.

19. Percy W. Ward (executive director, Province of Quebec Division, CCS) to Ralph Foster, February 11, 1949, NFB archives, *Challenge: Science Against Cancer*, production file 02-130, vol. 1.

20. Percy W. Ward to Ralph Foster, February 11, 1949, NFB archives, *Challenge: Science Against Cancer*, production file 02-130, vol. 1.

21. Ralph Foster to Alan Field, March 21, 1949; David S. Ruhe to Ralph Foster, March 28, 1949, April 11, 1948; Ralph Foster to David S. Ruhe, April 7, 1949, "Memorandum of Agreement," NFB archives, *Challenge: Science Against Cancer*, production file 02-130, vol. 1.

22. "Memorandum of Agreement," NFB archives, production file 02-130, vol. 1.

23. Morten Parker interview, March 26, 2008.

24. "Outline of Structure," May 5, 1949, NFB archives, *Challenge: Science Against Cancer*, production file 02-130, vol. 2; "Treatment for Film on Cancer Research," May 5, 1949, NFB archives, *Challenge: Science Against Cancer*, production file 02-130, vol. 2.

25. M. L. Constant, "A Story Outline for a Film on Cancer Research Titled THE SCIENTIST VS CANCER (THE MYSTERY OF THE RAMPANT GROWTH)," May 12, 1949, NFB archives, *Challenge: Science Against Cancer*, production file 02-130, vol. 2.

26. "Outline of Structure," May 5, 1949, NFB archives, *Challenge: Science Against Cancer*, production file 02-130, vol. 2.

27. "Outline of Structure," May 5, 1949, NFB archives, *Challenge: Science Against Cancer*, production file 02-130, vol. 2, p.9A.

28. "Outline of Structure," May 5, 1949, NFB archives, *Challenge: Science Against Cancer*, production file 02-130, vol. 2, p.9A.

29. It is unclear if this last statement is spoken by the reporter answering his own question, or by the scientist in answer to the reporter's query.

30. "Outline of Structure," May 5, 1949, NFB archives, *Challenge: Science Against Cancer*, production file 02-130, vol. 2, p. 9A.

31. "Outline of Structure," May 5, 1949, NFB archives, *Challenge: Science Against Cancer*, production file 02-130, vol. 2, p. 9A.

32. "Outline of Structure," May 5, 1949, NFB archives, *Challenge: Science Against Cancer*, production file 02-130, vol. 2, p 2.

33. "Outline of Structure," May 5, 1949, NFB archives, *Challenge: Science Against Cancer*, production file 02-130, vol. 2, p. 4.

34. "Treatment for Film on Cancer Research," May 5, 1949, NFB archives, *Challenge: Science Against Cancer*, production file 02-130, vol. 2, p. 3; M.L. Constant, "A Story Outline for a Film on Cancer Research Titled THE SCIENTIST VS CANCER (THE MYSTERY OF THE RAMPANT GROWTH)," May 12, 1949, NFB archives, *Challenge: Science Against Cancer*, production file 02-130, vol. 2, p. 3.

35. "Outline of Structure," May 5, 1949, NFB archives, *Challenge: Science Against Cancer*, production file 02-130, vol. 2, p. 1; "Treatment for Film on Cancer Research," May 5,1949, NFB archives, *Challenge: Science Against Cancer*, production file 02-130, vol. 2, p. 1.

36. "Outline of Structure," May 5, 1949, NFB archives, *Challenge: Science Against Cancer*, production file 02-130, vol. 2, p. 1; "Treatment for Film on Cancer Research," May 5,1949, NFB archives, *Challenge: Science Against Cancer*, production file 02-130, vol. 2, p. 1.

37. "Outline of Structure," May 5, 1949, NFB archives, *Challenge: Science Against Cancer*, production file 02-130, vol. 2, p. 1 (text in caps in the original); "Treatment for Film on Cancer Research," May 5, 1949, NFB archives, *Challenge: Science Against Cancer*, production file 02-130, vol. 2, p.1 (text in caps in the original).

38. "Outline of Structure," May 5, 1949, NFB archives, *Challenge: Science Against Cancer*, production file 02-130, vol. 2, p. 1; "Treatment for Film on Cancer Research," May 5, 1949, NFB archives, *Challenge: Science Against Cancer*, production file 02-130, vol. 2, p. 1.

39. "Outline of Structure," May 5, 1949, NFB archives, *Challenge: Science Against Cancer*, production file 02-130, vol. 2, p. 2; "Treatment for Film on Cancer Research," May 5, 1949, NFB archives, *Challenge: Science Against Cancer*, production file 02-130, vol. 2, p. 2. In the earlier script this is the alternative opening. Another superimposes the title over a flask containing tissue culture.

40. "Outline of Structure," May 5, 1949, NFB archives, *Challenge: Science Against Cancer*, production file 02-130, vol. 2, p. 2.

41. "Outline of Structure," May 5,1949, NFB archives, *Challenge: Science Against Cancer*, production file 02-130, vol. 2, title page (The whole picture); p. 10 (The broad picture).

42. "Treatment for Film on Cancer Research," May 5, 1949, NFB archives, *Challenge: Science Against Cancer*, production file 02-130, vol. 2, p. 2; M. L. Constant, "A Story Outline for a Film on Cancer Research Titled THE SCIENTIST VS CANCER (THE MYSTERY OF THE RAMPANT GROWTH)," May 12, 1949, NFB archives, *Challenge: Science Against Cancer*, production file 02-130, vol. 2, p. 3. The reference to the king here is to the king of beasts, the lion, portrayed as behind bars, symbolic of human dominion over nature. The Cabbage and King reference is to "The Walrus and The Carpenter" in Carroll, *Through the Looking-Glass*, 75.

43. "Treatment for Film on Cancer Research," May 5,1949, NFB archives, *Challenge: Science Against Cancer*, production file 02-130, vol. 2, p. 2.

44. "Treatment for Film on Cancer Research," May 5, 1949, NFB archives, *Challenge: Science Against Cancer*, production file 02-130, vol. 2, p. 2.

45. "Treatment for Film on Cancer Research," May 5, 1949, NFB archives, *Challenge: Science Against Cancer*, production file 02-130, vol. 2, p. 3.

46. "Treatment for Film on Cancer Research," May 5, 1949, NFB archives, *Challenge: Science Against Cancer*, production file 02-130, vol. 2, p. 3.

47. "Treatment for Film on Cancer Research," May 5, 1949, NFB archives, *Challenge: Science Against Cancer*, production file 02-130, vol. 2, p. 3.

48. "Treatment for Film on Cancer Research," May 5, 1949, NFB archives, *Challenge: Science Against Cancer*, production file 02-130, vol. 2, p. 11.

49. M. L. Constant, "A Story Outline for a Film on Cancer Research Titled THE SCIENTIST VS CANCER (THE MYSTERY OF THE RAMPANT GROWTH)," May 12, 1949, NFB archives, *Challenge: Science Against Cancer*, production file 02-130, vol. 2, p. 1.

50. M. L. Constant, "A Story Outline for a Film on Cancer Research Titled THE SCIENTIST VS CANCER (THE MYSTERY OF THE RAMPANT GROWTH)," May 12, 1949, NFB archives, *Challenge: Science Against Cancer*, production file 02-130, vol. 2, p. 11.

51. Three copies of this version of the script are discussed in this section. Two are in the Morten Parker collection, both bound with a black hard cover embossed with the NFB logo. One is a clean copy of the script (hereafter Shooting script, *Man Against Cancer* (clean version), n.d, Morten Parker Papers); the other is heavily annotated, re-ordered for the purposes of filming, and was used by Parker during the planning and shooting of the live-action sequences (hereafter Shooting script, *Man Against Cancer* [annotated version], n.d., Morten Parker Papers). The third is another annotated copy in the NFB archives (hereafter: Shooting script, *Man Against Cancer* [annotated version], June 1949, NFB archives, *Challenge: Science Against Cancer*, production file 02-130, vol 2. In all of these, the film begins with a shot of a symbolic photo, mural, or bas-relief of an unspecified scientific subject. For the purposes of this discussion, I will refer to the NFB archives copy.

52. Shooting script, *Man Against Cancer* [annotated version], June 1949, NFB archives, *Challenge: Science Against Cancer*, production file 02-130, vol. 2.

53. Shooting script, *Man Against Cancer* [annotated version], June 1949, NFB archives, *Challenge: Science Against Cancer*, production file 02-130, vol. 2, p. 1.

54. An earlier cancer education film, *Enemy X* (1942), produced for the American Cancer Society, had previously used a similar device of a film within the film to persuade men to seek early detection and treatment for cancer. Cantor, "Uncertain Enthusiasm"; Cantor, "Choosing to Live."

55. Shooting script, *Man Against Cancer* [annotated version], June 1949, NFB archives, *Challenge: Science Against Cancer*, production file 02-130, vol. 2, p. 5.

56. Shooting script, *Man Against Cancer* [annotated version], June 1949, NFB archives, *Challenge: Science Against Cancer*, production file 02-130, vol. 2, p. 6.

57. Shooting script, *Man Against Cancer* [annotated version], June 1949, NFB archives, *Challenge: Science Against Cancer*, production file 02-130, vol. 2, p. 6.

58. Shooting script, *Man Against Cancer* [annotated version], June 1949, NFB archives, *Challenge: Science Against Cancer*, production file 02-130, vol. 2, p. 8.

59. Shooting script, *Man Against Cancer* [annotated version], June 1949, NFB archives, *Challenge: Science Against Cancer*, production file 02-130, vol. 2, p. 8.

60. Shooting script, *Man Against Cancer* [annotated version], June 1949, NFB archives, *Challenge: Science Against Cancer*, production file 02-130, vol. 2, p. 8.

61. Shooting script, *Man Against Cancer* [annotated version], June 1949, NFB archives, *Challenge: Science Against Cancer*, production file 02-130, vol. 2, p. 8.

62. Shooting script, *Man Against Cancer* [annotated version], June 1949, NFB archives, *Challenge: Science Against Cancer*, production file 02-130, vol. 2, p. 9.

63. Shooting script, *Man Against Cancer* [annotated version], June 1949, NFB archives, *Challenge: Science Against Cancer*, production file 02-130, vol. 2, p. 12.

64. Shooting script, *Man Against Cancer* [annotated version], June 1949, NFB archives, *Challenge: Science Against Cancer*, production file 02-130, vol. 2, p. 12.

65. Shooting script, *Man Against Cancer* [annotated version], June 1949, NFB archives, *Challenge: Science Against Cancer*, production file 02-130, vol. 2, p. 15.

66. Shooting script, *Man Against Cancer* [annotated version], June 1949, NFB archives, *Challenge: Science Against Cancer*, production file 02-130, vol. 2, p. 15.

67. Shooting script, *Man Against Cancer* [annotated version], June 1949, NFB archives, *Challenge: Science Against Cancer*, production file 02-130, vol. 2, p. 17.

68. Shooting script, *Man Against Cancer* [annotated version], June 1949, NFB archives, *Challenge: Science Against Cancer*, production file 02-130, vol. 2, p. 18.

69. Shooting script, *Man Against Cancer* [annotated version], June 1949, NFB archives, *Challenge: Science Against Cancer*, production file 02-130, vol. 2, p. 17.

70. Shooting script, *Man Against Cancer* [annotated version], June 1949, NFB archives, *Challenge: Science Against Cancer*, production file 02-130, vol. 2, p. 24.

71. Shooting script, *Man Against Cancer* [annotated version], June 1949, NFB archives, *Challenge: Science Against Cancer*, production file 02-130, vol. 2, p. 25.

72. Shooting script, *Man Against Cancer* [annotated version], June 1949, NFB archives, *Challenge: Science Against Cancer*, production file 02-130, vol. 2, p. 25.

73. Shooting script, *Man Against Cancer* [annotated version], June 1949, NFB archives, *Challenge: Science Against Cancer*, production file 02-130, vol. 2, p. 25.

74. Shooting script, *Man Against Cancer* [annotated version], June 1949, NFB archives, *Challenge: Science Against Cancer*, production file 02-130, vol. 2, p. 28.

75. There are two copies of this version of the script. One is in the NCI archives (hereafter Shooting script, *Man Against Cancer*, NCI archives, AR-4900-010785). Another is in the NFB archives (hereafter Shooting script, *Man Against Cancer* (clean version), NFB archives, *Challenge: Science Against Cancer*, production file 02-130, vol. 2). For the purposes of this discussion, I will refer to the version in the NFB archives.

76. Dallas Johnson to Ralph Foster, August 25, 1949, NFB archives, *Challenge: Science Against Cancer*, production file 02-130, vol. 1. On Earle, see Evans, "Wilton R. Earle," vii; "Wilton Robinson Earle."

77. "*Challenge: Science Against Cancer*. Elgin Theatre, Ottawa, 3.00 p.m., Sunday, 19th March, Under the distinguished Patronage of His Excellency the Governor-General,"

produced by Information Services Division, Department of National Health and Welfare, c.1950, NCI archives, AR-4900-010785, p.1.

78. Shooting script, *Man Against Cancer* (clean version), NFB archives, *Challenge: Science Against Cancer,* production file 02-130, vol. 2, p. 4.

79. Ralph Foster to David S. Ruhe, August 29, 1949, NFB archives, *Challenge: Science Against Cancer,* production file 02-130, vol. 1.

80. For remembrances of Hundal and the South Asian community in Ottawa, see Bhandari, *How to Be a Diplomat,* 14; Dustoor, *American Days,* 129.

81. There are several versions of the commentary in the NFB files.

One version seems to date from the period when the film was called "Man Against Cancer" "Commentary. *Man Against Cancer,*" n.d., NFB archives, *Challenge: Science Against Cancer,* production file 02-130, vol. 2.

Two seem to be the versions of the commentary that Constant, Parker, and Dryer worked on and are both annotated. They have the same title (except for the punctuation), but one is lightly annotated, the other more heavily annotated:

a. "Commentary: *Challenge: Science Against Cancer,*" n.d. (lightly annotated), NFB archives, *Challenge—Science Against Cancer,* production file 02-130, vol. 2.

b. "Commentary. *Challenge—Science Against Cancer,*" n.d. (heavily annotated), NFB archives, *Challenge: Science Against Cancer,* production file 02-130, vol. 2.

A further version is a marked-up version of the commentary read by Massey: "Commentary. *Challenge—Science Against Cancer,*" February 6, 1950 (marked-up), NFB archives, *Challenge: Science Against Cancer,* production file 02-130, vol. 2.

A final version is a clean version of the commentary read by Massey: "Commentary. *Challenge—Science Against Cancer,*" February 6, 1950 (clean), NFB archives, *Challenge: Science Against Cancer,* production file 02-130, vol. 2.

This quotation is in "Commentary. *Challenge—Science Against Cancer,*" February 6, 1950 (clean), NFB archives, *Challenge: Science Against Cancer,* production file 02-130, vol. 2, reel 4, p. 9.

Chapter 5

1. Morten Parker interview, February 1, 2008.

2. Grierson, "The Documentary Producer," 8.

3. Colin Low interviews, February 16, 2007, and May 2, 2007.

4. For biographical information on Glover, see Waugh, *The Romance of Transgression,* 421–22; Dobson, *The Film Work of Norman McLaren.* Glover's biographical file in the NFB archives contains his CV and some biographical press releases. On Glover's radical background, see Khouri and Varga, *Working on Screen,* 53, 61. See also Fabre, *The Unfinished Quest,* 261; Grace, *Sursum Corda!* 186–87; Cavell, *Love, Hate, and Fear,* 200. On the creation of the animation unit see Dobson, *The Film Work of Norman McLaren,* 132–37.

5. Jones, *Movies and Memoranda,* 76.

6. Jones, *Movies and Memoranda,* 76. The combination of animation with documentary was noticed by Peter Harcourt, who suggested that this affinity was perhaps what made the NFB documentary unique. "Animation, then, might be said to represent the more introspective aspect of filmmaking. . . . Documentary, on the other hand, is always altered by the reality it encounters. One has to go out and get it. But perhaps the fact that so many people at the Film Board have worked both in animation and in documentary explains to a degree the moral seriousness and introspective quality of so many Canadian documentary films." Harcourt, "Some Relationships," 153.

7. Morten Parker interview, March 26, 2008.

8. Colin Low interview, February 16, 2007.

9. Morten Parker interview, February 1, 2008. But see Parker, "Animating Cartoons."

10. Biographical details from the NFB's biographical file on Morten Parker.

11. Morten Parker interview, March 26, 2008; Ramsey, "Cherry, Evelyn Spice."

12. Morten Parker interview, March 26, 2008.

13. Aitken, *Film and Reform.*

14. Aitken, *Film and Reform,* 60.

15. "*Challenge: Science Against Cancer.* Elgin Theatre, Ottawa, 3.00 p.m., Sunday, 19th March Under the distinguished Patronage of His Excellency the Governor-General," produced by Information Services Division, Department of National Health and Welfare, c.1950, NCI archives, AR-4900-010785, p. 2.

16. "*Challenge: Science Against Cancer.* Elgin Theatre, Ottawa, 3.00 p.m., Sunday, 19th March Under the distinguished Patronage of His Excellency the Governor-General," produced by Information Services Division, Department of National Health and Welfare, c.1950, NCI archives, AR-4900-010785, pp. 1–2.

17. Winston, *Claiming the Real,* 134.

18. "Commentary. *Challenge—Science Against Cancer,*" February 6, 1950 (clean), NFB archives, *Challenge: Science Against Cancer,* production file 02-130, vol. 2 reel 1, p. 1.

19. Aitken, *Film and Reform,* 58; see also Weckbecker, "Re-forming Vision"; Druick, *Projecting Canada,* 54.

20. Parker, "Taking Films to the People"; Parker, "Films for Trade Unions."

21. Aitken, *Film and Reform.*

22. Druick, *Projecting Canada,* 52.

23. Morten Parker interview, March 26, 2008.

24. Glover, "Film," 104, 108.

25. Glover, "Film," 105.

26. Glover, "Film," 105.

27. Glover, "Film," 105.

28. Glover, "Film," 105.

29. Glover, "Film," 105.

30. Aitken, *Film and Reform,* 60.

31. Waugh, "Cinemas, Nations, Masculinities."

32. Colin Low interview, May 2, 2007.

33. Ellis, *John Grierson*, 173.

34. Tchelitchew had designed for the ballet in 1930s and was part of a network of gay artists and cultural critics that included Lincoln Kirstein (1907–1996) and Parker Tyler (1904–1974), both of whom wrote extensively about him and his art. For Tchelitchew's homoerotic drawings and paintings see Leddick, *The Homoerotic Art of Pavel Tchelitchev*.

35. Johnson, *The Lavender Scare*; Cavell, *Love, Hate, and Fear*.

36. Morten Parker interview, February 1, 2008.

Chapter 6

1. "Commentary. *Challenge—Science Against Cancer*," February 6, 1950 (clean), NFB archives, *Challenge: Science Against Cancer*, production file 02-130, vol. 2, reel 4, p. 9.

2. Louis Applebaum, Score for *Challenge Science Against Cancer*, Toronto, January 20, 1950, Louis Applebaum Papers, Clara Thomas Archives and Special Collections, York University, call number 1979-002/020, file 324.

Graham, *Canadian Film Technology*, 158. On Schieman and Petty see: Arnold Schieman biography file, NFB archives. Anon. "Gordon Petty CSC."

3. Morten Parker interview, February 1, 2008.

4. Dobson, "Norman McLaren"; Dobson, *The Film Work of Norman McLaren*, 142–49.

5. On McLaren's status at the NFB see Dobson, *The Film Work of Norman McLaren*, 149–57.

6. A collection of most of McLaren's motion pictures was released as a seven-DVD set in 2006, *Norman McLaren: The Masters Edition*.

7. Colin Low interview, May 2, 2007.

8. On Evelyn Lambart see the Association Internationale du Film d'Animation. Special Issue. "Evelyn Lambart"; McArthur, "The Fine Touch." See also "Lambart, Evelyn Mary"; National Film Board of Canada, "Evelyn Lambart"; "Evelyn Lambart," biographical file, NFB archives.

9. Terence Dobson tells a slightly different story in which she volunteers when McLaren asked for extra help. Dobson, *The Film Work of Norman McLaren*, 1.

10. For a biography of Low see Lenburg, "Low, Colin." See also Colin Low interview, May 2, 2007.

11. Glassman and Wise, "Filmmaker of Vision."

12. Colin Low interview, May 2, 2007. Karen Mazurkewich has a different story. She notes that Low and his colleague George Dunning took a three-month leave of absence from the NFB in 1949 to work on an adaptation of *The Adventures of Baron*

Munchausen. But the production, utilizing metal cutouts and imaginative imagery, proved too ambitious and the film had to be abandoned. Mazurkewich, *Cartoon Capers.*

13. On Daly see Jones, *The Best Butler in the Business.*

14. Colin Low interview, May 2, 2007.

15. American Association of Medical Colleges, *Minutes of the Proceedings of the Sixtieth Annual Meeting*, 31. For Ruhe's earlier contacts with Bazilauskas see "Personnel Briefs," 32.

16. Ralph Foster to Dr R. A. Vonderlehr (medical director and chief medical officer, Communicable Disease Center, US Public Health Service, Atlanta, GA), June 22, 1949, NFB archives, *Challenge: Science Against Cancer*, production file 02-130, vol. 1.

17. Much of the biographical information comes from Randy Bazilauskas interview, March 10, 2008.

18. Huettner, *Fundamentals of Comparative Embryology*, xi, 117 (fig. 54), 137 (fig. 59), 150 (fig. 64), 236 (fig. 94), 324 (fig. 130), 350 (fig. 140), and 351 (fig. 141).

19. His films included *The Diagnosis of Tuberculosis with an Improved Culture Medium*, c. 1942 (film supervisor) and *The Embryology of Human Behavior*, 1950 (collaborator). See also American Association of Medical Colleges, *Minutes of the Proceedings of the Sixtieth Annual Meeting*, 30.

20. Dr R. A. Vonderlehr to Ralph Foster, June 24, 1949, NFB archives, *Challenge: Science Against Cancer*, production file 02-130, vol. 1.

21. Ralph Foster to Dr V. F. Bazilauskas, June 28, 1949, NFB archives, *Challenge: Science Against Cancer*, production file 02-130, vol. 1.

22. Telegram from Ralph Foster to Janet Scellen, (NFB, NYC), July 12, 1949, and V. F. Bazilauskas, telegram to Ralph Foster, July 14, 1949, NFB archives, *Challenge: Science Against Cancer*, production file 02-130, vol. 1.

23. Memorandum of agreement between the NFB and V. F. Bazilauskas, July 25, 1949, NFB archives, *Challenge: Science Against Cancer*, production file 02-130, vol. 1.

24. David S. Ruhe to Ralph Foster, August 10, 1949, NFB archives, *Challenge: Science Against Cancer*, production file 02-130, vol. 1.

25. Memorandum of agreement between the NFB and V. F. Bazilauskas, September 5, 1949, NFB archives, *Challenge: Science Against Cancer*, production file 02-130, vol. 1.

26. Memorandum of agreement between the NFB and V.F. Bazilauskas, November 3, 1949, NFB archives, *Challenge: Science Against Cancer*, production file 02-130, vol. 1.

27. Memorandum of agreement between the NFB and V. F. Bazilauskas, November 3, 1949, NFB archives, *Challenge: Science Against Cancer*, production file 02-130, vol. 1.

28. Ralph Foster to Bernard V. Dryer, November 12, 1949, NFB archives, *Challenge: Science Against Cancer*, production file 02-130, vol. 1.

29. Colin Low interview, May 2, 2007.

30. On the body as interstellar space see Petchesky, "Fetal Images"; Birke, *Feminism and the Biological Body*, chaps. 4, 8.

31. Guy Glover's account of *C'est l'aviron* in Graham, *Canadian Film Technology*, 108.

32. Colin Low interview, May 2, 2007.

33. Randy Bazilauskas interview, March 10, 2008.

34. Colin Low interview, May 2, 2007. See also Low's comments in Graham, *Canadian Film Technology*, 116.

35. "*Challenge: Science Against Cancer*. Elgin Theatre, Ottawa, 3.00 p.m., Sunday 19th March, Under the distinguished Patronage of His Excellency the Governor-General," produced by Information Services Division, Department of National Health and Welfare, c.1950, NCI archives, AR-4900-010785, p. 5.

36. "*Challenge: Science Against Cancer*. Elgin Theatre, Ottawa, 3.00 p.m., Sunday 19th March, Under the distinguished Patronage of His Excellency the Governor-General," produced by Information Services Division, Department of National Health and Welfare, c.1950, NCI archives, AR-4900-010785, p. 5.

37. Colin Low interview, May 2, 2007.

38. Shooting script, *Man Against Cancer* [annotated version], June 1949, p.5; Shooting script, *Man Against Cancer* (clean version), p. 5. Both in NFB archives, *Challenge: Science Against Cancer*, production file 02-130, vol. 2.

39. Shooting script, *Man Against Cancer* [annotated version], June 1949, p.6; Shooting script, *Man Against Cancer* (clean version), p. 6. Both in NFB archives, *Challenge: Science Against Cancer*, production file 02-130, vol. 2.

40. Shooting script, *Man Against Cancer* [annotated version], June 1949, p.6; Shooting script, *Man Against Cancer* (clean version), p. 6. Both in NFB archives, *Challenge: Science Against Cancer*, production file 02-130, vol. 2.

41. Compare this sequence with images in Smith, *Exploring Biology*, 426; Smith, *Exploring Biology*, 3rd ed., 267; Smallwood, Reveley, Bailey, and Dodge, *Elements of Biology*, 343; Weymouth, *Science of Living Things*, 466 (starfish cells).

42. For films see *Human Growth*, 1947; *Human Reproduction*, 1947.

43. The closest (but not that close) textbook images I could find were in Smith, *Exploring Biology*, 426; Smith, *Exploring Biology*, 3rd ed., 267; Weymouth, *Science of Living Things*, 466 (starfish blastula). Others bore no resemblance: see Smallwood, Reveley, Bailey, and Dodge, *Elements of Biology*, 343, 535; Curtis, Caldwell, and Sherman, *Everyday Biology*, 577.

44. Dubow, *Ourselves Unborn*, especially chap. 2. See also Morgan, *Icons of Life*; Cole, "Sex and Death on Display"; Noe, "The Human Embryo Collection"; Hopwood, *Haeckel's Embryos*.

45. Beck and Weinzirl, *Human Growth*.

46. Duden, *Disembodying Women*, 11–24; Jülich, "Fetal Photography"; Jülich, "Lennart Nilsson's A Child Is Born"; Jülich, "The Making of a Best-selling Book on Reproduction"; Jülich, "Lennart Nilsson's Fish-Eyes"; Jülich, "Colouring the Human Landscapes"; Jülich, "Picturing Abortion Opposition in Sweden."

47. Colin Low interview, May 2, 2007.

48. Glassman and Wise, "Filmmaker of Vision." Low repeats this point in Colin Low interview, May 2, 2007.

49. Colin Low interview, May 2, 2007. In addition to the paintings on permanent display at MoMA, Tchelitchew contributed paintings to a MoMA circulating exhibition, "Symbolism in Painting," which ran from 1947–48.

50. Colin Low interview, February 16, 2007.

51. Tyler, "Human Anatomy as the Expanding Universe," 8. For other contemporary discussions and images of Tchelitchew see Kirstein, "The Interior Landscapes of Pavel Tchelitchew"; Tyler, "Tchelitchew's World"; Kirstein, "The Position of Pavel Tchelitchew." The last two were part of a special Tchelitchew issue of *View*—series 2, no. 2 (May 1942)—published before his interior landscapes, and several of his interior landscapes appeared on the covers of later issues. See, for example, the covers of the December 1943 issue (series 3. no.4) and the Spring 1947 issue (series 6, no.3). On *View* see Nessen, "Surrealism in Exile," 218–341; Dimakopoulou, "Europe in America."

52. For example, Head, I, reproduced on the cover of *ART News* 49, no. 9 (January 1951).

53. Kirstein, "The Interior Landscapes of Pavel Tchelitchew," 52; see also Kirstein, *Tchelitchev*, 92.

54. Kirstein, "The Interior Landscapes of Pavel Tchelitchew," 52; see also Kirstein, *Tchelitchev*, 92.

55. Kirstein, "The Interior Landscapes of Pavel Tchelitchew," 51.

56. Kirstein, "The Interior Landscapes of Pavel Tchelitchew," 51.

57. Kirstein, "The Interior Landscapes of Pavel Tchelitchew," 52.

58. Colin Low interview, February 16, 2007.

59. Kirstein, "The Interior Landscapes of Pavel Tchelitchew," 52.

60. Callen, "Ideal Masculinities." On the variety of portrayals of Apollo in the movies see Winkler, "Neo-Mythologism."

61. However, in the completed film these suggestions of death and anatomy are counterbalance by the narration (which talks of the completeness of the body and is suggestive of the wonder of the various body systems and anatomies); by the music (which resolves into a calming harmony that the composer used to suggest completeness rather than death); and by the subsequent scene of the movie in which we are treated to a tour through the living functioning body.

62. Tyler, "Human Anatomy as the Expanding Universe," 8.

63. Tyler, "Human Anatomy as the Expanding Universe," 8.

64. Tyler, "Human Anatomy as the Expanding Universe," 8. For other contemporary discussions and images of Tchelitchew see Kirstein, "The Interior Landscapes of Pavel Tchelitchew"; Tyler, "Tchelitchew's World"; Kirstein, "The Position of Pavel Tchelitchew." The last two were part of a special Tchelitchew issue of *View*—series 2, no. 2 (May 1942)—published before his interior landscapes, and several of his interior landscapes appeared on the covers of later issues. See, for example, the covers of the December 1943 issue (series 3. no.4) and the Spring 1947 issue (series 6, no.3). On *View* see Nessen, "Surrealism in Exile," 218–341; Dimakopoulou, "Europe in America."

Chapter 7

1. Telephone interview with Morten Parker, February 1, 2008.

2. On the history of tissue culture research see Landecker, *Culturing Life*; Wilson, *Tissue Culture in Science and Society*.

3. Shooting script, *Man Against Cancer* [annotated version], June 1949, p. 9; Shooting script, *Man Against Cancer* (clean version), p. 9. Both in NFB archives, *Challenge: Science Against Cancer*, production file 02-130, vol. 2.

4. Shooting script, *Man Against Cancer* [annotated version], June 1949, p. 13; Shooting script, *Man Against Cancer* (clean version), p. 13. Both in NFB archives, *Challenge: Science Against Cancer*, production file 02-130, vol. 2.

5. Shooting script, *Man Against Cancer* [annotated version], June 1949, p. 13; Shooting script, *Man Against Cancer* (clean version), p. 13. Both in NFB archives, *Challenge: Science Against Cancer*, production file 02-130, vol. 2.

6. Shooting script, *Man Against Cancer* [annotated version], June 1949, p. 13; Shooting script, *Man Against Cancer* (clean version), p. 13. Both in NFB archives, *Challenge: Science Against Cancer*, production file 02-130, vol. 2.

7. Clarke Daprato, biographical file, NFB archives; Graham, *Canadian Film Technology*, p.93.

8. Grant McLean, biographical file, NFB archives.

9. Guy Glover to Ralph Foster, August 2, 1949; Ralph Foster to Dr. D. A. Keys (vice president, National Research Council Laboratories, Chalk River, Ontario), August 3, 1949; David S. Ruhe to Guy Glover, August 4, 1949, and David S. Ruhe to Ralph Foster, August 4, 1949, NFB archives, *Challenge: Science Against Cancer*, production file 02-130, vol. 1.

10. David S. Ruhe to Ralph Foster, August 4, 1949, NFB archives, *Challenge: Science Against Cancer*, production file 02-130, vol. 1.

11. Estimate signed by GCE[?], dated September 30, 1949, Rent-A-Car Ltd, 916 Yonge St., Toronto, NFB archives, *Challenge: Science Against Cancer*, production file 02-130, vol. 1.

12. For preparations for the Toronto visit see Ross McLean to G. D. W. Cameron, September 27, 1949, NFB archives, *Challenge: Science Against Cancer*, production file 02-130, vol. 1.

13. Memo to Guy Glover, October 11, 1949, insert in Shooting script, *Man Against Cancer* [annotated version], Morten Parker Papers.

14. Memo to Guy Glover, October 11, 1949, insert in Shooting script, *Man Against Cancer* [annotated version], Morten Parker Papers.

15. Memo to Guy Glover, October 11, 1949, insert in Shooting script, *Man Against Cancer* [annotated version], Morten Parker Papers.

16. "Shooting Schedule . . . Toronto locations," n.d., NFB archives, *Cancer (Theatrical), The Fight Against Cancer*, production file 16-001. Note that this document seems to have been misfiled.

17. Ralph Foster to Dallas Johnson, November 3, 1949, NFB archives, *Challenge: Science Against Cancer*, production file 02-130, vol. 1.

18. Ralph Foster to A. V. Deibert, November 3, 1949; H. E. Betts to L. G. Chance, November 1, 1949, NFB archives, *Challenge: Science Against Cancer*, production file 02-130, vol. 1.

19. Ralph Foster to A.V. Deibert, November 3, 1949, NFB archives, *Challenge: Science Against Cancer*, production file 02-130, vol. 1.

20. The Rochester team included director, Morten Parker; cameraman, Grant McLean; assistant cameraman, Jean Roy; sound recordist, Clarke Daprato; (assistant?) soundman, Geoffrey Taylor; stills photographer, Christian Lund; business manager, Allen Stark; technical adviser, Maurice Constant; electrician, John Cote; and transportation, Douglas Bradley. For the correspondence on this travel see Ralph Foster to L. G. Chance (chief of Consular Division, Department of External Affairs, Ottawa), September 28, 1949; A. D. P. Heeney (undersecretary of state for External Affairs) to Ralph Foster, October 6, 1949; Harold Betts (NFB production secretary), memo, "Personnel Participating in CANCER VS SCIENCE shooting in Rochester, NY, October 8, 1949; Ralph Foster to Guy Glover, October 11 [1949]; Allen Stark to Harold Betts, October 17, 1949; A. D. P. Heeney to Ralph Foster, October 19, 1949; Ralph Foster to A. D. P. Heeney, October 21, 1949; Harold Betts to Guy Glover, October 21, [1949]; Harold Betts to Allen Stark, October 21, 1949; Harold Betts to Dallas Johnson, October 21, 1949; Harold Betts to Bernard V. Dryer, October 21, 1949; Harold Betts to David Ruhe, October 21, 1949; Harold Betts to Bernard V. Dryer, October 24, 1949; H. E. Betts to L. G. Chance, November 1, 1949, all in NFB archives, *Challenge: Science Against Cancer*, production file 02-130, vol. 1.

21. Grant McLean, biographical file, NFB archives.

22. A. V. Deibert to Ralph Foster, November 10, 1949, NFB archives, *Challenge: Science Against Cancer*, production file 02-130, vol. 1.

23. Morten Parker interview, March 26, 2008. Born in Birmingham, England, Emerson Houghton emigrated to Canada in 1911. A silversmith by training, he settled in Toronto and until 1914 worked at Roden Brothers, a Canadian tableware design and manufacturing company. After service during the First World War, he returned to Toronto in 1917 and married. In 1919, he set up a stationery store in Toronto before opening Houghton's Silverware and Plating (in operation c. 1920–1980). The records of the last company are held at the Library and Archives, National Gallery of Canada, Houghton's Silverware and Plating Ltd. Fonds.

24. Mitchell and Mitchell, *W. O.*; Latham, *Magic Lies*; Harrison, *W. O. Mitchell*.

25. Morten Parker interview, March 26, 2008; "In Memoriam, Larry McCance."; "Larry M'Cance."

26. Morten Parker interview, March 26, 2008.

27. I am grateful to Lagrimas Ulanday, records archivist, University of Toronto Archives and Records Management Services, for newspaper clippings and photos of Rae from University of Toronto Archives (UTA), Department of Graduate Records, A73-0026/371 (53); UTA, Department of Information, A1978-0041/018 (03); and the UTA People File. On Rae and the chemistry department at the University of Toronto see Brook and McBryde, *Historical Distillates*, 117, 121, 123, 144, 170.

28. Hansen, *Picturing Medical Progress.*

29. Norman Camberlin, memo, "The Scientist Against Cancer," December 19, 1949, NFB archives, *Challenge: Science Against Cancer*, production file 02-130, vol. 1.

30. See the comments on one of the film's consultants—Dr. H. B. Andervant—who noted that this method was not used in his lab. Norman Camberlin, memo, "The Scientist Against Cancer," December 19, 1949, NFB archives, *Challenge: Science Against Cancer*, production file 02-130, vol. 1.

31. David S. Ruhe to Guy Glover, August 4, 1949, NFB archives, *Challenge: Science Against Cancer*, production file 02-130, vol. 1.

32. Lederer, "Hollywood and Human Experimentation."

33. Morten Parker interview, March 26, 2008.

34. Cantor, "Cancer Control and Prevention in the Twentieth Century"; Aronowitz, *Unnatural History*; Wailoo, *How Cancer Crossed the Color Line*; Gardner, *Early Detection*; Lerner, *The Breast Cancer Wars*; Hayter, *An Element of Hope*; Clow, *Negotiating Disease.*

35. This account of past triumphs is there in the Shooting script and the narration written later. Shooting script, *Man Against Cancer* [annotated version], June 1949, p.1; Shooting script, *Man Against Cancer* (clean version), p.1. "Commentary. *Challenge—Science Against Cancer,*" February 6, 1950 (clean), reel 1, p. 1. All in NFB archives, *Challenge: Science Against Cancer*, production file 02-130, vol. 2.

36. For a survey of gothic filmmaking see Kaye, "Gothic Film." See also Bunnell, "The Gothic"; Hopkins, *Screening the Gothic*; Klossner, "Horror on Film and Television" Kavka, "The Gothic on Screen"; Morris, "Metropolis and the Modernist Gothic" Schneider, "Mixed Blood Couples"; Scahill, "Invasion of the Husband Snatchers"; Tudor, *Monsters and Mad Scientists*; Skal, *The Monster Show.*

37. Morten Parker interview, March 26, 2008.

38. "*Challenge: Science Against Cancer.* Elgin Theatre, Ottawa, 3.00 p.m., Sunday 19th March, Under the distinguished Patronage of His Excellency the Governor-General," produced by Information Services Division, Department of National Health and Welfare, c.1950, NCI archives, AR-4900-010785, p. 2.

39. Shooting script, *Man Against Cancer* [annotated version], June 1949, p.7; Shooting script, *Man Against Cancer* (clean version), p.7. "Commentary. *Challenge—Science Against Cancer,*" February 6, 1950 (clean), NFB archives, reel 1, p. 2. All in *Challenge: Science Against Cancer*, production file 02-130, vol. 2.

40. "Commentary. *Challenge—Science Against Cancer,*" February 6, 1950 (clean), NFB archives, *Challenge: Science Against Cancer*, production file 02-130, vol. 2, reel 3, p. 7.

41. Shooting script, *Man Against Cancer* (clean version), Morten Parker Papers, p. 21.

42. Shooting script, *Man Against Cancer* (clean version), Morten Parker Papers, p. 22.

43. Shooting script, *Man Against Cancer* (clean version), Morten Parker Papers, p. 22.

44. Shooting script, *Man Against Cancer* (clean version), Morten Parker Papers, p. 19.

45. Shooting script, *Man Against Cancer* (clean version), Morten Parker Papers, p. 23.

46. "Commentary. *Challenge—Science Against Cancer,*" February 6, 1950 (clean), NFB archives, *Challenge: Science Against Cancer*, production file 02-130, vol. 2, reel 4, p. 8.

47. "Commentary. *Challenge—Science Against Cancer*," February 6, 1950 (clean), NFB archives, *Challenge: Science Against Cancer*, production file 02-130, vol. 2, reel 2, p. 4.

48. Bowser, *The Transformation of Cinema*, 93–4.

49. "Commentary. *Challenge—Science Against Cancer*," February 6, 1950 (clean), NFB archives, *Challenge: Science Against Cancer*, production file 02-130, vol. 2, reel 2, p. 3.

50. "Commentary. *Challenge—Science Against Cancer*," February 6, 1950 (clean), NFB archives, *Challenge: Science Against Cancer*, production file 02-130, vol. 2, reel 4, p. 8.

51. Shapin, *The Scientific Life*.

52. This description was included in both the June 1949 version of the shooting script and later versions. Shooting script, *Man Against Cancer* [annotated version], June 1949, p. 25; Shooting script, *Man Against Cancer* (clean version), p. 25. Both in NFB archives, *Challenge: Science Against Cancer*, production file 02-130, vol. 2.

53. "Commentary. *Challenge—Science Against Cancer*," February 6, 1950 (clean), NFB archives, *Challenge: Science Against Cancer*, production file 02-130, vol. 2, reel 4, p. 8.

54. Shooting script, *Man Against Cancer* [annotated version], June 1949, p. 17; Shooting script, *Man Against Cancer* (clean version), p. 17. Both in NFB archives, *Challenge: Science Against Cancer*, production file 02-130, vol. 2.

55. Shooting script, *Man Against Cancer* [annotated version], June 1949, p. 17; Shooting script, *Man Against Cancer* (clean version), p. 17. Both in NFB archives, *Challenge: Science Against Cancer*, production file 02-130, vol. 2.

56. Shooting script, *Man Against Cancer* [annotated version], June 1949, p. 17; Shooting script, *Man Against Cancer* (clean version), p. 17. Both in NFB archives, *Challenge: Science Against Cancer*, production file 02-130, vol. 2.

57. Shooting script, *Man Against Cancer* [annotated version], June 1949, p. 17; Shooting script, *Man Against Cancer* (clean version), p. 17. Both in NFB archives, *Challenge: Science Against Cancer*, production file 02-130, vol. 2.

58. "Commentary. *Challenge—Science Against Cancer*," February 6, 1950 (clean), NFB archives, *Challenge: Science Against Cancer*, production file 02-130, vol. 2, reel 3, p. 6.

59. Shooting script, *Man Against Cancer* [annotated version], Morten Parker Papers, p. 20.

60. "Commentary. *Challenge—Science Against Cancer*," February 6, 1950 (clean), NFB archives, *Challenge: Science Against Cancer*, production file 02-130, vol. 2, reel 4, p. 8.

61. "Commentary. *Challenge—Science Against Cancer*," February 6, 1950 (clean), NFB archives, *Challenge: Science Against Cancer*, production file 02-130, vol. 2, reel 4, p. 8.

62. Shooting script, *Man Against Cancer* [annotated version], June 1949, p. 10; Shooting script, *Man Against Cancer* (clean version), p. 10. Both in NFB archives, *Challenge: Science Against Cancer*, production file 02-130, vol. 2.

63. Shooting script, *Man Against Cancer* [annotated version], June 1949, p. 10; Shooting script, *Man Against Cancer* (clean version), p. 10. Both in NFB archives, *Challenge: Science Against Cancer*, production file 02-130, vol. 2.

64. Shooting script, *Man Against Cancer* [annotated version], June 1949, p. 10; Shooting script, *Man Against Cancer* (clean version), p. 10. Both in NFB archives, *Challenge: Science Against Cancer*, production file 02-130, vol. 2.

Chapter 8

1. Morten Parker interview, March 26, 2008.

2. On Applebaum see Pitman, *Louis Applebaum*. For a list of movies for which Applebaum composed the music see McCarty, *Film Composers in America*, 26–8.

3. Memorandum of agreement between Louis Applebaum and the NFB, December 22, 1949, NFB archives, *Challenge: Science Against Cancer*, production file 02-130, vo. 1.

4. Louis Applebaum, Score for *Challenge Science Against Cancer*, Toronto, January 20, 1950, Louis Applebaum Papers, Clara Thomas Archives and Special Collections, York University, call number 1979-002/020, file 324.

5. Invoice for CAN$1,684.12 from Camie Howard to the NFB, February 4, 1950, NFB archives, *Challenge: Science Against Cancer*, production file 02-130, vol. 1.

6. It was to comprise the following instruments: flute, clarinet, bass clarinet, cello, horn, trumpet, trombone, tuba, percussion, violin, violas, celeste, double bass, harp, piano, glockenspiel, timpani, piccolo, vibraphone, xylophone, tambourine, gong, wood block, and castanet. Louis Applebaum, Score for *Challenge Science Against Cancer*.

7. Invoice for CAN$1,684.12 from Camie Howard to the NFB, February 4, 1950.

8. Potvin, "Belland, Jean."

9. Poussart, "Delcellier, Joseph."

10. Papineau-Couture, "Baillargeon, Marcel."

11. Gorbman, *Unheard Melodies*.

12. Gorbman, *Unheard Melodies*.

13. Hayward, *Off the Planet*, especially the introduction. See also Bartkowiak, *Sounds of the Future*.

14. Berger, "Filming the Invisible," 13. For a photograph of this photomicrography equipment see Graham, *Canadian Film Technology*, 159. No such sequence appears in the film, so it was probably deleted. However, it is possible that the reference is to a shot in sequence 3, where the viewer sees a tissue culture image of cancer cells through microscope.

15. Clarke Daprato, biographical file, NFB archives.

16. Morten Parker interview, March 26, 2008.

17. Participants included (from the US) Bernard Dryer, Dr. David Ruhe, Dr. Austin Deibert, Dr. Andervant [*sic*], Dr. Bazilauski [*sic*], Dr. Chalkley, and Dallas Johnson; (from Canada) Dr. O. H. Warwick (executive director of the Canadian Cancer Society) and Dr. Raymond Parker. NFB representatives were Ralph Foster, Guy Glover, Maurice Constant, and Morten Parker. The Department of Health and Welfare was represented by Dr. Cameron (Deputy Minister of Health); Dr. Ansley (Director of Health Services); C. W. Gilchrist and Norman Camberlin (Information Services Division). Norman Camberlin, memo, "The Scientist Against Cancer," December 19, 1949, NFB archives, *Challenge: Science Against Cancer,* production file 02-130, vol. 1.

18. Norman Camberlin, memo "The Scientist Against Cancer," December 19, 1949, NFB archives, *Challenge: Science Against Cancer*, production file 02-130, vol. 1.

19. On Andervont see Shimkin, "Howard B. Andervont."

20. The subcommittee comprised Dallas Johnson, David Ruhe, Dr. Warwick, and C. W. Gilchrist. Norman Camberlin, memo "The Scientist Against Cancer," December 19, 1949, NFB archives, *Challenge: Science Against Cancer*, production file 02-130, vol. 1.

21. C. W. Gilchrist to Dallas Johnson, December 21, 1949, NFB archives, *Challenge: Science Against Cancer*, production file 02-130, vol. 1.

22. In the final cut three scientists are watching a slide of Mr. Davis's tumor when he enters the doctor's office. Mr. Davis's body then dissolves into the animated sequence, which then fades back into Mr. Davis where he is told that his cancer is 90 percent curable. This would also seem to fit the description in Massey's commentary. In the synopsis, however, Mr. Davis enters the doctor's office only after the first animation sequence. It is the slide of his tumor that the scientists are viewing before his entry that expands and develops into the first animation sequence on normal and abnormal growth. 'Challenge: Science Against Cancer. Elgin Theatre, Ottawa 3.00 p.m., Sunday 19th March Under the distinguished Patronage of His Excellency the Governor-General', Produced by Information Services Division, Department of National Health and Welfare, c.1950, p. 2. NCI archives, AR-4900-010785. Copy of the commentary and dialogue "*Commentary. Challenge—Science Against Cancer*," February 6, 1950 (clean), NFB archives, *Challenge: Science Against Cancer*, production file 02-130, vol. 2, reel 4, p. 9.

23. Bernard V. Dryer and Ralph Foster to Dr. Warwick, Dr. Deibert, Dr. Ruhe, Mr. Gilchrist, and Mr. Glover, January 29, 1950. See also Bernard V. Dryer to Miss Kay Brown (Music Corporation of America), January 29, 1950, both in NFB archives, *Challenge: Science Against Cancer*, production file 02-130, vol. 1. According to one article, this fund was based in New York: "Challenge! Science Against Cancer," 7.

24. Bernard V. Dryer to Miss Kay Brown (Music Corporation of America), January 29, 1950, NFB archives, *Challenge: Science Against Cancer*, production file 02-130, vol. 1.

25. Bernard V. Dryer and Ralph Foster to Dr. Warwick, Dr. Deibert, Dr. Ruhe, Mr. Gilchrist, and Mr. Glover, January 29, 1950, NFB archives, *Challenge: Science Against Cancer*, production file 02-130, vol. 1.

26. See especially "Commentary: *Challenge: Science Against Cancer*," n.d. (lightly annotated), NFB archives, *Challenge—Science Against Cancer*, production file 02-130, vol. 2. "Commentary. *Challenge—Science Against Cancer*," n.d. (heavily annotated), NFB archives, *Challenge: Science Against Cancer*, production file 02-130, vol. 2. Also see: "Commentary. *Challenge—Science Against Cancer*," February 6, 1950 (marked-up), NFB archives, *Challenge: Science Against Cancer*, production file 02-130, vol. 2, and "Commentary. *Challenge—Science Against Cancer*," February 6, 1950 (clean), NFB archives, *Challenge: Science Against Cancer*, production file 02-130, vol. 2.

27. In the June 1949 shooting script, the normal and abnormal growth sequence (2) starts with the comment: "It begins with the fertilized egg . . . a single cell 1/2000 of an inch in size," which appeared in the commentary and the film as: "It begins with a fertilized human egg—a single pinpoint fragment of life— a cell." Shooting script, *Man Against Cancer* [annotated version], June 1949, NFB archives, *Challenge: Science Against Cancer*, production file 02-130, vol. 2, p. 5, and "Commentary, *Challenge—Science Against Cancer*," NFB archives, *Challenge: Science Against Cancer*, production file

02-130, vol 2, reel 1, p. 2. "Commentary. *Challenge—Science Against Cancer*," February 6, 1950 (clean), NFB archives, *Challenge: Science Against Cancer*, production file 02-130, vol. 2, reel 4, p. 9. The phrase "when the centrosome divides in a quiver of creation," was changed in the cell-as-universe (genetics) sequence (6) to "when the astral body divides in a quiver of creation." "Commentary. Challenge—Science Against Cancer," February 6, 1950 (clean), NFB archives, *Challenge: Science Against Cancer*, production file 02-130, vol. 2, reel 2, p. 4. In one of the annotated drafts of the commentary the word "centrosome" has also been crossed out at line 140, and the words "astral body" written in "Commentary. *Challenge—Science Against Cancer*," n.d. (heavily annotated), NFB archives, *Challenge: Science Against Cancer*, production file 02-130, vol. 2.

28. Bernard V. Dryer and Ralph Foster to Dr. Warwick, Dr. Deibert, Dr. Ruhe, Mr. Gilchrist, and Mr. Glover, January 29, 1950, NFB archives, *Challenge: Science Against Cancer*, production file 02-130, vol. 1.

29. "Commentary. *Challenge—Science Against Cancer*," February 6, 1950 (marked-up), NFB archives, *Challenge: Science Against Cancer*, production file 02-130, vol. 2. "Commentary. *Challenge—Science Against Cancer*," February 6, 1950 (clean), NFB archives, *Challenge: Science Against Cancer*, production file 02-130, vol. 2.

30. "Challenge! Science Against Cancer," 7.

31. Morten Parker interview, February 1, 2008.

32. On Bobet see Canadian Film Encyclopedia, "Jacques Bobet." Dorland, "Creation Myth."

33. "Commentary. *Challenge—Science Against Cancer*," February 6, 1950 (clean), NFB archives, *Challenge: Science Against Cancer*, production file 02-130, vol. 2, reel 1, p. 1.

34. "Commentaire. *Alerte—Science Contre Cancer*," NFB archives, *Challenge: Science Against Cancer*, production file 02-130, vol. 2, bobine 1, p. 1.

35. In the heavily annotated version of the English commentary, this phrase from Ecclesiastes is crossed out, and the "houses of healing" introduction written in at lines 1 and 2: "Commentary. Challenge—Science Against Cancer," n.d. (heavily annotated), NFB archives, *Challenge: Science Against Cancer*, production file 02-130, vol. 2.

36. See Jacques Bobet's order, March 9, 1950, NFB archives, *Challenge: Science Against Cancer*, production file 02-130, vol. 2.

37. See Jacques Bobet's order, February 7, 1950, NFB archives, *Challenge: Science Against Cancer*, production file 02-130, vol. 2.

Chapter 9

1. David S. Ruhe to Ralph Foster, July 8, 1949, NFB archives, *Challenge: Science Against Cancer*, production file 02-130, vol. 1.

2. David S. Ruhe to Ralph Foster, July 8, 1949, NFB archives, *Challenge: Science Against Cancer*, production file 02-130, vol. 1.

3. Hansen, *Picturing Medical Progress*, chap. 9.

4. David S. Ruhe to Ralph Foster, August 10, 1949, NFB archives, *Challenge: Science Against Cancer*, production file 02-130, vol. 1.

5. David S. Ruhe to Ralph Foster, August 10, 1949, NFB archives, *Challenge: Science Against Cancer*, production file 02-130, vol. 1.

6. Dallas Johnson to Col. C. W. Gilchrist, August 15, 1949, NFB archives, *Challenge: Science Against Cancer*, production file 02-130, vol. 1.

7. Dallas Johnson to Col. C. W. Gilchrist, August 15, 1949, NFB archives, *Challenge: Science Against Cancer*, production file 02-130, vol. 1.

8. Ralph Foster to Jack Hughes, October 27, [1949], NFB archives, *Challenge: Science Against Cancer*, production file 02-130, vol. 1.

9. Ralph Foster to Dallas Johnson, November 3, 1949, NFB archives, *Challenge: Science Against Cancer*, production file 02-130, vol. 1.

10. Payne, *The Official Picture*, 33 (reference to *Life* magazine).

11. Dallas Johnson to Col. C. W. Gilchrist, August 15, 1949, NFB archives, *Challenge: Science Against Cancer*, production file 02-130, vol. 1.

12. Albert J. Rosenberg to Hugh Jackson, March 7, 1950, NCI archives, no reference number, full text PDF 4780.4. On McGraw Hill's Text Film Department see "Tenth Anniversary." On Rosenberg and the market in text-films see Acland, "Classrooms, Clubs, and Community Circuits," esp. 158.

13. Dallas Johnson to Ralph Foster, October 28, 1949, NFB archives, *Challenge: Science Against Cancer*, production file 02-130, vol. 1.

14. For the provisional approval for a film on cancer, see United Nations Film Board, *Summary Record of the Eleventh Quarterly Session held at Lake Success, NY, 12 October 1949 and 26 October 1949*, United Nations Archives and Records Section, DAG 12/3.1, box 18, series-0540-0073, box title, "Sessions of the Visual Information Board/United Nations Film Board, Summary Records of Sessions," 1947-67, p. 3. Rendueles attended this meeting—other films submitted for approval focused on civil aviation, human rights, land utilization, and the life of the schoolchild.

15. The records meetings of the UN Film Board at available in United Nations Archives and Records Section, DAG 12/3.1, box 2, series-0540-0057 and United Nations Archives and Records Section, DAG 12/3.1, box 3, series-0540–0058.

16. Dallas Johnson, undated and unattributed MSS, 1950[?], [Listed as "Cancer Research Educational Program/Challenge: Science Against Cancer Documentary Film/ Challenge Of Cancer Book" in the finding aid], NCI archives, AR-5000-010683, p. 2.

17. Biographical information on Grant from Melissa Ludtke (editor, *Nieman Reports*), email message to author, January 21, 2009; Fiore, "Lester Grant."

18. John R. Heller to Mrs. [Helen] Ogden Reid (President, *New York Herald Tribune*), April 5, 1949, NFB archives, *Challenge: Science Against Cancer*, production file 02-130, vol. 1.

19. Grant, *The Challenge of Cancer*.

20. National Cancer Institute, *A Teaching Guide*, 2.

21. Dallas Johnson to Ralph Foster, August 19, 1949, NFB archives, *Challenge: Science Against Cancer*, production file 02-130, vol. 1; Dallas Johnson to Col. C. W. Gilchrist, September 6, 1949, NFB archives, *Challenge: Science Against Cancer*, production file 02-130, vol. 1.

22. "Morris Meister"; Lacey, "In Memoriam. Morris Meister." For Meister and science education see Terzian, *Science Education and Citizenship*.

23. Dallas Johnson to Ralph Foster, August 26, 1949, NFB archives, *Challenge: Science Against Cancer*, production file 02-130, vol. 1.

24. Dallas Johnson to Ralph Foster, August 26, 1949, NFB archives, *Challenge: Science Against Cancer*, production file 02-130, vol. 1.

25. Dallas Johnson to Ralph Foster, August 26, 1949, NFB archives, *Challenge: Science Against Cancer*, production file 02-130, vol. 1.

26. Ralph Foster to Dallas Johnson, August 30, 1949, NFB archives, *Challenge: Science Against Cancer*, production file 02-130, vol. 1.

27. Dallas Johnson to Ralph Foster, September 6, 1949, NFB archives, *Challenge: Science Against Cancer*, production file 02-130, vol. 1.

28. Draft of publicity leaflet "Presenting *The Challenge of Cancer*," n.d. (probably early September 1949), NFB archives, *Challenge: Science Against Cancer*, production file 02-130, vol. 1.

29. Dallas Johnson to Ralph Foster, November 15, 1949, NFB archives, *Challenge: Science Against Cancer*, production file 02-130, vol. 1.

30. Dallas Johnson to Ralph Foster, November 15, 1949, NFB archives, *Challenge: Science Against Cancer*, production file 02-130, vol. 1.

31. Dallas Johnson to Ralph Foster, November 15, 1949, NFB archives, *Challenge: Science Against Cancer*, production file 02-130, vol. 1.

32. Dallas Johnson to John Heller, "Relations between Cancer Report Section and Research Branch," May 19, 1949, box 19, folder 3, Harold Leroy Stewart Papers, MSC 228.

33. Dallas Johnson to John Heller, "Relations between Cancer Report Section and Research Branch," May 19, 1949, Harold Leroy Stewart Papers, MSC 228, p. 3; Hueper, *Environmental Cancer*.

34. Dallas Johnson to Ralph Foster, August 19, 1949, NFB archives, *Challenge: Science Against Cancer*, production file 02-130, vol. 1.

35. Dallas Johnson to Ralph Foster, August 19, 1949, NFB archives, *Challenge: Science Against Cancer*, production file 02-130, vol. 1.

36. Dallas Johnson to Ralph Foster, August 26, 1949, NFB archives, *Challenge: Science Against Cancer*, production file 02-130, vol. 1.

37. Draft of publicity leaflet "Presenting *The Challenge of Cancer*," n.d. (probably early September 1949), NFB archives, *Challenge: Science Against Cancer*, production file 02-130, vol. 1.

38. Shooting script, *Man Against Cancer* [annotated version], June 1949, NFB archives, *Challenge: Science Against Cancer*, production file 02-130, vol. 2, p. 19.

39. Dallas Johnson to Ralph Foster, August 19, 1949, NFB archives, *Challenge: Science Against Cancer*, production file 02-130, vol. 1.

40. Dallas Johnson to Ralph Foster, August 19, 1949, NFB archives, *Challenge: Science Against Cancer*, production file 02-130, vol. 1.

41. Dallas Johnson to Ralph Foster, August 19, 1949, NFB archives, *Challenge: Science Against Cancer*, production file 02-130, vol. 1. For an endorsement of the tissue culture section by Morris Meister see Dallas Johnson to Ralph Foster, August 26, 1949, NFB archives, *Challenge: Science Against Cancer*, production file 02-130, vol. 1.

42. Dallas Johnson to Ralph Foster, August 25, 1949, NFB archives, *Challenge: Science Against Cancer*, production file 02-130, vol. 1. Baker, "Jesse P. Greenstein."

43. Jesse Greenstein quoted in Dallas Johnson to Ralph Foster, August 25, 1949, NFB archives, *Challenge: Science Against Cancer*, production file 02-130, vol. 1.

44. Jesse Greenstein quoted in Dallas Johnson to Ralph Foster, August 25, 1949, NFB archives, *Challenge: Science Against Cancer*, production file 02-130, vol. 1.

45. Evans, "Wilton R. Earle"; "Wilton Robinson Earle."

46. Dallas Johnson to Ralph Foster, August 25, 1949, NFB archives, *Challenge: Science Against Cancer*, production file 02-130, vol. 1.

47. Dallas Johnson to Ralph Foster, August 25, 1949, NFB archives, *Challenge: Science Against Cancer*, production file 02-130, vol. 1.

48. "Commentary. *Challenge—Science Against Cancer*," February 6, 1950 (clean), NFB archives, *Challenge: Science Against Cancer*, production file 02-130, vol. 2, reel 3, p. 1. In the heavily annotated version of the commentary the phrase "complicated industrial factory," is crossed out and "complex industrial organism" written in at line 186: "Commentary. *Challenge—Science Against Cancer*," n.d. (heavily annotated), NFB archives, *Challenge: Science Against Cancer*, production file 02-130, vol. 2.

49. Mr. Davis's cancer cost CAN$50 for the reproduction—a moulage of carcinomatous lesions for lip and cheek. Apparently, this moulage could be applied either to the lip or cheek depending on the filmmakers' preference. It was made by H. Louise Gordon of 104 Brentcliffe Road, Leaside, Ontario. Invoice from H. Louise Gordon (medical artist) to Morten Parker, NFB, Ottawa, October 27, 1949, NFB archives, *Challenge: Science Against Cancer*, production file 02-130, vol. 1 For a history of the moulage in medical teaching see Schnalke, *Diseases in Wax*.

Chapter 10

1. Dallas Johnson to Ralph Foster, December 2, 1949, NFB archives, *Challenge: Science Against Cancer*, production file 02-130, vol. 1.

2. J. R. Heller to Branch, Section and Unit Heads, NCI, "Appointment of Chief, Cancer Reports Section," December 16, 1950, box 19, folder 3, Harold Leroy Stewart Papers, MSC 228.

3. See, for example, Dallas Johnson to Hugh Jackson, March 17, 1950, NCI archives, no reference number, full text PDF 4780.4.

4. "Newspaperman Named."

5. Dallas Johnson, "Production, Promotion and Distribution Schedule for CHAL-LENGE— SCIENCE AGAINST CANCER," January 23, 1950, NCI archives, AR-4900–010785.

6. On science writers in the 1940s and 1950s see Krieghbaum, "The Background and Training of Science Writers"; Krieghbaum, "American Newspaper Reporting of Science News"; Johnson, "Status and Attitudes of Science Writers"; See also Hoyle, "British Scientists Also Write"; Nieman Fellows, "Science in the Press"; Bryson, *Science and Freedom*; Davis, "Science and the Press"; Friedwald, *Man's Last Choice*; Herzberg, *Late City Edition*, 101–8; Kaempffert, *Science Today and Tomorrow*.

7. Blantz, *George N. Shuster*.

8. Farley, *Brock Chisholm*. Dowbiggin, "Prescription for Survival."

9. Dallas Johnson, "Production, Promotion and Distribution Schedule for CHAL-LENGE– SCIENCE AGAINST CANCER," January 23, 1950, NCI archives, AR-4900-010785, p. 5.

10. Dallas Johnson, "Production, Promotion and Distribution Schedule for CHAL-LENGE– SCIENCE AGAINST CANCER," January 23, 1950, NCI archives, AR-4900-010785, pp. 5–7, For a later list of people see Dallas Johnson, "List of Invitees," February 17, 1950, NCI archives, AR-4900-010785.

11. Johnson listed him as Radio City Corporation, but it seems more likely she meant Radio Corporation of America (RCA) which had created the National Broadcasting Company (NBC).

12. Dallas Johnson, "Production, Promotion and Distribution Schedule for CHAL-LENGE– SCIENCE AGAINST CANCER," January 23, 1950, NCI archives, AR-4900-010785, p. 8.

13. Dallas Johnson, "Production, Promotion and Distribution Schedule for CHAL-LENGE– SCIENCE AGAINST CANCER," January 23, 1950, NCI archives, AR-4900-010785, p. 12. On Winchell see Gabler, *Winchell*.

14. "Matthew Gordon." For more generally on the UN and UNESCO and film see Langlois, "And Action!" and Druick, "UNESCO, Film, and Education."

15. "Sympathy for Chief."

16. United Nations Film Board 27/28 June 1950, United Nations Department of Public Information Films and Visual Information Division, *Report covering period March 1, 1950, to June 1, 1950,* United Nations Archives and Records Section, DAG 12/3.1, box 3, series-0540-0058. File title: "United Nations Film Board. Thirteenth Session."

17. Dallas Johnson, "Production, Promotion and Distribution Schedule for CHAL-LENGE– SCIENCE AGAINST CANCER," January 23, 1950, NCI archives, AR-4900-010785, p. 9.

18. Dallas Johnson, "Production, Promotion and Distribution Schedule for CHAL-LENGE– SCIENCE AGAINST CANCER," January 23, 1950, NCI archives, AR-4900-010785, p. 10.

19. Dallas Johnson, "Production, Promotion and Distribution Schedule for CHAL-LENGE– SCIENCE AGAINST CANCER," January 23, 1950, NCI archives, AR-4900-010785, p. 10.

20. Nourie, "*Look*."

21. Wright, "His Name High in Two Mastheads."

22. Dallas Johnson, "Production, Promotion and Distribution Schedule for CHAL-LENGE– SCIENCE AGAINST CANCER," January 23, 1950, NCI archives, AR-4900-010785, p. 10. On *Collier's*, see Vogt, "Collier's."

23. Maisel, "Bedlam 1946"; Deutsch, *The Shame of the States*.

24. Dallas Johnson, "Production, Promotion and Distribution Schedule for CHAL-LENGE – SCIENCE AGAINST CANCER," January 23, 1950, NCI archives, AR-4900-010785, p. 12.

25. Dallas Johnson, "Production, Promotion and Distribution Schedule for CHAL-LENGE– SCIENCE AGAINST CANCER," January 23, 1950, NCI archives, AR-4900-010785, pp.14–20.

26. Judson Hardy addition to memorandum from Jack Fletcher to Judson Harvey, February 15, 1950, NCI archives, no reference number, full text PDF 4780.4.

27. Zilpha C Franklin to Hugh Jackson, February 21, 1950, NCI archives, no reference number, full text PDF 4780.4.

28. Hugh Jackson to Dallas Johnson, February 24, 1950, NCI archives, no reference number, full text PDF 4780.4.

29. Huggins and Cameron are both mentioned as speakers in Zilpha C. Franklin to Hugh Jackson, February 21, 1950, NCI archives, no reference number, full text PDF 4780.4.

30. Brock Chisholm, "World Health," speech given at the Hunter College Premiere of *Challenge*, March 13, 1950, NCI archives, AR-4900–010785.

31. C. P. Rhoads, "Recent Trends in Cancer Research," speech given at the Hunter College premiere of *Challenge*, March 13, 1950, NCI archives, AR-4900–010785.

32. Paul Martin, "Canada's Crusade Against Cancer," speech given at the Hunter College premiere of *Challenge*, March 13, 1950, NCI archives, AR-4900–010785.

33. Oscar R. Ewing, "Teamwork Looks to the Future," speech given at the Hunter College premiere of *Challenge*, March 13, 1950, NCI archives, AR-4900–010785.

34. George D. Stoddard, "Science and UNESCO," speech given at the Hunter College premiere of *Challenge*, March 13, 1950, NCI archives, AR-4900–010785.

35. Leonard Scheele, "By-products of Cancer Research," speech given at the Hunter College premiere of *Challenge*, March 13, 1950, NCI archives, AR-4900–010785.

36. Dietz, *Science Battles Cancer*; Dietz, *The War on Cancer*. For a program see NCI archives, AR-4900–010785.

37. Bruno Gebhart to National Cancer Institute, March 15, 1950, NCI archives, AR-4900–010785.

38. Marsh, "Health Museum Acquires."

39. Bruno Gebhart to Dallas Johnson, March 15, 1950, NCI archives, AR-4900-010785. See also "Available—At Last!"

40. Announcement in NCI archives, AR-4900–010785.

41. "Challenge: Science Against Cancer."

42. Stillman K. Taylor (assistant librarian, Gary Public Library) to Dallas Johnson, April 18, 1950, NCI archives, AR-4900–010785.

43. Unknown correspondent from ACS, Minnesota Division, to Dallas Johnson, March 14, 1950, NCI archives, AR-4900–010785.

44. O. H. Warwick (executive director, Canadian Cancer Society) to Dallas Johnson, February 23, 1950, NCI archives, AR-4900–010785.

45. Mrs. Egmont L. Frankel (president, Toronto Branch, Canadian Cancer Society) to Dallas Johnson, March 27, 1950, NCI archives, AR-4900–010785. Heller's speech is "Address by Dr. J. F. Heller at the Premiere of *Challenge: Science Against Cancer*, to be held in Toronto, Ontario, April 2, 1950," March 30, 1950, NCI archives, AR-4900–010785.

46. Mrs. Egmont L. Frankel to Dallas Johnson, March 27, 1950, NCI archives, AR-4900–010785.

Chapter 11

1. Druick, *Projecting Canada*, 55–57.

2. Much of the following discussion is derived from my two interviews with Colin Low, February 16, 2007, and May 2, 2007. See also my interviews with Morten Parker, February 1, 2008, and March 26, 2008.

3. "Commentary, *Challenge—Science Against Cancer*," NFB archives, *Challenge: Science Against Cancer*, production file 02-130, vol. 2, reel 1, p. 2.

"Commentary. *Challenge—Science Against Cancer*," February 6, 1950 (clean), NFB archives, *Challenge: Science Against Cancer*, production file 02-130, vol. 2, reel 1, p. 2. "Commentary. *Challenge—Science Against Cancer*," line 140, n.d. (heavily annotated), NFB archives, *Challenge: Science Against Cancer*, production file 02-130, vol. 2.

4. R. E. Dyer, "Establishment of Office of Scientific Reports," September 29, 1948, NCI archives, AR-4809-000143. The office brought together a number of existing units within the NIH including the Editorial Section, Library Section, Translating Section, Color Reproduction Section, Photographic and Research Section, and the Medical Art and Scientific Exhibits Section, all of which predated the Office of Scientific Reports.

5. Wiegand, "John E. Fletcher."

6. Don Reed to Jack Fletcher, March 17, 1950, NCI archives, no reference number, full text PDF 4780.4.

7. "Thousands See," 3.

8. Don Reed to Jack Fletcher, March 17, 1950, NCI archives, no reference number, full text PDF 4780.4.

9. Don Reed to Jack Fletcher, March 17, 1950, NCI archives, no reference number, full text PDF 4780.4.

10. *Attitudes and Health* (1949); *Rest and Health* (1949).

11. D.F. Smiley to David Ruhe, March 24, 1950, NFB archives, *Challenge: Science Against Cancer*, production file 02-130, vol. 1.

12. D. F. Smiley to David Ruhe, March 24, 1950, NFB archives, *Challenge: Science Against Cancer*, production file 02-130, vol. 1.

13. D. F. Smiley to David Ruhe, March 24, 1950, NFB archives, *Challenge: Science Against Cancer*, production file 02-130, vol. 1.

14. D. F. Smiley to David Ruhe, March 24, 1950, NFB archives, *Challenge: Science Against Cancer*, production file 02-130, vol. 1.

15. D. F. Smiley to David Ruhe, March 24, 1950, NFB archives, *Challenge: Science Against Cancer*, production file 02-130, vol. 1.

16. D. F. Smiley to David Ruhe, March 24, 1950, NFB archives, *Challenge: Science Against Cancer*, production file 02-130, vol. 1.

17. D. F. Smiley to David Ruhe, March 24, 1950, NFB archives, *Challenge: Science Against Cancer*, production file 02-130, vol. 1.

18. D. F. Smiley to David Ruhe, March 24, 1950, NFB archives, *Challenge: Science Against Cancer*, production file 02-130, vol. 1.

19. D. F. Smiley to David Ruhe, March 24, 1950, NFB archives, *Challenge: Science Against Cancer*, production file 02-130, vol. 1.

20. D. F. Smiley to David Ruhe, March 24, 1950, NFB archives, *Challenge: Science Against Cancer*, production file 02-130, vol. 1.

21. American Association of Medical Colleges, Medical Audio-Visual Institute, "Selection of Medical Films for Use by the Department of State," memo on *Challenge: Science Against Cancer*, c.1950–2, Nichtenhauser Papers, MSC277, box 20, folder reviews, R-S.

22. American Association of Medical Colleges, Medical Audio-Visual Institute, "Selection of Medical Films for Use by the Department of State Order No., 14547-(14)-52," memo on *Challenge: Science Against Cancer*, March 27, 1952, Nichtenhauser Papers, MSC277, box 20, folder reviews, R-S.

23. American Association of Medical Colleges, Medical Audio-Visual Institute, "Selection of Medical Films for Use by the Department of State," memo on *Challenge: Science Against Cancer*, c.1950–2, Nichtenhauser Papers, MSC277, box 20, folder reviews, R-S.

24. American Association of Medical Colleges, Medical Audio-Visual Institute, "Selection of Medical Films for Use by the Department of State," memo on *Challenge: Science Against Cancer*, c.1950–2, Nichtenhauser Papers, MSC277, box 20, folder reviews, R-S.

25. American Association of Medical Colleges, Medical Audio-Visual Institute, "Selection of Medical Films for Use by the Department of State," memo on *Challenge: Science Against Cancer*, c.1950–2, Nichtenhauser Papers, MSC277, box 20, folder reviews, R-S.

26. American Association of Medical Colleges, Medical Audio-Visual Institute, "Selection of Medical Films for Use by the Department of State," memo on *Challenge: Science Against Cancer*, c.1950–2, Nichtenhauser Papers, MSC277, box 20, folder reviews, R-S.

27. American Association of Medical Colleges, Medical Audio-Visual Institute, "Selection of Medical Films for Use by the Department of State," memo on *Challenge: Science Against Cancer*, c.1950–2, Nichtenhauser Papers, MSC277, box 20, folder reviews, R-S.

28. American Association of Medical Colleges, Medical Audio-Visual Institute, "Selection of Medical Films for Use by the Department of State," memo on *Challenge: Science Against Cancer*, c.1950–2, Nichtenhauser Papers, MSC277, box 20, folder reviews, R-S.

29. American Association of Medical Colleges, Medical Audio-Visual Institute, "Selection of Medical Films for Use by the Department of State," memo on *Challenge: Science Against Cancer*, c.1950–2, Nichtenhauser Papers, MSC277, box 20, folder reviews, R-S.

30. Erik Cripps and Marie L. Coleman, memo to Drs. Ruhe and Nichtenhauser, Medical Audio-Visual Institute, "Cancer Film Recommendations to State Department," February 4, 1952, Nichtenhauser Papers, MSC277, box 19, folder reviews, C-D.

31. American Association of Medical Colleges, Medical Audio-Visual Institute, "Selection of Medical Films for Use by the Department of State Order No., 14547-(14)-52," memo on *Challenge: Science Against Cancer*, March 27, 1952, Nichtenhauser Papers, MSC277, box 20, folder reviews, R-S.

32. Keller, Review of *"Challenge: Science against Cancer."*

33. Keller, Review of *"Challenge: Science against Cancer."*

34. Keller, Review of *"Challenge: Science against Cancer."*

35. Keller, Review of *"Challenge: Science against Cancer."*

36. Keller, Review of *"Challenge: Science against Cancer."*

37. Bill McClelland to Len Chatwin, Guy Glover, Paul Theriault, and Alan Field, May 1, 1950, NFB archives, *Challenge: Science Against Cancer*, production file 02-130, vol. 1.

38. Pierre Chaloult, "Report on the Preview in Quebec City, on Wednesday April 12, of the French version of the Cancer Film," April 15, 1950, NFB archives, *Challenge: Science Against Cancer*, production file 02-130, vol. 1.

39. Guy Glover to Jim [Beveridge?], September 22, 1950, NFB archives "Cancer (Theatrical), *The Fight Against Cancer*," production file 16–001.

40. Glover, "Film."

41. On Blakeslee, see Wilford, "Alton Blakeslee."

42. Blakeslee, *Polio Can be Conquered*. For more on this pamphlet see Rogers, "Polio Can be Cured," 91–93.

43. The two examples that Johnson provided were Blakeslee, "Pituitary Studies Aid Cancer Fight," and Blakeslee, "Rat Glands Grown in Glass." See NCI archives, AR-4900–010785.

44. Leonard Scheele, "By-products of Cancer Research," speech given at the Hunter College premiere of *Challenge*, March 13, 1950, NCI archives, AR-4900–010785.

45. There were some hopes of using ACTH in the treatment of leukemia, but this was not the focus of attention in Blakeslee's article. On cortisone see Haller, "Stress, Cortison und Homöostase"; Cantor, "Cortisone and the Politics of Empire"; Cantor, "Cortisone and the Politics of Drama"; Marks, "Cortisone, 1949"; Gaudillière, "From *Propaganda* to Scientific Marketing"; Rasmussen, "Steroids in Arms"; Quirke, "Making British Cortisone."

46. Blakeslee, "Rat Glands Grown in Glass."

47. Blakeslee, "Pituitary Studies Aid Cancer Fight."

48. Leonard Scheele, "By-products of Cancer Research," speech given at the Hunter College Premiere of *Challenge*, March 13, 1950, NCI archives, AR-4900–010785.

49. Dallas Johnson and C. W. Gilchrist, *"Challenge Science Against Cancer*: A Project Report on Promotion and Distribution," c.1950, NCI archives, AR-4900-010785, p. 27.

50. Dallas Johnson and C. W. Gilchrist, *"Challenge Science Against Cancer*: A Project Report on Promotion and Distribution," c.1950, NCI archives, AR-4900-010785, p. 31.

51. For example see Blakeslee, "Story of Cancer Fight." Other Blakeslee clippings from the Sunday papers are in Dallas Johnson and C. W. Gilchrist, "Challenge Science Against Cancer: A Project Report on Promotion and Distribution," c.1950, NCI archives, AR-4900-010785, pp. 31–34.

52. For example see Blakeslee, "Story of Cancer Fight."

53. Hunt, "Is Cancer Yielding."

54. Dallas Johnson and C. W. Gilchrist, *"Challenge: Science Against Cancer*: A Project Report on Promotion and Distribution," c.1950, NCI archives, AR-4900-010785, p. 35.

55. For more descriptive accounts see "Film Launches International Campaign on Cancer Research."

56. *"Challenge—Science Against Cancer," Educational Screen.*

57. *"Challenge Science Against Cancer," See and Hear.*

58. "You <u>Can</u> Teach About Cancer." See also Wells, "Science Teachers Join the Fight Against Cancer."

59. Erik Cripps and Marie L. Coleman, memo to Drs. Ruhe and Nichtenhauser, Medical Audio-Visual Institute, "Cancer Film Recommendations to State Department," February 4, 1952, Nichtenhauser Papers, MSC277, box 19, folder reviews, C-D. For a fuller condemnation see American Association of Medical Colleges, Medical Audio-Visual Institute, "Selection of Medical Films for Use by the Department of State Order No., 14547-(14)-52," memo on *From One Cell*, February 23, 1952, Nichtenhauser Papers, MSC277, box 19, folder reviews, C-D.

60. Starr, *"Challenge: Science Against Cancer."* See also Starr, "Films Everywhere . . ."

61. *"Challenge: Science Against Cancer," Film News.* See also "$200,000 Film Program to Help Fight Cancer."

62. Marsh, "Health Museum Acquires."

63. Marsh, "Health Museum Acquires."

64. Dallas Johnson and C. W. Gilchrist, *"Challenge Science Against Cancer*: A Project Report on Promotion and Distribution," c.1950, NCI archives, AR-4900-010785. For periodical articles on the film see *"Challenge—Science Against Cancer," Quick.*

65. "Real Progress on Cancer Cure."

66. Dallas Johnson and C. W. Gilchrist, "*Challenge Science Against Cancer*: A Project Report on Promotion and Distribution," c.1950, NCI archives, AR-4900-010785, p. 37.

67. Dallas Johnson and C. W. Gilchrist, "*Challenge Science Against Cancer*: A Project Report on Promotion and Distribution," c.1950, NCI archives, AR-4900-010785, p. 37. Johnson offered as an example one clipping, "Cancer News," *News-Sentinel* (Fort Wayne, IN) June 24, 1950, which included seven images.

68. William F. Bennett (chief, Acquisitions Section, Photographic Branch, International Press and Publications Division, State Department) to Dallas Johnson, June 23, 1950, NCI archives, AR-4900-010785.

69. The photograph was taken by Christian Lund in February 1950 after the live-action shoots were over. It is labeled "'Mr. Davis' worries about growth on cheek, decides to see doctor," NFB archives, publicity photos for *Challenge*, #51221.

70. Austin V. Deibert to David S. Ruhe, May 5, 1950, NFB archives, *Challenge: Science Against Cancer*, production file 02-130, vol. 1.

71. Austin V. Deibert to David S. Ruhe, May 5, 1950, NFB archives, *Challenge: Science Against Cancer*, production file 02-130, vol. 1.

72. Austin V. Deibert to David S. Ruhe, May 5, 1950, NFB archives, *Challenge: Science Against Cancer*, production file 02-130, vol. 1.

73. Austin V. Deibert to David S. Ruhe, May 5, 1950, NFB archives, *Challenge: Science Against Cancer*, production file 02-130, vol. 1. The Bethesda–Chevy Chase High School yearbook for 1950 does not mention this film show, nor does the student newspaper. My thanks to Sean W. Bulson, Brian Baczkowski, and John Virden for providing me with access to the yearbook and student newsletter, February 6, 2008.

Chapter 12

1. Austin V. Deibert, "Memorandum on Cancer Informational Material No. 14," April 11, 1950, NCI archives, AR-4900–010785.

2. Austin V. Deibert, "Memorandum on Cancer Informational Material No. 14," April 11, 1950, NCI archives, AR-4900–010785.

3. Austin V. Deibert, "Memorandum on Cancer Informational Material No. 14," April 11, 1950, NCI archives, AR-4900–010785.

4. For background see Hurewitz, *Bohemian Los Angeles*. On Ritchie see especially chap. 2.

5. Ritchie, *Printing and Publishing in Southern California*, 649; Ritchie, *The Ward Ritchie Press*.

6. Ritchie, *Printing and Publishing in Southern California*, 649.

7. National Cancer Institute, and American Cancer Society, *Proceedings of the First National Cancer Conference*. See also Ritchie, *The Ward Ritchie Press*, 131.

8. Ritchie, *Printing and Publishing in Southern California*, 650.

9. Ritchie, *Printing and Publishing in Southern California*, 651.

10. Hueper, *Environmental Cancer.*

11. Dallas Johnson to John Heller, "Relations between Cancer Report Section and Research Branch," May 19, 1949, box 19, folder 3, p. 5, Harold Leroy Stewart Papers, MSC 228.

12. Dallas Johnson to Ward Ritchie, n.d., box 31, folder 4, The Challenge of Cancer, Ward Ritchie Papers. Curiously, she signs this letter "Um" or "llm"

13. Dallas Johnson to Ward Ritchie, n.d., box 31, folder 4, The Challenge of Cancer, Ward Ritchie Papers.

14. Dallas Johnson to Ward Ritchie, n.d., box 31, folder 4, The Challenge of Cancer, Ward Ritchie Papers.

15. Hugh Jackson to Judson Hardy, "Matters For Discussion with Dallas Johnson," March 20, 1950, NCI archives, no reference number, full text PDF 4780.4.

16. The print run was 10,000 copies for distribution to among other groups science teachers, state health departments, Farm Service Agency regional offices, medical societies, public health educators, National Science Teachers Association, science departments of colleges, science writers, the NCI's National Advisory Cancer Council, *New York Herald Tribune* and for limited distribution at the 5th International Cancer Congress in Paris, July 1950; The cost breakdown for the book, including travel: Layout, design, typography (US$275); Art (US$300); printing of 10,000 copies (US$3,900)—total US$4,475. Hugh Jackson, chief, Cancer Reports Section, "Program and Project Report: Public Information, Publications and Public Relations Activities. National Cancer Institute, July–December, 1950," NCI archives, item number AR-5000–003912.

17. Dallas Johnson to Ward Ritchie, n.d., box 31, folder 4, The Challenge of Cancer, Ward Ritchie Papers.

18. Hugh Jackson, chief, Cancer Reports Section, "Program and Project Report: Public Information, Publications and Public Relations Activities, National Cancer Institute. July–December, 1950," NCI archives, item number AR-5000–003912.

19. Albert Tannenbaum to Dallas Johnson, March 9, 1951, NCI archives, AR-5100-010682. Tannenbaum was director of the Cancer Research Department, Medical Research Institute, Michael Reese Hospital, Chicago.

20. Howard B. Owens Science Center, "Who Was Howard B. Owens?" The committee comprised Howard B. Owens, chairman (Hyattsville High School); Mary E. Adams, Virginia C. Carney, Mary L. Davis; Thaddeus Elder Jr. (assistant in chemistry, University of Maryland College Park in 1948-9); Lillian Guis; Helena J. Haines (Greenbelt High School); James E. Lauer; Lucille M. Richmond; Pauline E. Saunders; and Mary A. Thompson.

21. "The Public's Health - Your First Concern No. 3. Cancer of the Stomach," NCI archives, AR-4808-006539. "Discussion between D. M. and Mrs. Dallas Johnson, in charge of film promotion for the National Cancer Institute, in Ralph Foster's office, 13.12.49," NFB archives, *What We Know About Cancer*, production file. On Karasik see Megan Rosenfeld, "'Government Girls.'" See also Karasik and Karasik, *The Ride Together.*

22. Teacher's guide: Production, distribution and promotional plans: 10,000 copies to be printed, and single copies will be made on special mailing lists to all state health officers, Farm Service Agency regional offices, science teachers, and health educators. Hugh Jackson, chief, Cancer Reports Section, "Program and Project Report: Public Information, Publications and Public Relations Activities, National Cancer Institute, July–December, 1950," NCI archives, Item Number AR-5000–003912.

23. National Cancer Institute. *Meeting the Challenge of Cancer.*

24. National Cancer Institute, *A Teaching Guide*, 2.

25. National Cancer Institute, *A Teaching Guide*, 8.

26. National Cancer Institute, *A Teaching Guide*, 2.

27. National Cancer Institute, *A Teaching Guide*, 3–6.

28. National Cancer Institute, *A Teaching Guide*, 7–11.

29. National Cancer Institute, *A Teaching Guide*, 8, 13.

30. Grant, *The Challenge of Cancer*, ii.

31. Grant, *The Challenge of Cancer*, 14, 22, 53, 77, 91, 94, 95, 97, 111.

32. Canadian research gets only one mention in the book in a chapter on environment and cancer (Grant, *The Challenge of Cancer*, 33), compared with the ten instances of the "National Cancer Institute" in the body of the book.

33. Grant, *The Challenge of Cancer*, 46, 51.

34. Grant, *The Challenge of Cancer*, 31–33.

35. Grant, *The Challenge of Cancer*, 20–21.

36. In the film some are identified by the narrator (such as the therapeutic technologies of X-rays, radium, and surgery, and research technologies such as [radio] isotopes, tissue culture), and others that were shown but not identified (Van Slyke apparatus, ultracentrifuge, Warburg apparatus, electron microscopes).

37. Hugh Jackson to Judson Hardy, "Matters for Discussion with Dallas Johnson," March 20, 1950, NCI archives, no reference number, full text PDF 4780.4.

38. "Discussion between D. M. and Mrs. Dallas Johnson, in charge of film promotion for the National Cancer Institute, in Ralph Foster's office, 13.12.49," NFB archives, *What We Know About Cancer*, production file.

39. Dallas Johnson to Dorothy McPherson, January 16, 1950, NFB archives, *What We Know About Cancer*, production file.

40. Dallas Johnson to Dorothy McPherson, January 23, 1950, NFB archives, *What We Know About Cancer*, production file.

41. Dallas Johnson to Dorothy McPherson, January 23, 1950, NFB archives, *What We Know About Cancer*, production file.

42. Storyboard, "*Challenge Science Against Cancer* Filmstrip," January 23, 1950, NFB archives, *What We Know About Cancer*, production file.

43. Dallas Johnson to Dorothy McPherson, January 23, 1950, NFB archives, *What We Know About Cancer*, production file.

44. Dallas Johnson, undated and unattributed MSS, 1950[?], p. 2. [Listed as "Cancer Research Educational Program/Challenge: Science Against Cancer Documentary Film/Challenge of Cancer Book" in the finding aid], NCI archives, AR-5000-010683.

45. Austin V. Deibert to Col. C. W. Gilchrist, February 28, 1950, NFB archives, *What We Know About Cancer*, production file.

46. Austin V. Deibert to Col. C. W. Gilchrist, February 28, 1950, NFB archives, *What We Know About Cancer*, production file.

47. Script, *Challenge–Science Against Cancer*, February 11, 1950, NFB archives, *What We Know About Cancer*, production file.

48. Dorothy McPherson, "CHALLENGE Filmstrip–U.S. Edition," June 21, 1951, NFB archives, *What We Know About Cancer*, production file.

49. "Meeting Re "Challenge" — May 25, 1950," NFB archives, *What We Know About Cancer*, production file.

50. "Meeting Re "Challenge" — May 25, 1950," NFB archives, *What We Know About Cancer*, production file.

51. Script, *Challenge–Science Against Cancer*, June 13, 1950, NFB archives, *What We Know About Cancer*, production file.

52. Dorothy McPherson, "CHALLENGE Filmstrip–U.S. Edition," June 21, 1951, NFB archives, *What We Know About Cancer*, production file.

53. Dorothy McPherson, "CHALLENGE Filmstrip–U.S. Edition," June 21, 1951, NFB archives, *What We Know About Cancer*, production file. See also F. W. Rouse to Dorothy McPherson, October 11, 1950, NFB archives, *What We Know About Cancer*, production file.

54. F. W. Rouse to Dorothy McPherson, March 29, 1951, NFB archives, *What We Know About Cancer*, production file.

55. Norman Chamberlin to Dorothy McPherson, April 9, 1951, NFB archives, *What We Know About Cancer*, production file.

56. On Kaiser's appointment and biography see Hugh Jackson, press release, February 14, 1951, NCI archives, AR-5102–000650.

57. Jack Olsen to Dorothy McPherson, July 31, 1951 "U.S. Version–WHAT WE KNOW ABOUT CANCER filmstrip"; Helen Marsh to Dorothy McPherson, June 18, 1951. Both in NFB archives, *What We Know About Cancer*, production file.

58. Dallas Johnson to Dorothy McPherson, January 16, 1950, NFB archives, *What We Know About Cancer*, production file.

59. F. W. Rouse to Dorothy McPherson, March 29, 1951, NFB archives, *What We Know About Cancer*, production file.

60. Dorothy McPherson, "CHALLENGE Filmstrip–U.S. Edition," June 21, 1951, NFB archives, *What We Know About Cancer*, production file.

61. Jack Olsen to Dorothy McPherson, December 4, 1951, "French Version of *What We Know about Cancer*," NFB archives, *What We Know About Cancer*, production file.

62 When the first announcements of its (impending) availability appeared (length: 30 to 50 frames) the specifications were: 35-mm black-and-white filmstrip, available with captions in English or French. "You Can Teach About Cancer," 106.

63. Scheele and Hilleboe, *Cancer Control*, 41.

64. "Notes on Short Version of Cancer Film," Ottawa, March 3, 1950, NFB archives: "Cancer (Theatrical), *The Fight Against Cancer*," Production file 16–001.

65. Ralph C. Ellis (theatrical distribution) to Don Mulholland and John Street, March 14, 1950, NFB archives: "Cancer (Theatrical). *The Fight Against Cancer*," production file 16–001.

66. Ralph C. Ellis (Theatrical Distribution) to Don Mulholland and John Street, March 14, 1950, NFB archives, "Cancer (Theatrical), *The Fight Against Cancer*," production file 16–001.

67. W. Arthur Irwin to Jim Beveridge, Guy Glover, Don Mulholland, and Len Chatwin, April 6, 1950, and W. Arthur Irwin to Guy Glover, April 11, 1950, NFB archives, "Cancer (Theatrical), *The Fight Against Cancer*," production file 16–001.

68. Guy Glover to David Ruhe, April 12, 1950, NFB archives, "Cancer (Theatrical), *The Fight Against Cancer*," production file 16–001.

69. RW Buckland(?), memo, "Advice of Production," April 17, 1950, NFB archives, "Cancer (Theatrical), *The Fight Against Cancer*," production file 16–001.]

70. Harold Betts to Guy Glover, April 13, 1950, NFB archives, "Cancer (Theatrical), *The Fight Against Cancer*," production file 16–001.

71. Guy Glover to Jim [Beveridge?], September 22, 1950, NFB archives, "Cancer (Theatrical), *The Fight Against Cancer*," production file 16–001.

72. W. A. Irwin, memo, "Production Request," April 12, 1950, NFB archives, "Cancer (Theatrical), *The Fight Against Cancer*," production file 16–001.

73. Invoice for CAN$18 from 104 Brentcliffe Road, Leaside, Ontario, June 23, 1950, and Requisition (#B-16077) for Simulating Healed Carcinamatous Lesion for Cancer Film for Mrs. Louise Gordon, 104 Brentcliffe Road, Leaside, Ontario, July 17, 1950, NFB archives, "Cancer (Theatrical), *The Fight Against Cancer*," production file 16–001. Note that the requisition includes the date April 18, 1950, shortly after production began.

74. Panda Photography invoice, April 29, 1950, NFB archives. "Cancer (Theatrical), *The Fight Against Cancer*," production file 16–001.

75. The orders for these tickets, dated April 14, 1950, and April 17, 1950, are in NFB archives, "Cancer (Theatrical), *The Fight Against Cancer*," production file 16–001.

76. Ross Millard, Clarkson, Ontario, Requisition #B-12272, April 24, 1950, NFB archives, "Cancer (Theatrical), *The Fight Against Cancer*," production file 16–001. On Millard and Ontario theater history see Saddlemyer and Plant, *Later Stages*, 52–53.

77. Draft letter to David Ruhe, September 26, 1950, NFB archives, "Cancer (Theatrical), *The Fight Against Cancer*," production file 16–001.

78. Morten Parker to David Ruhe, September 9, 1950, NFB archives, "Cancer (Theatrical), *The Fight Against Cancer*," production file 16–001.

79. Morten Parker to David Ruhe, September 9, 1950, NFB archives, "Cancer (Theatrical), *The Fight Against Cancer*," production file 16–001.

80. Draft letter to David Ruhe, September 26, 1950, NFB archives, "Cancer (Theatrical), *The Fight Against Cancer*," production file 16–001.

81. Morten Parker to David Ruhe, September 9, 1950, NFB archives, "Cancer (Theatrical), *The Fight Against Cancer*," production file 16–001.

82. Guy Glover to David Ruhe, April 12, 1950, NFB archives, "Cancer (Theatrical), *The Fight Against Cancer*," production file 16–001.

83. Raymond Massey to Paul Martin, May 4, 1950, file "Publicity Cancer," Morten Parker Papers.

84. Draft letter to David Ruhe, September 26, 1950, NFB archives, "Cancer (Theatrical), *The Fight Against Cancer*," production file 16–001.

85. Ralph Foster to Morten and Gudrun Parker, July 25, 1950, file "Publicity Cancer," Morten Parker Papers.

86. Draft letter to David Ruhe, September 26, 1950, NFB archives, "Cancer (Theatrical), *The Fight Against Cancer*," production file 16–001.

87. On Drainie see the biography written by his daughter Bronwyn Drainie, *Living the Part*. See also Fairbridge, "Drainie, John Robert Roy (1916–1966)."

88. Requisition (#B-16186) for CAN$157 (CAN$120 plus expenses) from John Drainie, 87 Harper Street, Toronto, October 16, 1950, NFB archives, "Cancer (Theatrical), *The Fight Against Cancer*," production file 16–001.

89. Commentary, "The Fight," October 12, 1950, NFB archives, "Cancer (Theatrical), *The Fight Against Cancer*," production file 16–001.

90. Guy Glover to Jim [Beveridge?], September 22, 1950, NFB archives, "Cancer (Theatrical), *The Fight Against Cancer*," production file 16–001.

91. Guy Glover to Jim [Beveridge?], September 22, 1950, NFB archives, "Cancer (Theatrical), *The Fight Against Cancer*," production file 16–001.

92. Guy Glover to Jim [Beveridge?], September 22, 1950, NFB archives, "Cancer (Theatrical), *The Fight Against Cancer*," production file 16–001.

93. T. V. Adams to Len Chatwin, "Re: *Challenge: Science Against Cancer*, English French," November 25, 1950, NFB archives, "Cancer (Theatrical), *The Fight Against Cancer*," production file 16–001.

94. L. Chatwin to Guy Glover, February 7, 1951, NFB archives, "Cancer (Theatrical), *The Fight Against Cancer*," production file 16–001.

95. Bill McClelland to W. Arthur Irwin, February 14, 1951, NFB archives, "Cancer (Theatrical), *The Fight Against Cancer*," production file 16–001.

96. Margaret Herrick (executive director, Academy of Motion Picture Arts and Sciences) to Clinton Kenny (NIH) and Donald Mulholland (NFB), March 13, 1951, NFB archives, "Cancer (Theatrical), *The Fight Against Cancer*," production file 16–001.

97. Margaret Herrick telegram to Donald Mulholland, March 22, 1951, NFB archives, "Cancer (Theatrical), *The Fight Against Cancer*," production file 16–001.

98. Penciled draft of telegram sent to Herrick, March 22, 1951, and penciled note to "Don" dated (curiously) March 31, 1951 (after the awards ceremony), NFB archives, "Cancer (Theatrical), *The Fight Against Cancer*," production file 16–001.

99. Goetz, "The Canadian Wartime Documentary."

100. O. H. Warwick (executive director of the CCS) to Mr. G. M. McClelland, February 22, 1951, and Don Mulholland, memo, "Record of Telephone Conversation

between Mulholland & Dr. David S. Ruhe," February 23, 1951 (11:30 a.m.), NFB archives, *The Outlaw Within*, production file 02–170.

101. Don Mulholland to A. Irwin, February 23, 1951, NFB archives, *The Outlaw Within*, production file 02–170.

102. F. W. Rowse (Assistant ot the Director, Information Services Division, Department of Health and Welfare) to Mr. G. M. McClelland (liaison officer, NFB), February 27, 1951, NFB archives, *The Outlaw Within*, production file 02–170.

103. Don Mulholland, memo "Record of Telephone Conversation between Mulholland & Dr. David S. Ruhe," February 23, 1951 (11:30 a.m.), NFB archives, *The Outlaw Within*, production file 02–170.

104. Don Mulholland to A. Irwin, February 23, 1951, NFB archives, *The Outlaw Within*, production file 02–170.

105. David S. Ruhe to W. Arthur Irwin, February 28, 1951, NFB archives, *The Outlaw Within*, production file 02-170. The absence of this credit had been noted by the US surgeon general, Leonard Scheele, earlier in February. The credit had been left out deliberately—perhaps with Ruhe's agreement—and the NFB realized that if they got a distribution contract on *The Fight* that they would have to put in a small FSA credit. L. W. Chatwin to Guy Glover, February 7, 1951, NFB archives, "Cancer (Theatrical), *The Fight Against Cancer*," production file 16–001.

106. W. Arthur Irwin to David S. Ruhe, March 5, 1951, NFB archives, *The Outlaw Within*, production file 02–170.

107. Memo, "Background information. 'The Outlaw Within,'" (n.d.), NFB archives, *The Outlaw Within*, production file 02–170.

108. Memo beginning "Cut Dup neg. pix," n.d., NFB archives, *The Outlaw Within*, production file 02–170.

109. Memo, "Background information. "The Outlaw Within,"" (n.d.), NFB archives, *The Outlaw Within*, production file 02–170.

110. Various versions of the commentary are in NFB archives, *The Outlaw Within*, production file 02-170. The final version is titled "Commentary for The Outlaw Within,"

111. Translations of the script are available in NFB archives, "Cancer," production file 05-239. The final version is Jacques Bobet (Traducteur), Gérard Arthur (Narrateur), "Cancer", 10 mars 1951.

112. Ferguson, *And Now*; Ferguson, *The Unmuzzled Max*. "CBC Radio's Max Ferguson dies."

113. Invoice from Max Ferguson, 65 Charles St. W., Apt. 4, Toronto, Ontario, dated March 13, 1951, for a total of CAN$99.30 (CAN$60 + expenses), NFB archives, *The Outlaw Within*, production file 02-170. An earlier invoice dated March 10, 1951, in the same file suggests that the recording took place on March 10. The expenses are lower, the total coming to CAN$90.75. Invoice from Gérard Arthur, 2080 Lincoln, Apt. 2, Montreal, for CAN$82.50 (CAN$60.00 + expenses), n.d. NFB archives, "Cancer," production file 05-239.

114. Copy of this text in is NFB archives, *The Outlaw Within*, production file 02–170.

115. "Commentary for The Outlaw Within," NFB archives, *The Outlaw Within*, production file 02-170, p. 4.

116. Jacques Bobet (Traducteur), Gérard Arthur (Narrateur), "Cancer", 10 mars 1951, NFB archives, "Cancer," production file 05-239, p. 2.

117 "Commentary for The Outlaw Within," NFB archives, *The Outlaw Within*, production file 02-170, p. 4.

118. "Commentary for The Outlaw Within," NFB archives, *The Outlaw Within*, production file 02-170, p. 4.

119. Jacques Bobet (Traducteur), Gérard Arthur (Narrateur), "Cancer", 10 mars 1951, NFB archives, "Cancer," production file 05-239, p. 2.

Conclusion

1. James F. Kieley, curriculum vitae, December 1, 1965, NCI archives, AR-6512-004346

2. Donaghy, *Grit*, 130.

3. Glover, "Film"; Guy Glover and Colin Low in Graham, *Canadian Film Technology*, 116.

4. Glassman and Wise, "Filmmaker of Vision," 24.

5. Benson, *Space Odyssey*, 71.

6. Sellors, "What in the World," 116.

7. For a brief mention see Anderson and Langton, *Health Principles*, 413.

8. Patterson, *The Dread Disease*; Rettig, *Cancer Crusade*; Strickland, *Politics, Science, and Dread Disease*; Rushefsky, *Making Cancer Policy*.

9. The Cancer Reports Section at the NCI (the organization that would become the public education component of the NCI's Office of Communications and Public Liaison [OCPL]), and the Office of Scientific Reports at NIH, later Scientific Reports Branch.

10. Arnold Schieman, biography file, NFB archives; "Gordon Petty CSC."

11. Adler, "Reminiscences," 1-2. Contrast these with the role of reporters in newspapers; see, for example, Aucoin, *Evolution of American Investigative Journalism*.

12. Bernays, *Biography of an Idea*; Tye, *The Father of Spin*.

13. "Home Movies" (advertisement).

SOURCES

Archives

Canada

Library and Archives Canada, Ottawa
   Department of National Health and Welfare Archives on Cancer and Film.
National Film Board of Canada archives, National Film Board of Canada, Montreal.
   Production files: *Challenge: Science Against Cancer, Alerte: Science Contre Cancer,
      The Fight: Science Against Cancer, The Outlaw Within, Le Cancer,* and *Ce Que
      Nous Savons du Cancer/What We Know About Cancer.*
   Biographical files: Maurice Constant, Clarke Daprato, Ralph Foster, Guy Glover,
      Evelyn Lambart, Colin Low, Grant McLean, Morten Parker, Arnold Schieman.
National Gallery of Canada
   Houghton's Silverware and Plating Ltd. Fonds.
Clara Thomas Archives and Special Collections, York University
   Louis Applebaum Papers.
University of Toronto
   University of Toronto Archives and Records Management Services
   Lagrimas Ulanday, records archivist, email January 30, 2008. Biographical material
      on Maurice Constant
   Department of Graduate Records, A73-0026/371 (53); Department of Information,
      A1978-0041/018 (03); and the People File. JJ Rae: Newspaper clippings and pho-
      tographs of Rae.
University of Waterloo, Ontario
   Oral History by Linda Kellar of Maurice Constant.

United States

William Andrews Clark Memorial Library, University of California, Los Angeles
   Ward Ritchie papers.
National Archives
   Record group 443, box 6.
National Cancer Institute, Bethesda, MD
   NCI Archives on *Challenge* listed in the Lion database: https://lion.nci.nih.gov/
      (On access to the Lion database see Cantor, "Finding Historical Records.")

National Library of Medicine, Archives and Modern Manuscripts Collection, History of Medicine Division
  Adolph Nichtenhauser Papers.
  Harold Leroy Stewart Papers.
Morten Parker papers. This is a private collection of material on *Challenge* held by the film's director, Morten Parker. Parker died after I viewed this collection, and its current location is unknown.
  Parker's copies of the shooting script.
  Correspondence and clippings files.
United Nations Archives and Records Section, New York
  Papers and records of the United Nations Film Board.

Interviews by Author

Dallas Johnson Read	In person, Chevy Chase, MD	March 23, 2005
Colin Low	Phone	February 16, 2007
	In person, Montreal, Canada	May 2, 2007
Morten Parker	Phone	February 1, 2008
	In person, New York, NY	March 26, 2008
Randy Bazilauskas	Phone	March 10, 2008
Arnold Schieman	Phone	December 15, 2008

Filmography

Anderson, Robert, dir. *The Feeling of Hostility*. 1948; National Film Board of Canada.
Anderson, Robert, dir. *The Feeling of Rejection*. 1947; National Film Board of Canada.
Blais, Roger, dir. *It's Fun to Sing*. 1948; National Film Board of Canada.
Ce Que Nous Savons du Cancer (filmstrip). 1950; National Film Board of Canada for the Information Services Division of the Department of National Health and Welfare.
Cherry, Evelyn Spice, dir. *That They May Live*. 1942: College of Medicine, University of Saskatchewan, for the Saskatchewan Cancer Commission.
Director unknown. *Attitudes and Health*. 1949; Coronet Instructional Films.
Director unknown. *The Cancer Crusaders*. 1947; unknown production company, British Columbia branch of the Canadian Cancer Society.Director unknown.
Director unknown. *Human Growth: A Classroom Film*. 1947; Eddie Albert Productions.
Director unknown. *Human Reproduction*. 1947; McGraw Hill Text-Films, Audio Productions, Inc.

Director unknown. *Rays of Hope*. 1937; Unknown production company for Saskatchewan Cancer Commission.

Director unknown. *Rest and Health*. 1949; Coronet Instructional Films.

Director unknown. Title unknown. c.1947; Canadian Cancer Society, London Unit.

Director unknown. Title unknown. 1947; produced by J. Ernest Ayres.

Director unknown. Title unknown (trailer). 1942–3; screened in Manitoba.

Director unknown. Title unknown (trailer). C. April 1946; unknown producer for the Canadian Cancer Society.

The Embryology of Human Behavior. 1950; Medical Film Institute of the Association of American Medical Colleges in cooperation with the Bureau of Medicine and Surgery and Office of Naval Research, Department of the Navy, from the studios of C.L. Welch.

Gansell, Alexander, dir. *Breast Self Examination*. 1950; New York: Audio Productions Inc. for the American Cancer Society and the National Cancer Institute of the US Public Health Service, Federal Security Agency.

Holm, Johannes, and V. F. Bazilauskas, dir. *The Diagnosis of Tuberculosis with an Improved Culture Medium*. C. 1942; Communicable Disease Center in cooperation with the Tuberculosis Control Division, US Public Health Service.

Hurtz, William T., dir. *Man Alive!* 1952; United Productions of America for the American Cancer Society.

Jackson, Stanley, dir. *Feelings of Depression*. 1950; National Film Board of Canada.

Kroitor, Roman, and Colin Low, dir. *Universe*. 1960; National Film Board of Canada.

Kubrick, Stanley, dir. *2001: A Space Odyssey*. 1968; Stanley Kubrick Productions/Distributed by Metro-Goldwyn-Mayer.

Lambart, Evelyn, and Norman McLaren, dir. *Begone Dull Care*. 1949; National Film Board of Canada.

Low, Colin, dir. *The Romance of Transportation in Canada*. 1952; National Film Board of Canada.

Low, Colin, dir. *Time and Terrain*. 1948; National Film Board of Canada.

Luey, W. Allen, dir. *Choose to Live*. 1940; United States Department of Agriculture Extension Service for the US Public Health Service and the American Society for the Control of Cancer.

McCorquodale, Claribel, producer. *A Nurse Looks at Radiology*. c. 1941; Department of Radiology, Toronto General Hospital.

McLaren, Norman, dir. *C'est l'aviron*. 1944; National Film Board of Canada.

McLaren, Norman, dir. *Fiddle-De-Dee*. 1947; National Film Board of Canada.

McLaren, Norman, dir. *Hoppity Pop*. 1946; National Film Board of Canada.

McLaren, Norman, dir. *Là-Haut sur ces montagnes*. 1945; National Film Board of Canada.

McLaren, Norman, dir. *A Little Phantasy on a Nineteenth-century Painting*. 1946; National Film Board of Canada.

McLaren, Norman. *Norman McLaren: The Masters Edition*. 2006; Montreal: National Film Board of Canada (DVD set).

McLaren, Norman, dir. *La Poulette grise*. 1947; National Film Board of Canada.

McLean, Grant, dir. *The People Between*. 1947; National Film Board of Canada for the United Nations Relief and Rehabilitation Agency.

Murphy, Owen, dir. *Enemy X*. 1942; Eagle Pictures for the American Society for the Control of Cancer and US Public Health Service.

Parker, Gudrun, dir. *Maps We Live By*. 1947; National Film Board of Canada.

Parker, Morten, dir. *Alerte: Science Contre Cancer*. 1950; National Film Board of Canada (in cooperation with the Medical Film Institute of the Association of American Medical Colleges) for the Department of National Health and Welfare, Canada, and the National Cancer Institute of the US Public Health Service, Federal Security Agency.

Parker, Morten, dir. *Cancer*. 1951; National Film Board of Canada (in cooperation with the Medical Film Institute of the Association of American Medical Colleges).

Parker, Morten, dir. *Challenge: Science Against Cancer*. 1950; National Film Board of Canada (in cooperation with the Medical Film Institute of the Association of American Medical Colleges) for the Department of National Health and Welfare, Canada, and the National Cancer Institute of the US Public Health Service, Federal Security Agency.

Parker, Morten, dir. *Family Circles*. 1949; National Film Board of Canada.

Parker, Morten, dir. *The Fight: Science Against Cancer*. 1951; National Film Board of Canada.

Parker, Morten, dir. *The Home Town Paper*. 1948; National Film Board of Canada in cooperation with Canadian Weekly Newspapers Association.

Parker, Morten, dir. *The Outlaw Within*. 1951; National Film Board of Canada (in cooperation with the Medical Film Institute of the Association of American Medical Colleges).

Parker, Morten, dir. *The Postman*. 1947; National Film Board of Canada.

Parker, Morten, dir. *The Stratford Adventure*. 1954; National Film Board of Canada.

Pichel, Irving, dir. *Destination Moon*. 1950; George Pal Productions, Inc.

Sturgis, Warren, dir. *From One Cell*. 1950; Sturgis-Grant Productions for the American Cancer Society.

Wellman, William A., dir. *The Story of G.I. Joe*. 1945; Lester Cowan Productions, distributed by United Artists.

Werker, Alfred L., dir. *Lost Boundaries*. 1949; Louis de Rochemont Associates and RD-DR Productions.

What We Know About Cancer (filmstrip). 1950; National Film Board of Canada for the National Cancer Institute of the US Public Health Service, Federal Security Agency.

Bibliography

Primary Sources

"3 New Health Movies Use Novel Technique." *Winnipeg Free Press*, January 24, 1948, 1.

"$200,000 Film Program to Help Fight Cancer." *Film News* 10, no. 5 (February 1950): 12–13.

American Association of Medical Colleges. *Minutes of the Proceedings of the Sixtieth Annual Meeting Held in Colorado Springs, Colo. November 7, 8 and 9, 1949*. Chicago: Office of the Secretary AAMC, c.1950.

American Cancer Society, National Education Association of the United States, and United States Office of Education. *Teaching about Cancer: Thoughts for School Administrators*. New York: American Cancer Society, 1950.

American Cancer Society. *1952 Annual Report*. New York: American Cancer Society, 1953.

———. *A Statement of Principles as a Guide to Cancer Education in the Schools*. New York: American Cancer Society, 1949.

———. *Suggestions on What to Teach About Cancer*. New York: American Cancer Society, 1949.

———. *Why Learn About Cancer?* New York: American Cancer Society, 1957.

American Society for the Control of Cancer. *Catalog of Educational Material*. New York: American Society for the Control of Cancer, c.1941 to c.1944.

Anderson, C. L., and Clair Van Norman Langton. *Health Principles and Practice*. Saint Louis: Mosby,

ART News 49, no. 9 (January 1951).

"Association of American Medical Colleges Opens Its Medical Film Unit." *Journal of the Association of American Medical Colleges* 24 (1949): 245–46.

"Available—At Last!" *Tone: The News Letter for Members and Friends of the Cleveland Health Museum* 11, no. 3 (April 1950): 2.

Berger, Monty. "Filming the Invisible." *C-I-L [Canadian Industries Limited] Oval* (April 1950): 12–13.

Blakeslee, Alton L. "Pituitary Studies Aid Cancer Fight." *New York Times*, March 14, 1950, 27.

———. *Polio Can be Conquered*. New York: Public Affairs Committee, 1949.

———. "Rat Glands Grown in Glass to Produce Scarce Hormones." *Richmond Times and Dispatch*, March 14, 1950, 27.

———. "Story of Cancer Fight Told in Biological 'Gangster' Film." *Oakland Tribune*, April 2, 1950, 22A.

Bloedorn, W. A., Joe E. Markee, and Robt. P. Walton. "Report of the Committee on Audiovisual Aids." *Journal of the Association of American Medical Colleges* 22 (1947): 129–36.

Brinkley, Samuel. "Industrial Research vs. Cancer Research." *Bulletin of the American Society for the Control of Cancer* 23, no. 8 (August 1941): 2.

Bryson, Lyman. *Science and Freedom*. New York: Columbia University Press, 1947.

Canadian Cancer Society. *Newsletter* no. 8 (February 10, 1947): 2–3, copy in Library and Archives Canada: RG 29, National Health and Welfare, Volume 189, File 311-C1-29.

"Cancer Committee Opens Drive to Raise $40,000 in County." *The Herald Statesman* (Yonkers, NY), November 6, 1942, 7.

Cancer Control Letter 10 (September 1, 1948): 3.

Cancer Control Letter 11 (October 22, 1948): 1–2.

Cancer Control Letter 19 (July 1, 1949): 2.

"Cancer: The Great Darkness." *Fortune*, March 15, 1937, 112–14, 162–79.

"Cancer: Health Education Film Shows Battle Being Waged Against This Dread Disease." *The Standard* (Montreal), April 1, 1950, 4–7.

"Cancer News." *News-Sentinel* (Fort Wayne, Indiana), June 24, 1950.

"Cancer Research Film is Studied." *Gazette* (Montreal), March 20, 1950.

Carroll, Lewis. *Through the Looking-Glass, and What Alice Found There*. London: Macmillan, 1872.

"Challenge! Science Against Cancer." *Canada's Health and Welfare* 5, no. 6 (March 1950): 6–7.

"Challenge: Science Against Cancer." *Film News* 10, no. 6 (March 1950): 8.

"Challenge: Science Against Cancer." *Films in Chicago* 1, no. 1 (March 1950): [1].

"Challenge—Science Against Cancer." *Educational Screen* 29, no. 4 (April 1950): 184.

"Challenge—Science Against Cancer." *Quick* (March 20, 1950): 16–17.

"Challenge Science Against Cancer." *See and Hear* 7, no. 5 (April 1950): 16.

Charlton, H. Richard. "Taking Cancer to School." *Bulletin of the American Society for the Control of Cancer* 23, no. 7 (July 1941): 3–5.

Clarkson, Adrienne. "Speech on the Occasion of the Unveiling of the MacKenzie-Papineau Battalion Monument." Ottawa, October 20, 2001. https://archive.gg.ca/media/doc.asp?lang=e&DocID=1331.

Curtis, Francis D., Otis W. Caldwell, and Nina Henry Sherman. *Everyday Biology*. Boston: Ginn, 1946.

Dallas, Helen. *The Consumer and the Anti-Chain Taxes*. Columbia, MO.: Institute for Consumer Education, Stephens College, 1939.

Davis, Watson. "Science and the Press." *Annals of the American Academy of Political and Social Science* 219 (January 1942): 100–106.

Deutsch, Albert. *The Shame of the States*. New York: Harcourt, Brace, 1948.

Dietz, David. *Science Battles Cancer: Reprints of a Series of Timely Articles*. Cleveland, OH: Cleveland Press, 1945.

———. *The War on Cancer*. Cleveland, OH: Cleveland Press, 1950.

Elias, Hans. "Principles of Scientific Teaching Film Production with Special Reference to the Medical Film." *Journal of the Association of American Medical Colleges* 25 (1950): 333–37.

Ellsey, D. M. "What Science is Doing to Combat Cancer." *Canadian Doctor* 16 (March 16, 1950): 36–39.

"Face the Facts about Cancer." Editorial, *Herald Statesman* (Yonkers, NY), April 30, 1946, 6.

"Film Launches International Campaign on Cancer Research." *Film World* (May 1950): 236.

Fish, H. D. "The Situation Confronting the Proposed Development of a Secondary School Cancer Control Study Program." *Bulletin of the American Society for the Control of Cancer* 25, no. 5 (May 1943): 51–54.

Friedwald, Eugene M. *Man's Last Choice; A Survey of Political Creeds and Scientific Realities*. New York: Viking, 1948.

Gerster, John C. A., and Susan M. Wood. "Cancer Education in New York City." *American Journal of Cancer* 15 (1931): 286–98.

Gilchrist, Lt. Col. C. W. "Canada Sees New Horizons for Health Education." *American Journal of Public Health* 37 (1947): 1415–20.

———. "Health Education in Canada." *Hospital Health Management* 11 (1948): 252–55.

Gilmour, Clyde. "Cancer Battle Film Draws Top Praise." *Vancouver Sun*, March 20, 1950, 6.

Glover, Guy. "Film." In *The Arts in Canada: A Stock-taking at Mid-century*, edited by Malcolm Ross, 104–13. Toronto: Macmillan, 1958.

Grant, Lester. *The Challenge of Cancer: A Research Story That Involves the Secret of Life Itself*. Bethesda MD: Federal Security Agency, US Public Health Service, National Institutes of Health, 1950.

Grierson, John. "The Documentary Producer." *Cinema Quarterly*, 2, no. 1 (Autumn 1933): 7–9.

Herzberg, Joseph G. *Late City Edition: An Account of the Organization and Preparation of a Newspaper*. New York: Holt, 1947.

Hill, Vernon R. "The Canadian Way of Life." *Progressive Education* 22, no.7 (May 1945): 26–29.

"Home Movies" (advertisement). *Popular Photography* 28, no. 4 (April 1951): 94.

Hoyle, Fred. "British Scientists Also Write." *The Saturday Review*, May 7, 1955, 30–31, 44–45.

Hueper, W. C. *Environmental Cancer*. Washington: Federal Security Agency, US Public Health Service, National Institutes of Health, National Cancer Institute, Cancer Control Branch, 1948.

Huettner, Alfred. *Fundamentals of Comparative Embryology of the Vertebrates*. New York: Macmillan, 1941.

Hunt, Morton M. "Is Cancer Yielding," *Parade* (April 16, 1950): 10–11.

"Idealists Fought the Good Fight in International Brigades." *Montreal Gazette*, November 4, 1996, A11.

Johnson, Dallas. *Facing the Facts about Cancer*. New York: Public Affairs Pamphlet No 38, 1951.

——— and Clarence C. Little. *Facing the Facts about Cancer*. New York: Public Affairs Pamphlet No 38, 1947.

——— and Elizabeth Bass Golding. *Don't Underestimate Woman Power: A Blueprint for Intergroup Action*. New York: Public Affairs Committee, 1951.

Johnson, Lee Z. "Status and Attitudes of Science Writers." *Journalism Quarterly* 34 (1957): 247–51.

Kaempffert, Waldemar. *Science Today and Tomorrow.* New York: Viking, 1939.

Keller, Caroline. Review of *"Challenge: Science Against Cancer* by National Film Board of Canada, Medical Film Institute of the Association of American Medical Colleges for the Department of National Health and Welfare and National Cancer Institute of the US Public Health Service." *American Journal of Nursing* 50, no. 12 (December 1950): 34.

"The King George the Fifth Silver Jubilee Cancer Fund for Canada." *Canadian Medical Association Journal* 32, no.2 (February 1935): 117–18.

Kirstein, Lincoln. "The Interior Landscapes of Pavel Tchelitchew." *Magazine of Art* 41 (February 1948): 49–53.

———. "The Position of Pavel Tchelitchew." *View: The Modern Magazine Series* 2, No.2 (May 1942).

Krieghbaum, Hillier. "American Newspaper Reporting of Science News." *Kansas State College Bulletin* 25, no. 5 (August 15, 1941): 1–73.

———. "The Background and Training of Science Writers." *Journalism Quarterly* 17 (1940): 15–18.

Lawrence, M. C. "Challenge: Science Against Cancer." *Health: Canada's National Health Magazine* (March-April 1950): 10–11, 31.

"Learning to Live." *Cancer News* 9, no. 4 (Fall 1955): 3, 9.

Little, Clarence Cook. *The Fight on Cancer.* New York: Public Affairs Committee, 1939.

———. (As C.C.L.) "Development of the Society's Secondary School Educational Program." *Bulletin of the American Society for the Control of Cancer* 25, no.9 (September 1943): 101.

———. "Schools and Cancer Education." *Bulletin of the American Society for the Control of Cancer* 23, no. 7 (July 1941): 2–3

Maisel, Albert Q. "Bedlam 1946: Most US Mental Hospitals are a Shame and a Disgrace. *Life* 20, no. 18 (May 6, 1946): 102–18.

"Maple Leaf Appears on German Streets." *Evening Citizen* (Ottawa), November 23, 1945. 12.

Marsh, W. Ward. "Health Museum Acquires a New, Excellent, 'Hopeful' Film on Subject of Cancer." *Cleveland Plain Dealer*, March 15, 1950.

Marshino, Ora. "The Expanded Federal Cancer Program." *Medical Woman's Journal* 55, no. 4 (April 1948): 21–24.

McCorquodale, Claribel. "A Nurse Looks at Radiology." *Canadian Nurse* 37, no. 9 (September 1941): 605–10.

———. "The Patient and Radiotherapy." *Canadian Nurse* 37, no. 10 (October 1941): 681–87.

McLaughlin, Will. "Films Reveal How Science Winning Fight Against Disease." *Ottawa Journal*, March 20, 1950.

Meader, R. G., and W. W. Payne. "Cancer Research Facilities Construction Grants." *Public Health Reports* 66, no. 24 (June 15, 1951): 762–68.

———, O. Malcolm Ray, and Donald T. Chalkley. "The Research Grants Branch of the National Cancer Institute." *Journal of the National Cancer Institute* 19, 2 (August 1957): 225–58.

Mider, G. B. "Research at the National Cancer Institute." *Journal of the National Cancer Institute* 19, 2 (August 1957): 191–223.

Moon, Truman J., Paul B. Mann, and James H. Otto. *Modern Biology*. New York: Holt, 1947.

National Cancer Institute. *Annual Report, Fiscal Year 1949. (July 1, 1948–June 30, 1949)*. NCI archives: AR-4900–010824.

———. *Annual Report, Fiscal Year 1950 (July 1, 1949–June 30, 1950)*.

———. *Meeting the Challenge of Cancer. (*A Supplement to *The Challenge of Cancer*, by Lester Grant). US Public Health Service Publication no.419. Washington: US Department of Health, Education and Welfare, Public Health Service, National Cancer Institute, 1955.

———. "National Cancer Act of 1937." https://www.cancer.gov/about-nci/overview/history/national-cancer-act-1937.

———. *A Summary Progress Report, Cancer Control Branch, National Cancer Institute, 1946-1949*. Bethesda[?]: National Cancer Institute, 1949.

———. *A Teaching Guide to the Challenge of Cancer*. Bethesda, MD.: Federal Security Agency, US Public Health Service, National Cancer Institute, 1950.

———, and American Cancer Society. *Proceedings of the First National Cancer Conference*. New York: American Cancer Society, 1949.

National Institute of Health. *The U.S. Fights Cancer: The Cancer Program of the National Cancer Institute*. Bethesda, MD: National Institute of Health, US Public Health Service and Health Education Institute (Raleigh, NC), August 1947.

"National Cancer Institute of Canada." *Canadian Medical Association Journal* 56 (1947): 325–26.

"New Educational Film—Challenge: Science Against Cancer." *Canadian Hospital* 27, no. 3 (March 1950): 36.

"Next Step—Teacher Training." *ACS Bulletin* 6, no. 1 (October 15, 1956): 3

Nieman Fellows. "Science in the Press." *Nieman Reports* 1 (April 1947): 11–12.

"90,000 Letters Carry Appeal of County Cancer Committee." *Herald Statesman* (Yonkers, NY), October 29, 1943, 11.

"Ontario." *Canadian Nurse* 41, no. 4 (April 1945): 321–22.

Parker, Morten. "Animating Cartoons Involves Precise Technique." *Saturday Night* 60 (June 9, 1945): 5, 23.

———. "Films for Trade Unions." *Canadian Forum* 24 (February 1945): 258–59.

———."Taking Films to the People." *Adult Education Journal* 4 (April 1945): 59–62.

"Personnel Briefs." *CDC Bulletin* 6, no. 1 (January-February-March 1947): 31-2.

"The Program of the National Cancer Institute." *Public Health Reports* 63 (1948): 501–28.

"Real Progress on Cancer Cure: Success in Two to Five Years." *U.S. News and World Report* 27, no. 17 (April 28, 1950): 13–15.

"A Project in Cancer Education." *Science Teachers News Bulletin* 9, no. 1 (April 1944): 19.

Ruhe, David S., and Trawick H. Stubbs. "A Method for the Curriculum Integration of Audiovisual Aids in Preventive Medicine and Public Health." *Journal of the Association of American Medical Colleges* 24 (1949): 10–20.

Saskatchewan Legislature. *Journals and Speeches, Saskatchewan Legislature-Session 1937.* 35 no. 25 March 31, 1937.

Scheele, Leonard. "The Cancer Problem of the United States Health Service." *Southern Medical Journal* 41 (1948): 237–45.

———. and Herman A Hilleboe. *Cancer Control: A Manual for Public Health Officers.* Albany: New York State Department of Health, 1952.

"Secondary Schools." *Bulletin of the American Society for the Control of Cancer* 25, no. 10 (October 1943): 115.

Smallwood, William M., Ida L. Reveley, Guy A. Bailey, and Ruth A. Dodge. *Elements of Biology.* Boston: Allyn and Bacon, 1948.

Smith, Ella T. *Exploring Biology.* New York: Harcourt and Brace, 1938.

———. *Exploring Biology.* 3rd ed. New York: Harcourt and Brace, 1949.

"Spanish-speaking Vets See ACS Films." *ACS Bulletin* 3, no. 2 (October 19, 1953): 2.

St. Maurice, Laurence. "Cancer Research in Pictures." *Canadian Nurse* 46, no. 3 (March 1950): 173–76.

Starr, Cecile. "Challenge: Science Against Cancer." *Saturday Review of Literature* 33 (October 28, 1950): 49.

———. "Films Everywhere . . ." *Saturday Review of Literature* 33 (July 8, 1950): 29–30.

Steelman, John Roy. *Science and Public Policy: A Report to the President.* Vol. 1, *A Program for the Nation.* Washington: The President's Scientific Research Board,1947.

Stewart, Helen R. "A Psychological Approach to the Problem of Lay Education in Cancer Control." *Bulletin of the American Society for the Control of Cancer* 23, no. 9 (September 1941): 7–11.

"Tenth Anniversary for McGraw-Hill's Text-Film Department." *Journal of Business Education* 33, no. 3 (December 1957): 131.

"Thousands See First Showing of Cancer Film." *NIH Record* 2, no. 5 (March 27, 1950): 3–4.

Tyler, Parker. "Human Anatomy as the Expanding Universe." *View: The Modern Magazine* series 6, no.3 (March/ Spring 1947): 7–8.

———. "Tchelitchew's World." *View: The Modern Magazine* series 2, no.2 (May 1942): n.p.

US Congress, Senate, *Cancer Research; Joint Hearings Before a Subcommittee of the Committee on Commerce, Senate and Subcommittee of the Committee on Interstate and Foreign Commerce.* 75th Congress, 1st Session, July 8, 1937. Washington.: US Government Printing Office, 1937.

———. Senate Committee on Foreign Relations, *Cancer Research; Hearings Before a Subcommittee of the Committee on Foreign Relations, United States Senate.* 75th Congress, 2nd session, *on S. 1875.* Washington: United States Government Printing Office, 1946.

"Unusual Film Is Screened in Ottawa." *Evening Citizen* (Ottawa), March 20, 1950.

"Unusual Film Is Screened in Ottawa." *Ottawa Citizen*, March 20, 1950.

Wells, Harrington. "Science Teachers Join the Fight Against Cancer." *The Science Teacher* (October 1950): 121–22, 145.

Westchester Cancer Committee. *Detectives Wanted!* Bronxville, NY: Westchester Cancer Committee, 1942.

———. *Youth Looks at Cancer.* New York: Brookville Press, 1940.

Weymouth, Clinton G. *Science of Living Things.* New York: Holt, 1941.

"You Can Teach about Cancer." *School Life* 32, no. 7 (April 1950): 104–6.

Biographical Sources

See also Biographical files in the NFB archives.

"Adelaide Brewster is Cancer Victim." *ACS Bulletin* 1, no. 23 (September 15, 1952): 4.

Adler, Alexander. "Reminiscences from the *NIH Record's* First Editor." *NIH Record* 51, no. 10 (May 18, 1999): 1–2.

Association Internationale du Film d'Animation. Special Issue. "Evelyn Lambart." *ASIFA Canada* 15, No. 3 (January 1988).

Bahaikipedia. "David Ruhe." *Bahaikipedia.* http://bahaikipedia.org/David_Ruhe.

Baker, Carl G. "Jesse P. Greenstein, Ph.D. (1902–1959)." *Cancer* 12, no. 4 (1959): i.

Beeching, William. *Canadian Volunteers, Spain, 1936–1939.* Regina: Canadian Plains Research Center, University of Regina, 1989.

Bernays, Edward. *Biography of an Idea: Memoirs of Public Relations Counsel Edward L. Bernays.* New York: Simon & Schuster, 1965.

Bhandari, P. L. *How to Be a Diplomat: Adventures in the Indian Foreign Service Post-Independence.* London: Quince Tree Publishing, 2013.

Blantz, Thomas E. *George N. Shuster: On the Side of Truth.* Notre Dame: University Press of Notre Dame, 1993.

Brook, Adrian G., and W. A. E. McBryde, *Historical Distillates: Chemistry at the University of Toronto Since 1843.* Toronto: Dundurn Press, 2007. Canadian Film Encyclopedia. "Jacques Bobet." Accessed January 4, 2021. https://cfe.tiff.net/canadianfilmencyclopedia/content/bios/jacques-bobet.

Connolley, Greg. "Ralph Foster Developed Australia's Film Board," *Ottawa Citizen,* August 28, 1948.

"CBC Radio's Max Ferguson dies." *CBC News* Posted: Mar 07, 2013. http://www.cbc.ca/news/arts/cbc-radio-s-max-ferguson-dies-1.1414648.

"David S. Ruhe, 1914–2005." *Bahá'í World News Service.* September 7, 2005. http://news.bahai.org/story/388.

"Dr. David S. Ruhe." *The Morning Call.* September 8, 2005. https://www.mcall.com/news/mc-xpm-2005-09-08-3617239-story.html

Dobson, Terence. "Norman McLaren: His UNESCO Work in Asia." *Animation Journal* 8, no. 2 (Spring 2000): 4–17.

———. *The Film Work of Norman McLaren.* Eastleigh: John Libbey Publishing, 2006.

Donaghy, Greg. *Grit: The Life and Politics of Paul Martin Sr.* Vancouver: University of British Columbia Press, 2015.

Dorland, Michael. "The Creation Myth: Jacques Bobet and the Birth of a National Cinema." *Cinema Canada* no. 106 (April 1984): 7–12.

Dowbiggin, Ian. "Prescription for Survival: Brock Chisholm, Sterilization and Mental Health in the Cold War Era." In *Mental Health and Canadian Society*, edited by James E. Moran and David Wright, 176–92. Montreal: McGill-Queen's University Press, 2006.

Drainie, Bronwyn. *Living the Part: John Drainie and the Dilemma of Canadian Stardom.* Toronto: Macmillan. 1988.

Dustoor, Phiroze Edulji. *American Days; A Traveller's Diary.* Bombay: Orient Longmans, 1952.

Ellis, Jack. *John Grierson: Life, Contributions, Influence.* Carbondale: Southern Illinois University Press, 2000.

Ervin, Randy G. "Men of the Mackenzie-Papineau Battalion: A Case Study in the Involvement of the International Communist Movement in the Spanish Civil War." Master's thesis, Carleton University, 1972.

Evans, Virginia J. "Wilton R. Earle 1902–1964." *In Vitro* 1, no. 1 (1965): vii.

Fairbridge, Jerry. "Drainie, John Robert Roy (1916–1966)." Canadian Communications Foundation in association with Ryerson University website on Canadian Broadcasting History, April 2003. https://broadcasting-history.com/personalities/drainie-john-robert-roy.

Farley, John. *Brock Chisholm, the World Health Organization, and the Cold War.* Vancouver: University of British Columbia Press, 2008.

Ferguson, Max. *And Now . . . Here's Max: A Funny Kind of Autobiography.* New York: McGraw-Hill, 1967.

———. *The Unmuzzled Max.* New York: McGraw-Hill Ryerson, 1971.

Fiore, Lois. "Lester Grant." *Nieman Reports* 59, no. 1 (Spring 2005): 113.

Gabler, Neal. *Winchell: Gossip, Power, and the Culture of Celebrity.* New York: Knopf, 1994.

Glassman, Marc, and Wyndham Wise. "Filmmaker of Vision; *Take One's* Interview with Colin Low, Pt.1." *Take One*, no. 23 (Spring 1999): 18–24, 29–31.

"Gordon Petty CSC." *Canadian Cinematography* 1, no. 4 (May-June 1962): 13.

Harrison, Dick. *W. O. Mitchell and His Works.* Toronto: ECW Press, 1991.

Howard B. Owens Science Center. "Who Was Howard B. Owens? The Life of Howard B. Owens PPT." https://offices.pgcps.org/Howard-B-Owens/Docs/Howard-b-owens-himself-photos/History-of-Howard-B-Owens/.

Howard, Victor, and Mac Reynolds. *The Mackenzie-Papineau Battalion: The Canadian* "In Memoriam, Larry McCance." *Canadian Labour* 15 (1970).

Karasik, Paul, and Judy Karasik. *The Ride Together: A Brother and Sister's Memoir of Autism in the Family.* New York: Washington Square Press, 2003.

Kirstein, Lincoln. *Tchelitchev*. Santa Fe, NM: Twelvetrees Press, 1994.

Lacey, Archie L. "In Memoriam Morris Meister (1895–1975): Scientist, Educator, Humanitarian—A Venerable Pillar of Science Education." *Science Education* 60 (1976): 289–90.

"Lambart, Evelyn Mary." In *Canadian Who's Who*, edited by Kieran Simpson and Elizabeth Lumley, 660. Toronto: University of Toronto Press, 1995.

"Larry M'Cance." *New York Times*, January 7, 1970, 43.

Latham, Sheila, and David Latham. *Magic Lies: The Art of W. O. Mitchell*. Toronto: University of Toronto Press, 1997.

Leddick, David. *The Homoerotic Art of Pavel Tchelitchev, 1929–1939*. North Pomfret, VT: Elysium Press, 1999.

Lenburg, Jeff. "Low, Colin." In *Who's Who in Animated Cartoons: An International Guide to Film and Television's Award-Winning and Legendary Animators*, by Jeff Lenburg, 216. New York: Applause Theatre & Cinema Books, 2006.

"Lieut.-Col. C. W. Gilchrist, O.B.E., E.D." *Canadian Medical Association Journal* 55 (1946): 424.

LoBrutto, Vincent. *Stanley Kubrick: A Biography*. New York: D. I. Fine Books, 1997.

"Matthew Gordon, News Executive, 84." *New York Times*, September 16, 1994.

Mazurkewich, Karen. *Cartoon Capers: The Adventures of Canadian Animators*. Toronto: McArthur & Company, 1999.

McArthur, Kerry. "The Fine Touch of the 'Country Mouse': Evelyn Lambart at the National Film Board." *Animation Journal* 22 (2014): 27–45.

McCarty, Clifford. *Film Composers in America: A Filmography, 1911–1970*. 2nd ed. New York: Oxford University Press, 2000 [1953].

Mitchell, Barbara, and Ormond Mitchell. *W. O.: The Life of W. O. Mitchell: Beginnings to Who Has Seen the Wind, 1914–1947*. Toronto.: McClelland & Stewart, 1999.

"Morris Meister." *Science Education* 50 (1966): 401–06.

National Film Board of Canada. "Evelyn Lambart." https://web.archive.org/web/20111001133334/http://www.onf-nfb.gc.ca/eng/portraits/evelyn_lambart.

"Newspaperman Named." *La Crosse Tribune*, March 7, 1950, 5.

Papineau-Couture, Isabelle. "Baillargeon, Marcel." https://www.thecanadianencyclopedia.ca/en/article/marcel-baillargeon-emc.

Petrou, Michael. *Renegades: Canadians in the Spanish Civil War*. Vancouver: University of British Columbia Press, 2008.

Pitman, Walter. *Louis Applebaum: A Passion for Culture*. Toronto: Dundurn Press, 2002.

Potvin, Gilles. "Belland, Jean." https://www.thecanadianencyclopedia.ca/en/article/jean-belland-emc.

Poussart, Annick. "Delcellier, Joseph." https://www.thecanadianencyclopedia.ca/en/article/delcellier-joseph-emc.

Pratley, Gerald. "Close-Up on Ralph Foster." *Canadian Television and Motion Picture Review* (June 1955): 17, 20.

Ramsay, Christine. "Cherry, Evelyn Spice (1906–90)." In *The Encyclopedia of Saskatchewan.* Regina: Canadian Plains Research Center, University of Regina. https://esask.uregina.ca/entry/cherry_evelyn_spice_1906-90.jsp.

Ritchie, Ward. *Printing and Publishing in Southern California,* Completed under the auspices of the Oral History Program, University of California, Los Angeles, The Regents of the University of California, 1969.

Rosenfeld, Megan. "'Government Girls': World War II's Army of the Potomac." *Washington Post,* May 10, 1999, A1.

Shimkin, Michael B. "Howard B. Andervont: An Appreciation." *Journal of the National Cancer Institute* 40, No, 6 (1968): xiii–xxv.

Sugarman, Martin. "Jews Who Served in the Spanish Civil War." In Jewish Virtual Library. http://www.jewishvirtuallibrary.org/jsource/History/spanjews.pdf.

"Sympathy for Chief: Ralph Foster Resigns Post on Film Board." *Toronto Globe and Mail,* December 21, 1949.

Wiegand, Ginny. "John E. Fletcher, 73; Was A Retired Merck Executive." *Philadelphia Inquirer,* February 15, 1988, B04.

Wilford, John Noble. "Alton Blakeslee, 83, Is Dead; A.P. Science Writer and Editor." *New York Times,* May 13, 1997.

"Wilton Robinson Earle: 1902–1964." *Journal of the National Cancer Institute* 35, no. 3, Supplement (September 1965): 3–13.

Wright, Harold H. *"His Name High in Two Mastheads:* Youthful Woodrow Wirsig, Occidental Alumnus, Is Editor of *Quick* and Executive Editor of the Equally-Famed *Look." The Phi Gamma Delta* 74, No. 1 (1951): 20–22.

Zuehlke, Mark. *The Gallant Cause: Canadians in the Spanish Civil War, 1936–1939.* Vancouver: Whitecap Books, 1996.

Secondary Sources

Acland, Charles R. "National Dreams, International Encounters: The Formation of Canadian Film Culture in the 1930s." *Canadian Journal of Film Studies* 3, no.1 (1994): 3–26.

Acland, Charles R, and Haidee Wasson, eds. *Useful Cinema.* Durham, NC: Duke University Press, 2011.

Aitken, Ian. *Film and Reform. John Grierson and the Documentary Film Movement.* London and New York, Routledge, 1990.

Aronowitz, Robert A. *Unnatural History: Breast Cancer and American Society.* New York: Cambridge University Press, 2007.

Aucoin, James. *The Evolution of American Investigative Journalism.* Columbia: University of Missouri Press, 2005.

Barnouw, Erik. *Mass Communication: Television, Radio, Film, Press; The Media and Their Practice in the United States of America.* New York: Rinehart, 1956.

Bartkowiak, Mathew J., ed. *Sounds of the Future: Essays on Music in Science Fiction Film.* Jefferson, NC: McFarland, 2010.

Beaulieu, Martin. "L'incursion de l'ONF dans la thérapie psychiatrique: Genèse, réalisation et pérennité de la série *Mental Mechanisms*." *Canadian Journal of Film Studies* 25 (2016): 46–66

Beers, Diane L. *For the Prevention of Cruelty: The History and Legacy of Animal Rights Activism in the United States.* Athens: Swallow Press/Ohio University Press, 2006.

Benson, Michael. *Space Odyssey: Stanley Kubrick, Arthur C. Clarke, and the Making of a Masterpiece.* New York: Simon & Schuster, 2018.

Birke, Lynda. *Feminism and the Biological Body.* Edinburgh: Edinburgh University Press, 1999.

Bonah, Christian, David Cantor, and Anja Laukötter, eds. *Health Education Films in the Twentieth Century.* Rochester: University of Rochester Press, 2018.

———, "Introduction." In *Health Education Films in the Twentieth Century.*

Boon, Tim. *Films of Fact: A History of Science in Documentary Films and Television.* London and New York: Wallflower Press, 2008.

Bowser, Eileen. *The Transformation of Cinema, 1907–1915.* Vol. 2, *History of the American Cinema.* New York: Scribner, 1990.

Breslow, Lester, Daniel Wilner, Larry Agran et al. *A History of Cancer Control in the United States, with Emphasis on the Period 1946–1971.* 4 vols. Bethesda, MD: Division of Cancer Control and Rehabilitation, National Cancer Institute, Department of Health, Education, and Welfare, Public Health Service, National Institutes of Health, 1977.

Brian, J. L. "'The New Generation': Mental Hygiene and the Portrayals of Children by the National Film Board of Canada, 1946–1967." *History of Education Quarterly* 43, no. 4 (Winter 2003): 540–70.

Buckner, Phillip A., ed. *Canada and the British Empire.* Oxford: Oxford University Press, 2008.

Bunnell, Charlene. "The Gothic: A Literary Genre's Transition to Film." In *Planks of Reason: Essay on the Horror Film*, edited by Barry Keith Grant, 79–100. Metuchen, NJ: Scarecrow, 1984.

Callen, Anthea. "Ideal Masculinities: An Anatomy of Power." In *The Visual Culture Reader*, 2nd ed., edited by Nicholas Mirzoeff, 603–16. London and New York: Routledge, 2002.

Cantor, David. "Cancer Control and Prevention in the Twentieth Century." *Bulletin of the History of Medicine* 81 (2007): 1–38.

———. "Choosing to Live: Cancer Education, Movies, and the Conversion Narrative in America, 1921–1960." *Literature and Medicine* 28 (2009): 278–332.

———. "Cortisone and the Politics of Drama, 1949–55." In *Medical Innovations in Historical Perspective*, edited by John V. Pickstone, 165–84. Basingstoke & London: Macmillan in association with the Centre for the History of Science, Technology and Medicine, 1992.

———. "Cortisone and the Politics of Empire: Imperialism and British Medicine, 1918–1955." *Bulletin of the History of Medicine* 67 (1993): 463–93.

———. "Finding Historical Records at the National Institutes of Health," *Social History of Medicine*, 28 (2015): 617–37.

———. "*Inside Magoo* (1960): Cancer and Comedic Commentary on 1950s America." In *Body, Capital, and Screens: Visual Media and the Healthy Self in the 20th Century*, edited by Christian Bonah and Anja Laukötter, 181–203. Amsterdam: Amsterdam University Press, 2020.

———. *Man Alive! (1952): Cartoon Fun with Cancer, Cars and Companionate Marriage in Suburban America*. Bethesda, MD: National Library of Medicine, 2014.

———. *The Reward of Courage (1921). A Rediscovered Cancer Film of the Silent Era.* Bethesda, MD: National Library of Medicine, 2013.

———. "Uncertain Enthusiasm: The American Cancer Society, Public Education, and the Problems of the Movie, 1921–1960." *Bulletin of the History of Medicine* 81 (2007): 39–69.

Cavell, Richard, ed. *Love, Hate, and Fear in Canada's Cold War.* Toronto: University of Toronto Press, 2004.

Clow, Barbara. *Negotiating Disease: Power and Cancer Care, 1900–1950.* Montreal: McGill–Queen's University Press, 2001.

Cole, Catherine. "Sex and Death on Display: Women, Reproduction and Fetuses at Chicago's Museum of Science and Industry." *The Drama Review* 37, no. 1 (1993): 43–60.

Colwell, Stacie. "*The End of the Road*: Gender, the Dissemination of Knowledge, and the American Campaign Against Venereal Disease during World War I." *Camera Obscura*, 10 (May 1992): 91–129.

Cromier, Jeffery. *The Canadianization Movement.* Toronto: University of Toronto Press, 2004.

Dimakopoulou, Stamatina. "Europe in America. Remapping Broken Cultural Lines: *View* (1940–7) and *VW* (1942–4)." In *The Oxford Critical and Cultural History of Modernist Magazines.* Vol. 2, *North America 1894–1960*, edited by Peter Brooker and Andrew Thacker, 737–58. Oxford: Oxford University Press, 2012.

Dorland, Michael. *So Close to the State/s: The Emergence of Canadian Feature Film Policy.* Toronto: University of Toronto Press, 1998.

Druick, Zoë. *Projecting Canada: Government Policy and Documentary Film at the National Film Board.* Montreal: McGill-Queen's University Press, 2007.

———. "UNESCO, Film, and Education." In Acland and Wasson, *Useful Cinema*, 81–102.

———and Gerda Cammaer, eds. *Cinephemera: Archives, Ephemeral Cinema, and New Screen Histories in Canada.* Montreal: McGill-Queen's University Press, 2014.

Dubow, Sara. *Ourselves Unborn: Fetal Meanings in Modern America.* Oxford: Oxford University Press, 2011.

Duden, Barbara. *Disembodying Women: Perspectives on Pregnancy and the Unborn*, translated by Lee Hoinacki. Cambridge, MA.: Harvard University Press, 1993.

Duflour, Paul. "'Eggheads' and Espionage: The Gouzenko Affair in Canada." *Journal of Canadian Studies* 16 (Fall/Winter 1981): 188–98.

Edwardson, Ryan. *Canadian Content: Culture and the Quest for Nationhood*. Toronto: University of Toronto Press, 2008.

Ellis, Jack C. *John Grierson: Life, Contributions, Influence*. Carbondale: Southern Illinois University Press, 2000.

Elston, Mary Ann. "Women and Anti-Vivisection in Victorian England, 1870–1900." In *Vivisection in Historical Perspective*, edited by Nicolaas A. Rupke, 259–94. London and New York: Croom Helm, 1987.

Evans, Gary. *In the National Interest: A Chronicle of the National Film Board of Canada from 1949 to 1989*. Toronto: University of Toronto Press, 1991.

———. *John Grierson and the National Film Board: The Politics of Wartime Propaganda*. Toronto: University of Toronto Press, 1984.

Evans, Joyce A. *Celluloid Mushroom Clouds: Hollywood and the Atomic Bomb*. Boulder, CO: Westview Press, 1998.

Ewen, Stuart. *P.R!: A Social History of Spin*. New York: Basic Books, 1996.

Fabre, Michel. *The Unfinished Quest of Richard Wright*. New York: Morrow, 1973.

Finkel, Alvin. *Social Policy and Practice in Canada: A History*. Waterloo: Wilfrid Laurier University Press, 2006.

Forsyth, Scott. "The Failures of Nationalism and Documentary: *Grierson and Gouzenko*." *Canadian Journal of Film Studies* 1, no. 1 (1991): 74–82.

Gaarder, Emily. *Women and the Animal Rights Movement*. New Brunswick, NJ: Rutgers University Press, 2011.

Gardner, Kirsten E. *Early Detection: Women, Cancer, and Awareness Campaigns in the Twentieth-Century United States*. Chapel Hill: University of North Carolina Press, 2006.

Gaudillière, Jean-Paul. "From *Propaganda* to Scientific Marketing: Schering, Cortisone, and the Construction of Drug Markets." *History and Technology* 29 (2013): 188–209.

Gittings, Christopher E. *Canadian National Cinema: Ideology, Difference Representation*. London and New York: Routledge, 2002.

Goetz, William. "The Canadian Wartime Documentary: 'Canada Carries On' and 'The World in Action.'" *Cinema Journal* 16 (1977): 59–80.

Gorbman, Claudia. *Unheard Melodies: Narrative Film Music*. London: BFI Publishing; Bloomington, Indiana: Indiana University Press, 1987.

Grace, Sherrill E. *Sursum Corda!: The Collected Letters of Malcolm Lowry*, Vol. 2, *1947–1957*. Toronto: University of Toronto Press, 1995–1997.

Graham, Gerald G. *Canadian Film Technology, 1896–1986*. Newark: University of Delaware Press; London: Associated University Presses, 1989.

Haller, Lea. "Stress, Cortison und Homöostase. Künstliche Nebennierenrindenhormone und physiologisches Gleichgewicht,1936–1960." *NTM Zeitschrift für Geschichte der Wissenschaften, Technik und Medizin* 18 (2010): 169–95.

Hansen, Bert. *Picturing Medical Progress from Pasteur to Polio: A History of Mass Media Images and Popular Attitudes in America*. New Brunswick, NJ: Rutgers University Press, 2009.

Harcourt, Peter. "Some Relationships between the NFB Animation Department and the Documentary." In *John Grierson and the NFB*, compiled by The John Grierson Project, McGill University,152–62. Toronto: ECW Press. 1984.

Harrison, Helen Elizabeth. "In the Picture of Health: Portraits of Health, Disease and Citizenship in Canada's Public Health Advice Literature, 1920–1960." PhD diss., Queen's University, 2001.

Hayter, Charles. *An Element of Hope: Radium and the Response to Cancer in Canada, 1900–1940*. Montreal: McGill-Queen's University Press, 2005.

Hayward, Philip, ed. *Off the Planet: Music, Sound and Science Fiction Cinema*. London: John Libbey, 2004.

Hediger, Vinzenz and Patrick Vondrau, eds. *Films That Work: Industrial Film and Productivity of Media*. Amsterdam: Amsterdam University Press, 2009.

———. "Introduction." In *Films That Work*, 9–16.

Hopkins, Lisa. *Screening the Gothic*. Austin: University of Texas Press, 2005.

Hopwood, Nick. *Haeckel's Embryos: Images, Evolution, and Fraud*. Chicago: University of Chicago Press, 2015.

Hurewitz, Daniel. *Bohemian Los Angeles and the Making of Modern Politics*. Berkeley: University of California Press, 2007.

James, C. Rodney. *Film as a National Art: The National Film Board of Canada and the Film Board Idea*. Dissertations on Film Series. New York: Arno, 1977.

Johnson, David K. *The Lavender Scare: The Cold War Persecution of Gays and Lesbians in the Federal Government*. Chicago: University of Chicago Press, 2004.

Jones, D. B. *The Best Butler in the Business: Tom Daly of the National Film Board of Canada*. Toronto: University of Toronto Press, 1996.

———. *Movies and Memoranda: An Interpretive History of the National Film Board of Canada*. Canadian Film Series. Ottawa: Canadian Film Institute/ Deneau, 1981

Jülich, Solveig. "Colouring the Human Landscapes: Lennart Nilsson and the Spectacular World of Scanning Electron Micrographs." *Nuncius: Annali di Storia della Scienza* 29 (2014): 464–97.

———. "Fetal Photography in the Age of Cool Media." In *History of Participatory Media: Politics and Publics, 1750–2000*, edited by Anders Ekström, Solveig Jülich, Frans Lundgren, and Per Wisselgren, 125–41. New York: Routledge, 2011.

———. "Lennart Nilsson's *A Child Is Born*: The Many Lives of a Best-Selling Pregnancy Advice Book." *Culture Unbound: Journal of Current Cultural Research* 7 (2015): 627–48.

———. "Lennart Nilsson's Fish-Eyes: A Photographic and Cultural History of Views from Below." *Konsthistorisk Tidskrift* 84 (2015): 75–92.

———. "The Making of a Best-selling Book on Reproduction: Lennart Nilsson's A Child Is Born." *Bulletin of The History of Medicine* 89 (2015): 491–525.

———. "Picturing Abortion Opposition in Sweden: Lennart Nilsson's Early Photographs of Embryos and Fetuses." *Social History of Medicine* 31 (2018): 278–307.

Kaiser, David. "Cold War Requisitions, Scientific Manpower, and the Production of American Physicists after World War II." *Historical Studies in the Physical and Biological Sciences* 33 (2002): 131–59.

———. "The Postwar Suburbanization of American Physics." *American Quarterly* 56 (2004): 851–88.

Kavka, John. "The Gothic on Screen." In *The Cambridge Companion to Gothic Fiction*, edited by Jerrold E. Hogle, 209–28. Cambridge: Cambridge University Press, 2002.

Kaye, Heidi. "Gothic Film." In *A Companion to the Gothic*, edited by David Punter, 180–92. Oxford and Malden, MA.: Blackwell, 2000.

Kevles, Daniel J. *The Physicists: The History of a Scientific Community in Modern America*. New York: Knopf, 1978.

Khouri, Malek and Darrell Varga. *Working on Screen: Representations of the Working Class in Canadian Cinema*. Toronto: University of Toronto Press, 2006.

Kirby, David A. *Lab Coats in Hollywood: Science, Scientists, and Cinema*. Cambridge, MA: MIT Press, 2011.

———. "Scientists on the Set: Science Consultants and the Communication of Science in Visual Fiction." *Public Understanding of Science*, 12 (2003): 261–73.

Klossner, Michael. "Horror on Film and Television." In *Horror Literature: A Reader's Guide*, edited by Neil Barron, 426–49. New York: Garland, 1990.

Knight, Amy. *How the Cold War Began: The Gouzenko Affair and the Hunt for Soviet Spies*. Toronto: McClelland and Stewart, 2005.

Kristmanson, Mark. "Love Your Neighbor: The Royal Canadian Mounted Police and the National Film Board, 1948–1953." *Film History* 10 (1998): 254–74.

Kuhn, Annette. *Cinema, Censorship, and Sexuality*, 1909–1925. London and New York: Routledge, 1988).

Kuo, Liangwen. *Migration Documentary Films in Postwar Australia*. Amherst, NY: Cambria, 2010.

Landecker, Hannah. *Culturing Life: How Cells Became Technologies*. Cambridge, MA: Harvard University Press, 2007.

Landsbury, Coral. *The Old Brown Dog: Women, Workers, and Vivisection in Edwardian England*. Madison: University of Wisconsin Press, 1985.

Langlois, Suzanne. "And Action! UN and UNESCO Coordinating Information Films, 1945–1951." In *A History of UNESCO: Global Actions and Impacts*, edited by Poul Duedahl, 73–96. New York: Palgrave Macmillan, 2016.

Lebas, Elizabeth. "*'Where There's Life, There's Soap'*: Municipal Public Health Films and Municipal Cinema in Britain between the Wars." In *Health Education Films in the Twentieth Century*, edited by Christian Bonah, David Cantor, and Anja Laukötter, 225–42. Rochester: University of Rochester Press, 2018.

Lederer, Susan E. "Hollywood and Human Experimentation. Representing Medical Research in Popular Film." In *Medicine's Moving Pictures: Medicine, Health, and Bodies in American Film and Television*, edited by Leslie J. Reagan, Nancy Tomes, and Paula A. Treichler, 282–306. Rochester: University of Rochester Press, 2007.

———. *Subjected to Science: Human Experimentation in America before the Second World War*. Baltimore: Johns Hopkins University Press, 1997.

Lerner, Barron H. *The Breast Cancer Wars: Hope, Fear, and the Pursuit of a Cure in Twentieth-century America*. New York: Oxford University Press, 2001.

Low, Brian J. *NFB Kids. Portrayals of Children by the National Film Board of Canada, 1939–1989*. Waterloo: Wilfrid Laurier University Press, 2006.

Macbeth, Robert A. "The Origin of the Canadian Cancer Society." *Canadian Bulletin of Medical History* 22 (2005): 155–73.

Macdonald, Shannon. "The History of Cancer Treatment in Nova Scotia." *Dalhousie Medical Journal* (Spring 2003). http://medjournal.medicine.dal.ca/DMJONLIN/spring03/history%20ccns.htm.

Marks, Harry. "Cortisone, 1949: A Year in the Political Life of a Drug." *Bulletin of the History of Medicine* 66 (1992): 419–39.

Marsh, Bill. "Visual Education in the United States and the 'Fly Pest' Campaign of 1910." *Historical Journal of Film, Radio and Television* 30 (2010): 21–36.

McCurdy, Howard E. *Space and the American Imagination*. 2nd ed. Baltimore: Johns Hopkins University Press, 2011.

Morgan, Lynn. *Icons of Life: A Cultural History of Human Embryos*. Berkeley: University of California Press, 2009.

Morris, Nigel. "Metropolis and the Modernist Gothic." In *Gothic Modernisms*, edited by Andrew Smith and Jeff Wallace, 188–206. Houndmills, Basingstoke and New York: Palgrave Macmillan, 2001.

Morris, Peter. "After Grierson: The National Film Board, 1945–1953." *Journal of Canadian Studies* 16 (1981): 3–12.

National Library of Medicine. Mary Lasker Papers. https://profiles.nlm.nih.gov/TL/

Nessen, Susan. "Surrealism in Exile: The Early New York Years." PhD diss., Boston University, 1986.

Noe, Adrienne. "The Human Embryo Collection." In *Centennial History of the Carnegie Institution of Washington*. Vol. 5, The Department of Embryology, edited by Jane Maienschein, Marie Glitz, and Garland E. Allen, 21–61. Cambridge: Cambridge University Press, 2004.

Nourie, Alan. "*Look*." In *American Mass-Market Magazines*, edited by Alan Nourie and Barbara Nourie, 225–33. Westport, CT: Greenwood Press, 1990.

O'Donnell, Victoria. "Science Fiction Films and Cold War Anxiety." In *Transforming the Screen: 1950–1959*, edited by Peter Lev, 169–96. Berkeley: University of California Press, 2007.

Orgeron, Devin, Marsha Orgeron, and Dan Streible, eds. *Learning with the Lights Off: Educational Film in the United States*. Oxford and New York: Oxford University Press, 2012.

Ostherr, Kirsten. "Cinema as Universal Language of Health Education: Translating Science in Unhooking the Hookworm (1920)." In *The Educated Eye: Visual Culture and Pedagogy in the Life Sciences*, edited by Nancy Anderson and Michael R Dietrich, 121–40. Hanover, NH: Dartmouth College Press, 2012.

———. *Medical Visions: Producing the Patient through Film, Television, and Imaging Technologies*. Oxford and New York: Oxford University Press, 2013.

Parry, Manon. *Broadcasting Birth Control: Mass Media and Family Planning*. New Brunswick, NJ: Rutgers University Press, 2013.

———. "'Pictures with a Purpose': The Birth Control Debate on the Big Screen." *Journal of Women's History* 23 (2011): 108–30.

Patterson, James T. *The Dread Disease: Cancer and Modern American Culture*. Cambridge, MA: Harvard University Press, 1987.

Payne, Carol. *The Official Picture: The National Film Board of Canada's Still Photography Division and the Image of Canada, 1941–1971*. Montreal: McGill-Queen's University Press, 2013.

Pernick, Martin S. *The Black Stork: Eugenics and the Death of "Defective" Babies in American Medicine and Motion Pictures Since 1915*. New York: Oxford University Press, 1996.

———. "More than Illustrations: Early Twentieth-Century Health Films as Contributors to the Histories of Medicine and of Motion Pictures." In *Medicine's Moving Pictures: Medicine, Health, and Bodies in American Film and Television*, edited by Leslie J. Reagan, Nancy Tomes, and Paula A. Treichler, 19-35. Rochester: University of Rochester Press, 2007.

———. "Thomas Edison's Tuberculosis Films: Mass Media and Health Propaganda." *The Hastings Center Report* 8, no. 3 (June 1978): 21–27.

Petchesky, Rosalind Pollack. "Fetal Images: The Power of Visual Culture in the Politics of Reproduction." *Feminist Studies* 13, no. 2 (1987): 263–63.

Posner, Miriam. "Communicating Disease: Tuberculosis, Narrative, and Social Order in Thomas Edison's Red Cross Seal Films." In *Learning with the Lights Off: Educational Film in the United States*, edited by Orgeron, Devin, Marsha Orgeron, and Dan Streible, 90-106. Oxford and New York: Oxford University Press, 2012.

———. "Prostitutes, Charity Girls, and *The End of the Road*: Hostile Worlds of Sex and Commerce in an Early Sexual Hygiene Film." In *Health Education Films in the Twentieth Century*, edited by Christian Bonah, David Cantor, and Anja Laukötter, 173-87. Rochester: University of Rochester Press, 2018.

Quirke, Viviane. "Making British Cortisone: Glaxo and the Development of Corticosteroid Drugs in the UK in the 1950s and 1960s." *Studies in History and Philosophy of Science Part C: Studies in History and Philosophy of Biological and Biomedical Sciences* 36 (2005): 645–74.

Rasmussen, Nicolas. "Steroids in Arms: Science, Government, Industry, and the Hormones of the Adrenal Cortex in the United States, 1930–1950." *Medical History* 46 (2002): 299–234.

Reagan, Leslie J. "Engendering the Dread Disease: Women, Men, and Cancer." *American Journal of Public Health* 87 (1997): 1779–87.

———. "Projecting Breast Cancer: Self-Examination Films and the Making of a New Cultural Practice." In *Medicine's Moving Pictures: Medicine, Health, and Bodies in American Film and Television*, edited by Leslie J. Reagan, Nancy Tomes, and Paula A. Treichler, 163-96. Rochester: University of Rochester Press, 2007.

Reagan, Nancy J., Nancy Tomes, and Paula A Treichler. *Medicine's Moving Pictures: Medicine, Health, and Bodies in American Film and Television*. Rochester.: University of Rochester Press, 2007.

Rettig, Richard. *Cancer Crusade; The Story of the National Cancer Act of 1971*. Washington: Joseph Henry Press, 1977.

Ritchie, Ward. *The Ward Ritchie Press, and Anderson, Ritchie & Simon*. Los Angeles: Anderson, Ritchie & Simon, 1961.

Robinson, Judith. *Noble Conspirator: Florence S. Mahoney and the Rise of the National Institutes of Health*. Washington: Francis Press, 2001.

Rodney, James, C. *Film as National Art: The NFB of Canada and the Film Board Idea*. New York: Arno, 1977.

Rogers, Naomi. "Polio Can be Cured: Science and Health Propaganda in the United States from Polio Polly to Jonas Salk." In *Silent Victories: The History and Practice of Public Health in Twentieth-Century America*, edited by John Ward and Christopher Warren, 81–101. New York: Oxford University Press, 2007.

Rudolph, John L. *Scientists in the Classroom: The Cold War Reconstruction of American Science Education*. New York: Palgrave Macmillan, 2002.

Rushefsky, Mark E. *Making Cancer Policy*. Albany: State University of New York Press, 1986.

Saddlemyer, Ann, and Richard Plant. *Later Stages: Essays in Ontario Theatre from World War I to the 1970s*. Toronto: University of Toronto Press, 1997.

Scahill, Andrew. "Invasion of the Husband Snatchers: Masculine Crisis and the Lavender Menace in *I Married a Monster from Outer Space*." In *Horrifying Sex: Essays on Sexual Difference in Gothic Literature*, edited by Ruth Bienstock Anolik, 188–200. Jefferson, NC: McFarland, 2007.

Schaefer, Eric. *Bold! Daring! Shocking! True! A History of Exploitation Films, 1919–1959* (Durham, NC: Duke University Press, 1999).

Scheffler, Robin Wolfe. *A Contagious Cause: The American Hunt for Cancer Viruses and the Rise of Molecular Medicine*. Chicago: University of Chicago Press, 2019.

Schneider, Steven J. "Mixed Blood Couples: Monsters and Miscegenation in U.S. Horror Cinema." In *The Gothic Other: Racial and Social Constructions in the Literary Imagination*, edited by Ruth Bienstock Anolik and Douglas L. Howard, 72–89. Jefferson, NC: McFarland, 2004.

Sellors, C. Paul. "What in the World Distinguishes Fiction from Nonfiction Film?" *Film and Philosophy* 18 (2014): 105–23.

Shapin, Steven. *The Scientific Life: A Moral History of a Late Modern Vocation*. Chicago: University of Chicago Press, 2008

———. "Who is the Industrial Scientist? Commentary from Academic Sociology and from the Shop-Floor in the United States, ca. 1900– ca. 1970." In *The Science-Industry Nexus: History, Policy, Implications: Nobel Symposium 123*, edited by Karl Grandin, Nina Wormbs, and Sven Widmalm, 337–63. Sagamore Beach, MA: Science History Publications, 2004.

Shephard, David A. E. "First in Fear and Dread: Cancer Control in Saskatchewan, the First Decade." *Canadian Bulletin of Medical History* 20 (2003): 323–42.

Skal, David J. *The Monster Show: A Cultural History of Horror*. rev. ed. New York: Faber and Faber, 2001.

Spottiswoode, Raymond. *Film and Its Techniques*. Berkeley: University of California Press, 1951.

Strickland, Stephen. *Politics, Science, and Dread Disease: A Short History of United States Medical Research Policy*. Cambridge, MA: Harvard University Press, 1972.

Stuart, Reginald C. *Dispersed Relations: Americans and Canadians in Upper North America*. Washington: Woodrow Wilson Center Press; Baltimore: Johns Hopkins University Press, 2007.

Sumpf, Alexandre. "Film and Anti-alcohol Campaigns in the Soviet Union of the 1920s." In *Health Education Films in the Twentieth Century*, 188–224.

Tedlow, Richard S. *Keeping the Corporate Image: Public Relations and Business, 1900–1950*. Greenwich, CT: JAI, 1979.

———. *New and Improved: The Story of Mass Marketing in America*. New York: Basic Books, 1990.

Thompson, John Herd, and Stephen J. Randall. *Canada and the United States: Ambivalent Allies*. Athens: University of Georgia Press, 2008.

Tippett, Maria. *Making Culture: English-Canadian Institutions and the Arts before the Massey Commission*. Toronto: University of Toronto Press, 1990.

Tudor, Andrew. *Monsters and Mad Scientists: A Cultural History of the Horror Movie*. Oxford: Blackwell, 1989.

Tye, Larry. *The Father of Spin: Edward L. Bernays and the Birth of Public Relations*. New York: Crown, 1998.

Vogt, Norman. *"Collier's."* In *American Mass-Market Magazines,* 53–8.

Von Heyking, Amy. "Talking About Americans: The Image of the United States in English–Canadian Schools, 1900–1965." *History of Education Quarterly* 46 (2006): 382–408.

Wailoo, Keith. *How Cancer Crossed the Color Line.* Oxford and New York: Oxford University Press, 2011.

Waugh, Thomas. "Cinemas, Nations, Masculinities: The Martin Walsh Memorial Lecture (1998)." *Canadian Journal of Film Studies* 8, no.1 (1999): 8–44.

——. *The Romance of Transgression in Canada: Queering, Sexualities, Nations, Cinemas.* Montreal: McGill-Queen's University Press, 2006.

Weckbecker, Lars. "Re-forming Vision: On the Governmentality of Griersonian Documentary Film." *Studies in Documentary Film* 9 (2015): 172–85.

Whitaker, Reg, and Gary Marcuse. *Cold War Canada: The Making of a National Insecurity State, 1945–1957.* Toronto: University of Toronto Press, 1994.

Williams, Deane, and Zoë Druick, eds. *The Grierson Effect: Tracing Documentary's International Movement.* London: British Film Institute I/Palgrave Macmillan, 2014.

Wilson, Duncan. *Tissue Culture in Science and Society: The Public Life of a Biological Technique in Twentieth Century Britain.* Basingstoke and New York: Palgrave Macmillan, 2011.

Winkler, Martin M. "Neo-Mythologism: Apollo and the Muses on the Screen." *International Journal of the Classical Tradition* 11 (2005): 383–423.

Winston, Brian. *Claiming the Real: The Griersonian Documentary and Its Legitimations.* London: British Film Institute, 1995.

——. *Claiming the Real II: Documentary: Grierson and Beyond.* London: British Film Institute, 2008.

Page numbers in italics indicate figures; those with a *t* indicate tables.

Printed in the United States
by Baker & Taylor Publisher Services